guidelines for
PERINATAL CARE

Fifth Edition

American Academy
of Pediatrics

The American College
of Obstetricians
and Gynecologists

Supported in part by

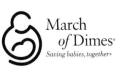

Guidelines for Perinatal Care was developed through the cooperative efforts of the American Academy of Pediatrics (AAP) Committee on Fetus and Newborn and the American College of Obstetricians and Gynecologists (ACOG) Committee on Obstetric Practice. The guidelines should not be viewed as a body of rigid rules. They are general and intended to be adapted to many different situations, taking into account the needs and resources particular to the locality, the institution, or type of practice. Variations and innovations that improve the quality of patient care are to be encouraged rather than restricted. The purpose of these guidelines will be well served if they provide a firm basis on which local norms may be built.

Copyright © October 2002 by the American Academy of Pediatrics and the American College of Obstetricians and Gynecologists

Library of Congress Cataloging-in-Publication Data

American Academy of Pediatrics.
 Guidelines for perinatal care.— 5th ed. / American Academy of Pediatrics
  [and] the American College of Obstetricians and Gynecologists.
  p. ; cm.
 Rev. ed. of: Guidelines for perinatal care. 4th ed. c1997.
 Includes bibliographical references and index.
 ISBN 0-915473-89-5 (alk. paper)
 1. Perinatology—Standards—United States.
 [DNLM: 1. Perinatal Care—standards—United States. WQ 210 A512g
 2002] I. American College of Obstetricians and Gynecologists. II.
 Title.
 RG600 .G85 2002

               2002010741

ISBN 1-58110-074-4   AAP
ISBN 0-915473-89-5   ACOG

Single copy price is $75 for nonmembers and $69 for ACOG/AAP members. Quantity prices available on request. Orders or inquiries regarding content may be directed to the respective organizations.

American Academy of Pediatrics
141 Northwest Point Boulevard
PO Box 927
Elk Grove Village, IL 60009-0927

The American College of Obstetricians and Gynecologists
409 12th Street, SW
PO Box 96920
Washington, DC 20090-6920

12345/65432

EDITORIAL COMMITTEE

Editors
Larry C. Gilstrap, MD, FACOG
William Oh, MD, FAAP

Associate Editors
Michael F. Greene, MD, FACOG
James A. Lemons, MD, FAAP

Staff
ACOG
Stanley Zinberg, MD, MS, FACOG
Beth Steele
Debra A. Hawks, MPH
Rebecca Carlson, MS

AAP
Jim Couto, MA

ACOG COMMITTEE ON OBSTETRIC PRACTICE

Members, 1999–2000
Michael F. Greene, MD, FACOG (Chair)
Robert Resnik, MD, FACOG (Vice Chair)
Raul Artal, MD, FACOG
Janice L. Bacon, MD, FACOG
Richard Depp, III, MD, FACOG
Patricia Grabauskas, CNM
Charles J. Lockwood, MD, FACOG
Allan T. Sawyer, MD, FACOG

Liaison Representatives
Marianna Crowley, MD
James A. Lemons, MD

Members, 2000–2001
Charles J. Lockwood, MD, FACOG (Chair)
Richard Depp III, MD, FACOG (Vice Chair)
Raul Artal, MD, FACOG
Janice L. Bacon, MD, FACOG
Jeanne M. Coulehan, CNM
James G. Quirk, MD, FACOG
Laura E. Riley, MD, FACOG
Allan T. Sawyer, MD, FACOG
Richard K. Wagner, Maj, MC USA

Liaison Representatives
Marianna Crowley, MD
James A. Lemons, MD

Members, 2001–2002
Charles J. Lockwood, MD, FACOG (Chair)
Raul Artal, MD, FACOG (Vice Chair)
Jeanne M. Coulehan, CNM
Judith U. Hibbard, MD, FACOG
Wilma I. Larsen, Ltc, MC USA
James G. Quirk, MD, FACOG
Laura E. Riley, MD, FACOG
Jone E. Sampson, MD, FACOG
Richard K. Wagner, Maj, MC USA

Liaison Representatives
David J. Birnbach, MD
Lillian Blackmon, MD

AAP Committee on Fetus and Newborn

Members, 1999–2000

James A. Lemons, MD, FAAP (Chairperson)
Lillian R. Blackmon, MD, FAAP
William P. Kanto, Jr, MD, FAAP
Hugh M. MacDonald, MD, FAAP
Carol A. Miller, MD, FAAP
Warren Rosenfeld, MD, FAAP
Craig T. Shoemaker, MD, FAAP
Michael E. Speer, MD, FAAP
Jane E. Stewart, MD, FAAP

Liaison Representatives
Michael F. Greene, MD, FACOG
Solomon Iyasu, MBBS, MPH
Jenny Ecord, MS, RNC, NNP, PNP
Arne Ohlsson, MD, FAAP
Linda L. Wright, MD
Jacob C. Langer, MD, FAAP
Richard Molteni, MD, FAAP

Members, 2000–2001

James A. Lemons, MD, FAAP (Chairperson)
William A. Engle, MD, FAAP
William P. Kanto, Jr, MD, FAAP
Hugh M. MacDonald, MD, FAAP
Carol A. Miller, MD, FAAP
Warren Rosenfeld, MD, FAAP
Michael E. Speer, MD, FAAP
Ann Stark, MD, FAAP
Jane E. Stewart, MD, FAAP

Liaison Representatives
Jenny Ecord, MS, RNC, NNP, PNP
Solomon Iyasu, MBBS, MPH
Charles J. Lockwood, MD, FACOG
Arne Ohlsson, MD, FAAP
Linda L. Wright, MD
Jacob C. Langer, MD, FAAP

Members, 2001–2002

Lillian Blackmon, MD, FAAP (Chairperson)
Edward F. Bell, MD, FAAP
William A. Engle, MD, FAAP
William P. Kanto, Jr, MD, FAAP
Gilbert I. Martin, MD, FAAP
Carol A. Miller, MD, FAAP
Warren Rosenfeld, MD, FAAP
Michael E. Speer, MD, FAAP
Ann Stark, MD, FAAP

Liaison Representatives
Jenny Ecord, MS, RNC, NNP, PNP
Solomon Iyasu, MBBS, MPH
Charles J. Lockwood, MD, FACOG
Keith J. Barrington, MD
Linda L. Wright, MD

The committee would like to express its appreciation to the following consultants:

Patricia Johnson, RN, MS, NNP
David A. Nagey, MD
Ronald Gibbs, MD
Barbara Stoll, MD
Larry Pickering, MD
Sebastian Faro, MD
David Stevenson, MD

Dale Phelps, MD
Charles Bauer, MD
Lu-Ann Papile, MD
Richard A. Ehrenkranz, MD
Jon Tyson, MD
Charles G. Prober, MD
Renee Wachtel, MD

CONTENTS

CHAPTER **8**
Neonatal Complications   237

CHAPTER **9**
Perinatal Infections   285

CHAPTER **10**
Infection Control   331

APPENDIXES
A. ACOG Antepartum Record and Discharge/ Postpartum Form   355

B. Early Pregnancy Risk Identification for Consultation   365

PREFACE

The fifth edition of *Guidelines for Perinatal Care* is a user-friendly guide that provides updated and expanded information from the fourth edition. This edition maintains the focus of the fourth edition on reproductive awareness, regionally based prenatal care services, and the philosophy of the March of Dimes Birth Defects Foundation's publication, *Toward Improving the Outcome of Pregnancy: The 90s and Beyond.*

Guidelines for Perinatal Care represents a cross section of different disciplines within the perinatal community. It is designed for use by all personnel who are involved in the care of pregnant women, their fetuses, and their neonates in community programs, hospitals, and medical centers. An intermingling of information in varying degrees of detail is provided to address their collective needs. The result is a unique resource that complements the educational documents listed in Appendix G, which provide more specific information. Readers are encouraged to refer to the appendix for related documents to supplement those listed at the end of each chapter.

The fifth edition of Guidelines has been reorganized to include a specific chapter regarding the care of the neonate. Maternal postpartum considerations have been combined with intrapartum care in this edition. Also, maternal and newborn nutrition has been separated and included in chapters that focus on care of the newborn and maternal prenatal and postpartum issues. New information has been added on vaginal birth after cesarean delivery, human immunodeficiency virus (HIV), cystic fibrosis, circumcision, air travel during pregnancy, exercise during pregnancy, breastfeeding, and newborn hearing screening. There also is a new and revised ACOG Antepartum Record and Discharge/ Postpartum Form in Appendix A.

Both the American Academy of Pediatrics (AAP) and the American College of Obstetricians and Gynecologists (ACOG) will continue to update information presented here through policy statements and recommendations that both organizations issue periodically, particularly with regard to rapidly evolving technologies and areas of practice, such as genetics, treatment of HIV infection, and prophylaxis of neonatal group B streptococcal disease.

Guidelines for Perinatal Care is published as a companion document to ACOG's *Guidelines for Women's Health Care*, which is in its second edition. Although each book is developed with the aid of a separate committee, their contents are coordinated to provide a comprehensive reference to all aspects of women's health care—gynecologic, obstetric, and neonatal—with minimal duplication.

The most current scientific information, professional opinions, and clinical practices have been used to create this document, which is intended to offer guidelines, not strict operating rules. Local circumstances must dictate the way in which these guidelines are best interpreted to meet the needs of a particular hospital, community, or system. For instance, the term *readily available*, used to designate acceptable levels of care, should be defined by each institution within the context of its resources and geographic location. Emphasis has been placed on identifying those areas to be covered by specific, locally defined protocols rather than on promoting rigid recommendations.

The content of this newest edition of Guidelines has undergone careful review to ensure accuracy and consistency with the policies of both groups. The guidelines are not meant to be exhaustive, nor do they always agree with those of other organizations; however, they reflect the latest recommendations of AAP and ACOG in areas that are subject to constant updating. The recommendations of AAP and ACOG are based on the best understanding of the data and consensus among authorities in the discipline. The text was written, revised, and reviewed by members of the AAP Committee on Fetus and Newborn and the ACOG Committee on Obstetric Practice; consultants in a variety of specialized areas also contributed to the content. The pioneering efforts of those who developed the previous editions also must be acknowledged. To each and every one of them, our sincere appreciation is extended.

Editorial Committee

INTRODUCTION

As the new millennium begins, it is important to reflect on the progress that was achieved during the 20th century, which brought unprecedented advancement and improvement in maternal and infant health in the United States. The result of this progress is a marked reduction in both maternal and infant mortality. In 1913, the U.S. Children's Bureau began to study factors influencing infant mortality based on each factor's "fundamental social importance." The results of these early studies indicated that many pregnant women did not receive appropriate prenatal, birth, and postpartum services. Expanded public health services, new knowledge of the causes of maternal mortality, and increased use of hospital-based labor and delivery services led to improvements in pregnancy outcome during the first half of the century.

In the 1960s and 1970s, there was a focus on new technology and the delivery of inpatient care. A regional perinatal care structure emerged, reflecting increased interest in addressing the management of preterm birth and the care of low-birth-weight infants. With the development of neonatal intensive care units, new professional roles were created. From local models, a national framework for the organization of perinatal care evolved. These interwoven trends were part of a broader effort to maximize the efficiency and cost-effectiveness of several new types of "intensive care" medicine. For maternal and infant health, these culminated in the concept of "regionalized perinatal care."

In the early 1970s, the March of Dimes Birth Defects Foundation assembled a multidisciplinary group of professionals representing all aspects of perinatal care. The group, called the Committee on Perinatal Health, developed the 1976 publication, *Toward Improving the Outcome of Pregnancy*, in which a model system for regionalized perinatal care was proposed and three levels of inpatient hospital care were defined.

That approach, which focused primarily on inpatient levels of emergency neonatal care, has served newborns well for two decades. It fostered a continuation of improved perinatal outcome and survival for high-risk infants, although the quality of long-term survival of these infants has not been significantly altered.

In the 1990s, as reported recently by the Neonatal Research Network of the National Institute of Child Health and Human Development, the application of new knowledge and technology in the care of low-birthweight infants resulted in further reduction of their mortality rates; unfortunately, the incidence of major morbidity (intraventricular hemorrhage, chronic lung disease, necrotizing enterocolitis) remained high (Figs. I–1 to I–3).

To further the goals of regionalized perinatal care, there is a need to continue the efforts of risk identification, care in a setting appropriate for the level of risk, and transport when necessary. Specifically, preterm infants born in subspecialty hospitals with neonatal care have better survival rates, even after controlling for interhospital differences in birth-weight distribution, race, gestational age, and multiple births. The greatest impact has been in reducing the mortality of very low-birthweight neonates (weighing <1,500 g at birth).

In the 1990s, it became apparent that there was a need to refine and augment the levels of care designated in a regionalized system of care. At the request of the American Academy of Pediatrics and the American College of Obstetricians and Gynecologists, a new Committee on Perinatal Health was assembled by the March of Dimes Birth Defects Foundation to respond to a changing environment and to make further recommendations for the regional coordination of perinatal care in the 1990s and beyond. Charged with updating the vision of content and organization developed by the original Committee on Perinatal Health, the group focused on what it considered to be four key areas: 1) care before and during pregnancy, 2) care during birth and beyond, 3) data documentation and evaluation, and 4) financing. The recommendations broadened the concept of regionalized services to address perinatal care from before conception through infancy, proposing practical strategies for implementation on a national basis. These recommendations are presented in *Toward Improving the Outcome of Pregnancy: The 90s and*

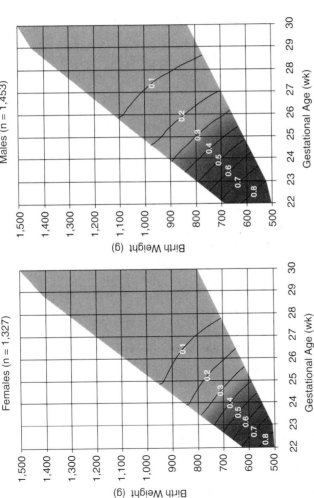

Fig I-1. Estimated mortality risk by birth weight and gestational age based on singleton infants born in NICHD Neonatal Research Network Centers between January 1, 1995 and December 31, 1996. (Used with permission of the American Academy of Pediatrics. Lemons JA, Bauer CR, Oh W, Korones SB, Papile LA, Stoll BJ, et al. Very low birth weight outcomes of the National Institute of Child Health and Human Development Neonatal Research Network, January 1995 through December 1996. NICHD Neonatal Research Network. Pediatrics 2001;107:E1.)

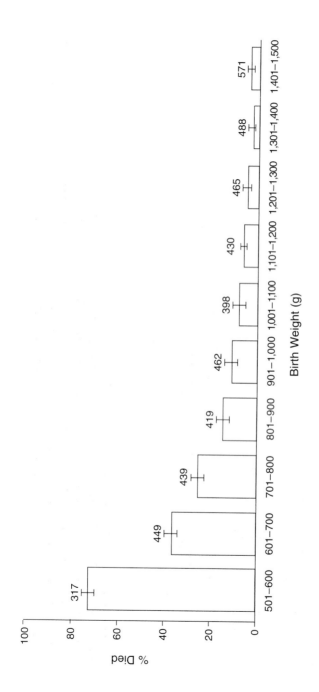

Fig. I–2. Mortality before discharge by birth weight among infants born in NICHD Neonatal Research Network Centers between January 1, 1995 and December 31, 1996. Data expressed as percentage died and 95% confidence intervals for each 100-g birth weight interval. (Used with permission of the American Academy of Pediatrics. Lemons JA, Bauer CR, Oh W, Korones SB, Papile LA, Stoll BJ, et al. Very low birth weight outcomes of the National Institute of Child Health and Human Development Neonatal Research Network, January 1995 through December 1996. NICHD Neonatal Research Network. Pediatrics 2001;107:EI.)

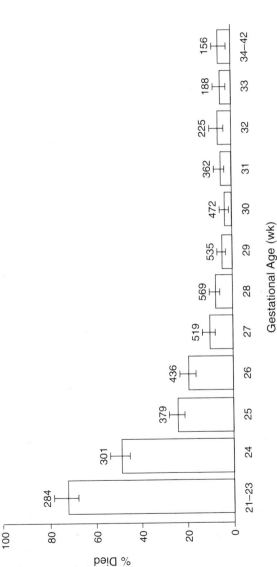

Fig. I–3. Mortality before discharge by gestational age as estimated by best obstetric estimate among infants born in NICHD Neonatal Research Network Centers between January 1, 1995 and December 31, 1996. Data expressed as percentage died and 95% confidence intervals for each gestational age group. (Used with permission of the American Academy of Pediatrics. Lemons JA, Bauer CR, Oh W, Korones SB, Papile LA, Stoll BJ, et al. Very low birth weight outcomes of the National Institute of Child Health and Human Development Neonatal Research Network, January 1995 through December 1996. NICHD Neonatal Research Network. Pediatrics 2001;107:EI.)

Beyond published in 1993, and some aspects of these recommendations have been incorporated into the fifth edition of *Guidelines for Perinatal Care*. A guide to the functional organization of individual regional programs is described in *Toward Improving the Outcome of Pregnancy: The 90s and Beyond*, and can be modified according to local needs and resources. Because the contents cited are valuable for the implementation of excellent management of women and their infants, they are retained in this edition.

At the beginning of the 21st century, the technologic revolution of communication and information systems is being harnessed to improve not only the ability to provide comprehensive and state-of-the-art health care, but also to assess the outcomes of such efforts. Only with such reassessment and quality management can our health care systems continue to evolve so that they are comprehensive, current, fiscally efficient and responsible, and sensitive to the particular needs of individual women and infants. It is encouraging to note that there is increasing use of single and multicenter trials to assess the efficacy and safety of therapeutic interventions in both maternal–fetal medicine and neonatology. Examples include evaluation of the safety of prenatal diagnostic techniques, use of antenatal steroids to accelerate fetal maturation, intrapartum antibiotic chemoprophylaxis to prevent neonatal group B streptococcal sepsis, antibiotics for preterm premature rupture of membranes, and surfactant therapy for newborn respiratory distress syndrome. Use of well-designed randomized clinical trials will improve the ability to provide the most appropriate care to women and their newborns.

guidelines for

PERINATAL CARE

Fifth Edition

CHAPTER 1

Organization of Perinatal Health Care

Health Care Delivery System

Innovation in health care organization was demonstrated by the perinatal provider community when regionally coordinated systems focusing on hospital-based services as recommended by an ad hoc Committee on Perinatal Health (COPH) of the March of Dimes Birth Defects Foundation were implemented and shown to be effective in the 1970s and 1980s. In the 1990s, an increased emphasis on ambulatory care, especially in the preconceptional and early prenatal intervals, was recommended by the second COPH. In recent years, a number of national reports have documented gaps in the organization and delivery of perinatal health care. A health care system that is responsive to the needs of families, and especially women, requires strategies to:

- Improve access to services
- Identify risks early
- Provide linkage to the appropriate level of care
- Ensure compliance, continuity, and comprehensiveness

Structural, financial, and cultural barriers need to be identified and eliminated. However, the regional organization must continue to develop and improve within the reality of a continuing evolution of the general health care delivery system while avoiding unnecessary duplication of services. Essential within this development are four basic principles: 1) access to comprehensive care services, 2) heightened reproductive awareness, 3) family-centered care, and 4) accountability for all components of the care delivery system.

Comprehensive Care Services

The integration of clinical activities, basic through subspecialty levels, within one geographic region potentially provides immediate access to comprehensive care at the appropriate level for the entire population. The primary goal of providing the appropriate level of care is facilitated by early and ongoing risk assessment to prevent, recognize, and treat conditions associated with morbidity and mortality and to improve linkages between levels of care through more effective mechanisms for referral and consultation. When populations needing reproductive health care are widely dispersed, both geographically and economically, a carefully structured, well-organized system of supportive services becomes necessary to ensure access. Networks and other forms of vertically integrated systems should be structured to provide all the necessary services, including social supports, transportation, public and professional education, research, and outcome evaluations. All components of service provision are necessary to meet the principle goal of maximal reduction of perinatal mortality and morbidity while using resources efficiently.

Reproductive Awareness

Insight into the broad social and medical implications of pregnancy and awareness of reproductive risks, health-enhancing behaviors, and family planning options are essential to improving the outcome of pregnancy. Reproductive awareness must be integrated more effectively into the health care system and society at large. An Institute of Medicine report, *The Best Intentions, Unintended Pregnancy and the Well-Being of Children and Families*, emphasizes that in the United States:

- Almost 60% of pregnancies are unintended, either mistimed or unwanted altogether
- Unintended pregnancies occur in all segments of society
- A woman with an unintended pregnancy is less likely to seek early prenatal care and is more likely to expose the fetus to noxious substances

- An unwanted pregnancy is at higher risk of producing a low-birth-weight neonate with other complications throughout childhood
- About one half of unintended pregnancies end in abortion

That less than one half of pregnancies in the United States are planned suggests the need for a new approach to reproductive awareness. Because unintended pregnancies and reproductive health hazards—including the use of alcohol, tobacco, and other drugs—occur across all socioeconomic groups, the target group for reproductive awareness must include all women of childbearing age. Reproductive health screening should be implemented by all health care providers serving women in their reproductive years. A sample form that may be useful in facilitating appropriate selective reproductive health screening is shown in Table 1–1.

Every encounter with the health care system, including those with adolescents and men, as well as those with women of childbearing age should be viewed as an opportunity to reinforce reproductive awareness. New messages regarding responsible reproductive health practices and innovations in marketing techniques may be required to change attitudes and behaviors among women and men.

FAMILY-CENTERED CARE

The health care system should be oriented toward providing family-centered care, with the governing assumption being the family is the primary source of support for anyone receiving services. Health care providers should engage parents as co-providers and decision-making partners and seek to ensure that every encounter builds on the family's strengths, preserves their dignity, and enhances their confidence and competence. Such an approach incorporates family perspectives, offers real choices, and respects the decisions made for themselves and their children. All counseling should be sensitive to cultural diversity, and a skilled translator should be used when the primary language of women and their families is not that of the health care providers.

Hospital and program leaders should communicate the concepts of family-centered care consistently and clearly to staff, students, families, and communities through vision, mission, and philosophy statements.

Table 1–1. Health Screening for Women of Reproductive Age

Selective Reproductive Health Screening (Menarche to Menopause)	Done	Referred
Reproductive awareness		
Pregnancy prevention counseling	❏	❏
Prepregnancy and nutrition counseling	❏	❏
Medical diseases (counsel regarding effects on future pregnancies)		
Diabetes mellitus	❏	❏
Hypertension	❏	❏
Epilepsy	❏	❏
Other chronic illness	❏	❏
Infectious diseases (counsel, test, or refer)		
Sexually transmitted diseases, including human immunodeficiency virus (HIV)	❏	❏
Hepatitis A	❏	❏
Hepatitis B (immunize if at high risk)	❏	❏
Rubella (test; if nonimmune, immunize)	❏	❏
Varicella	❏	❏
Teratogens/genetics (counsel regarding effects on future pregnancies)		
Hemoglobinopathy	❏	❏
Medication and vitamin use (eg, isotretinoin/vitamin A [retinoic acid])	❏	❏
Self or prior child with congenital defect	❏	❏
Family history of genetic disease	❏	❏
Environmental exposure at home or in workplace	❏	❏
Behavior (counsel regarding effects on future pregnancies)		
Alcohol use	❏	❏
Tobacco use	❏	❏
Use of illicit substances (eg, cocaine, crack)	❏	❏
Social support		
Safety (eg, domestic violence)	❏	❏
Personal resources (eg, transportation, housing)	❏	❏

Modified from March of Dimes Birth Defects Foundation, Committee on Perinatal Health. Toward improving the outcome of pregnancy: the 90s and beyond. White Plains (NY): March of Dimes Birth Defects Foundation; 1993.

This includes respecting the choices, values, and cultural backgrounds of expectant and new mothers and other family members; communicating honestly and openly; promoting opportunities for mutual support and information sharing; and collaborating in the development and evaluation of services.

Family-centered practices can help expectant and new parents become nurturing caregivers. Efforts should be made throughout the neonatal course to minimize the separation of newborns and families. Economic interests and decisions should never take priority over the best interests of the newborn, the mother, the family, and the community in keeping the family together. When separation of the family unit is necessitated by the requirement for a higher level of care for the mother or newborn, the responsibility for maintaining communication and involvement of the family in care decisions should be shared by the entire care team. Staff interactions and unit policies at every level should consistently reinforce the importance of parents and other family members to the health and well-being of their newborns. Families' strengths and capabilities should be the foundation on which to build competency and confidence in caregiving abilities. Preserving an individual sense of personal responsibility and identity is important for the optimum outcome of pregnancy and family life.

ACCOUNTABILITY

Although often associated only with the care of individual patients by individual health care providers, accountability for actions is a fundamental principle of health care provision applicable to all components of a health care delivery system, and a valuable attribute of professional practice that benefits all patients. Within the perinatal health care delivery system, accountability must be required equally of all components, including perinatal health care programs and systems, government agencies, insurers, and health maintenance organizations whose actions and policies influence patient care delivery and thereby influence outcomes. Access to quality care for the total patient population is a responsibility that requires a coordinated system with involvement, commitment, and accountability of all parties.

Clinical Components of Regionalized Perinatal Services

A regionally coordinated system focusing on levels of hospital-based perinatal care has been shown to be effective and to result in improved outcomes for women and their newborns. Such a system can be extended to encompass preconceptional evaluation and early pregnancy risk assessment in both an ambulatory and a hospital-based setting.

PRECONCEPTIONAL CARE

Regional perinatal health care programs and systems should enhance the positive impact of antepartum care on outcomes by placing additional emphasis on preconceptional care through educational programs. Clinical details of preconceptional care for perinatal health care providers are presented in "Preconceptional Care" in Chapter 4. All women of childbearing age should be provided access, structure, and support for preconceptional care and family-planning consultation.

Pediatricians and other health care providers have an obligation to provide information and counseling about sexuality, medical and psychosocial risks of pregnancy, and reproductive health care options in accordance with state and federal statutes and regulations to all adolescents in their practices. In addition, every opportunity during preventive care visits should be taken to provide education to parents, especially mothers, emphasizing the adverse medical and social consequences of adolescent pregnancy.

AMBULATORY PRENATAL CARE

The overall goals for regional coordination of ambulatory prenatal care are to ensure appropriate care for all women, to better use available resources, and to improve the outcome of pregnancy. Prenatal care can be delivered more effectively and efficiently by defining the capabilities and expertise (basic, specialty, and subspecialty) of providers and ensuring that pregnant women receive risk-appropriate care (Table 1–2). Developments in maternal–fetal risk assessment and diagnosis, as well as interventions to change behavior, make early and continuous prenatal care more effective in improving pregnancy outcome.

Table 1–2. Ambulatory Prenatal Care Provider Capabilities and Expertise

Level of Prenatal Care	Capabilities	Provider Types
Basic (Level I)	Risk-oriented prenatal care record, physical examination and interpretation of findings, routine laboratory assessment, assessment of gestational age and normal progress of pregnancy, ongoing risk identification, mechanisms for consultation and referral, psychosocial support, childbirth education, and care coordination (including referral for ancillary services, such as transportation, food, and housing assistance)	Obstetricians, family physicians, certified nurse–midwives, and other advanced-practice nurses with experience, training, and demonstrated competence
Specialty (Level II)	Basic care plus fetal diagnostic testing (eg, biophysical tests, amniotic fluid analysis, basic ultrasonography), expertise in management of medical and obstetric complications	Obstetricians
Subspecialty (Level III)	Basic and specialty care plus advanced fetal diagnoses (eg, targeted ultrasonography, fetal echocardiology); advanced therapy (eg, intrauterine fetal transfusion and treatment of cardiac arrhythmias); medical, surgical, neonatal, and genetic consultation; and management of severe maternal complications	Maternal–fetal medicine specialists and reproductive geneticists with experience, training, and demonstrated competence

Modified from March of Dimes Birth Defects Foundation, Committee on Perinatal Health. Toward improving the outcome of pregnancy: the 90s and beyond. White Plains (NY): March of Dimes Birth Defects Foundation; 1993.

Early and ongoing risk assessment should be an integral component of perinatal care. The primary goals are to prevent or treat conditions associated with morbidity and mortality and to improve linkages to inpatient care by establishing effective mechanisms for referral and consultation. Risk assessment facilitates development of a specific plan of care, including referral and consultation as appropriate among providers of basic, specialty, and subspecialty levels of prenatal care on the basis of the individual woman's circumstances and the expertise of the individual provider. All prenatal health care providers should be able to identify a full range of medical and psychosocial risks and either provide appropriate care or refer to the appropriate level throughout pregnancy (see Appendixes B and C).

The content and timing of prenatal care should be varied according to the needs and risk status of the woman and her fetus. Use of community-based risk assessment tools, such as a standardized prenatal record (see "ACOG Antepartum Record" in Appendix A), by all providers, both public and private within a perinatal care region, helps to implement risk assessment and intervention activities.

Prenatal care may involve the services of many types of health care providers, including the early involvement of pediatricians and neonatologists as well as other specialists. Consultation with a neonatologist is particularly important when fetal risks or problems have been identified.

IN-HOSPITAL PERINATAL CARE

In 1976, the COPH designated three levels of perinatal care—levels I, II, and III. Although this designation remains in common usage among many institutions and public agencies, such as state maternal–child health programs, the second COPH in 1993 recommended replacing numerical designations with functional, descriptive designations of basic, specialty, and subspecialty care. Since then, financial and marketing pressures, as well as community demands, have encouraged some hospitals to raise their perinatal care service level designation, primarily with regard to patient care activities without attention to regional coordination concerns. This tendency conflicts with the classic concept of regional organization, in which single level III or subspecialty care centers had the sole capability to provide complex patient care and usually, but not always, assumed regional responsibilities for transport, outreach education, research, and quality improvement for a specific population or geographic area. Attempts to share responsibilities among hospitals have not been uniformly successful. Sometimes differing levels of perinatal care services have developed within a single hospital—usually a basic or specialty obstetric service in conjunction with a subspecialty neonatal service. This imbalance or lack of coordination in the provision of services may be a product of a growing competitive health care market and prepaid health plans with overlapping geographic areas. Such competitive forces frequently have led to the unnecessary duplication of services within a single community or geographic region with the potential to result in decreased complex patient care, increased patient morbidity and mortality, and increased cost.

Careful documentation of birth weight specific neonatal mortality rates by hospital of birth has substantiated that the survival of very low-birth-weight infants, in particular, was highest when birth occurred in hospitals with larger neonatal intensive care units. This finding has been reported both in the United States and other countries. In addition, there are multiple reports regarding the outcomes of surgery from complex single or multiorgan system anomalies that support the concentration of resources and patients to a few highly specialized centers for surgical repair. Given the weight of the evidence, it must be emphasized that inpatient perinatal health care services should be organized within individual regions or service areas in such a manner that there is a concentration of care for the most at-risk pregnant women and their fetuses in the highest level perinatal health care centers.

Distinction must be made between the perinatal care services level that characterizes an institution or hospital and the level of care provided within individual patient care units of a single hospital. The former applies to the total organization of perinatal health care service and the additional responsibilities associated with participation in a coordinated regional system of care. The latter is based on the individual needs of the perinatal patient, postpartum woman, and neonate (see "Physical Facilities" in Chapter 2 for a detailed description). The determination of the appropriate level of care to be provided by a given hospital should be guided by prevailing local health care regulations, national professional organization guidelines, and identified regional perinatal health care service needs.

Following are the responsibilities of basic, specialty, and subspecialty levels of inpatient perinatal health care services. In the fourth edition of *Guidelines for Perinatal Care*, the numerical designation of levels was deleted. However, the numerical designations are still widely used. Therefore, in this edition, we have used both functional and numerical designations for the various levels of care services.

1. Basic Care (Level I)

   - Surveillance and care of all patients admitted to the obstetric service, with an established triage system for identifying high-risk patients who should be transferred to a facility that provides specialty or subspecialty care

   - Proper detection and initial care of unanticipated maternal–fetal problems that occur during labor and delivery

   - Capability to begin an emergency cesarean delivery within 30 minutes of the decision to do so (see "Preface," and "Cesarean Delivery" in Chapter 5)

   - Availability of appropriate anesthesia, radiology, ultrasound, laboratory, and blood bank services on a 24-hour basis

   - Care of postpartum conditions

   - Resuscitation and stabilization of all neonates born in the hospital

   - Evaluation and continuing care of healthy neonates in a nursery or with their mothers until discharge

   - Adequate nursery facilities and support for stabilization of small or ill neonates before transfer to a specialty or subspecialty facility

   - Consultation and transfer arrangements

   - Parent–sibling–neonate visitation

   - Data collection and retrieval

Some basic care facilities may provide continuing care for neonates who have minor problems. Many basic care facilities provide care for convalescing neonates who have been transferred from specialty and subspecialty facilities.

2. Specialty Care (Level II)
   - Provision of some enhanced services as well as basic care services as described previously
   - Care of appropriate high-risk women and fetuses, both admitted and transferred from other facilities
   - Stabilization of severely ill newborns before transfer
   - Treatment of moderately ill larger preterm and term newborns
   - Data collection and retrieval

Care in a specialty level facility should be reserved for stable or moderately ill newborns that have problems that are expected to resolve rapidly and that would not be anticipated to need subspecialty level services on an urgent basis. These situations usually occur as a result of relatively uncomplicated preterm labor or preterm rupture of membranes at approximately 32 weeks of gestation or later.

Although some specialty care level hospitals also have neonatal intensive care units with subspecialty capability, the available perinatal subspecialty expertise often is neonatal medicine and not maternal–fetal medicine. Availability of pediatric subspecialists, such as in cardiology, surgery, radiology, and anesthesiology, in specialty care facilities with advanced neonatal care units is variable. Anticipatory planning and agreement on situations to be managed should be established and consideration should be given to regional or system needs and resources. Preterm labor and impending delivery at less than 32 weeks of gestation usually warrants maternal transfer to a subspecialty care center as do gestations of less than 32 weeks.

3. Subspecialty Care (Level III)
   - Provision of comprehensive perinatal care services for both admitted and transferred women and neonates of all risk categories, including basic and specialty care services as described previously
   - Evaluation of new technologies and therapies
   - Data collection and retrieval

The services provided by a subspecialty care facility vary markedly from those at a specialty facility. Subspecialty care services include expertise in neonatal and maternal–fetal medicine. Both usually are required for management of pregnancies with threatened maternal complications at less than 32 weeks of gestation. Fetuses that may require immediate complex care should be delivered at a subspecialty care center.

In circumstances where subspecialty level maternal care is needed, the level of care subsequently needed by the neonate may prove to be at the basic or specialty level. It is difficult to predict accurately all neonatal risk and outcomes before birth. Appropriate assessment and consultation should be used, considering the potential risks of the woman as well.

4. Regional Subspecialty Perinatal Health Care Center
    • Provision of comprehensive perinatal health care services at and above those of subspecialty care facilities
    • Responsibility for regional perinatal health care service organization and coordination including:
        — Maternal and neonatal transport
        — Outreach support and regional educational programs
        — Research support and initial evaluation of new technologies and therapies
        — Analysis and evaluation of regional data, including those on perinatal complications and outcomes

Not all subspecialty perinatal health care hospitals must act as regional centers; however, regional organization of perinatal health care services requires that there be coordination in the development of specialized services, professional continuing education to maintain competency, and the collection of data on long-term outcomes to evaluate both the effectiveness of delivery of perinatal health care services and the safety and efficacy of new therapies and technologies. Experience has shown that these functions usually are best achieved when responsibility is concentrated in a single center with both perinatal and neonatal subspecialty services within a region. In some cases, regional coordination may be provided adequately by the collaboration of a children's hospital with a subspecialty perinatal facility that is in close geographic proximity.

Maternal and Newborn Postdischarge Care

Perinatal health care at all levels should include ambulatory care of the woman and the neonate after hospital discharge. Increasing economic pressures for both early discharge and for decreasing length of hospital stays after delivery have increased the importance of organization and coordination of continuing care as well as the need for evaluation and monitoring of outcomes. Maternal–newborn follow-up and early intervention services are important components of care, especially after a complicated perinatal course. Service components for follow-up care for women are discussed in Chapter 5 and for neonates in Chapter 7 and Chapter 8.

Workforce: The Distribution and Supply of Perinatal Care Providers

The distribution and supply of physicians providing perinatal health care services has been changing. Although the number of physicians has increased substantially over the past 20 years, the percentage of all physicians who provide obstetric care has declined. Some published data indicate that there currently appears to be a sufficient number of physician specialists in neonatal care. However, perinatal health care providers are unevenly distributed among geographic areas and types of facilities. A team approach to perinatal health care delivery is essential to improving the outcome of pregnancy. Certified nurse–midwives, physicians assistants, advanced practice nurses, perinatal social workers, and other professionals also are important providers of perinatal services.

Strategies aimed at increasing recruitment of perinatal health care providers, particularly in rural and urban medically underserved areas, are needed. More than 2,000 federal health provider shortage areas have been designated, with most of the people in need of services in these areas being women of childbearing age and young children. Lack of sufficient funding to support perinatal health care services contributes to the number of underserved women.

Examples of regional programs that have been successfully used to increase access to care include liability cost relief, locum tenens programs (with physicians to serve as backup or relief), satellite practice models, financial incentives to establish or maintain a practice, innovative approaches to continuing education, and programs to provide technical support. The National Health Service Corps and state scholarship and loan repayment programs for the education of health care professionals, which include a special requirement for service in underserved areas, provide another important incentive. Such programs should be strengthened, give priority to perinatal health care providers, and be adequately funded.

Data Collection and Documentation

Outcomes have been a concern of perinatal health care providers for decades. Care has been monitored and improved by focusing on specific outcomes such as maternal, newborn, and neonatal mortality. The public, including the media, parents, government agencies, and interested parties, such as foundations, also have played an important and appropriate role in focusing concerns. The fact that the low-birth-weight rate is increasing, despite public funding of both research and patient care programs for several decades, points to the need for continual reassessment of care components and delivery systems.

A regional perinatal health care program must be able to track the courses of patient care and measure indicators and outcomes as a basis for evaluating success of service delivery. Significant progress has been made in methods for gathering vital statistics (eg, linked birth and death certificates) and in collecting data (eg, prenatal records). The concept of key indicators has been used to signal inadequate access to early and continuous perinatal care and to predict or measure poor pregnancy outcome. For example, rates of unintended pregnancy, prenatal care use, and fetal and neonatal mortality are possible measures of access and outcome at different points along the continuum of perinatal health care delivery. New and improved tools in evaluative clinical sciences applied to well-constructed data sets of concepts, such as quality improvement and evidence-based medicine, should be used to monitor performance and provide the basis for improvement in clinical care and outcomes. Perinatal health care providers and facilities must play an active role by participating in regional data collection, developing standard data collection tools, supporting analysis, and using the resulting information for individual, institutional, and professional quality improvement. Thorough and systematic collection of data on long-term outcomes is essential to evaluate changes in perinatal care delivery systems as well as new technologies and therapies.

Bibliography

Congressional Budget Office. Factors contributing to the infant mortality ranking of the United States. Washington, DC: Congressional Budget Office; 1992.

Evidenced-based quality improvement in neonatal and perinatal medicine. Pediatrics 1999;103(1 Suppl E):203–384.

Institute of Medicine (US). The best intentions, unintended pregnancy and the well-being of children and families. Washington, DC: National Academy Press; 1995.

Institute of Medicine. Including children and pregnant women in health care reform. Washington, DC: National Academy Press; 1992.

Makuc DM, Haglund B, Ingram DD, Kleinman JC, Feldman JJ. Health service areas for the United States. Vital Health Stat 1991;112:1–102.

March of Dimes Birth Defects Foundation, Committee on Perinatal Health. Toward improving the outcome of pregnancy: the 90s and beyond. White Plains, (NY): MDBDF; 1993.

National Foundation-March of Dimes, Committee on Perinatal Health. Toward improving the outcome of pregnancy: recommendations for the regional development of maternal and perinatal health services. White Plains (NY): NFMD; 1976.

Pollack LD. An effective model for reorganization of perinatal services in a metropolitan area: a descriptive analysis and historical perspective. J Perinatol 1996;16:13–8.

Public Health Service. Caring for our future: the content of prenatal care. Washington, DC: Department of Health and Human Services; 1989.

Richardson DK, Gray JE, Gortmaker SL, Goldmann DA, Pursley DM, McCormick MC. Pediatrics 1998;102:893–9.

Stevenson DK, Quaintance CC. The California Perinatal Quality Care Collaborative: a model for national perinatal care. J Perinatol 1999;19: 249–50.

CHAPTER 2

Inpatient Perinatal Care Services

This chapter outlines recommendations regarding medical expertise, nursing ratios, staffing guidelines, support services, perinatal outreach education, and physical facilities required for providing hospital-based perinatal care. These components have been defined for facilities providing basic, specialty, and subspecialty care.

Personnel

Factors critical to planning and evaluating the quality and level of personnel required to meet patients' needs in perinatal settings include the mission, philosophy, geographic location, and design of the facility; patient population; scope of practice; qualifications of staff; and obligations for education or research. Perinatal care programs at basic, specialty, and subspecialty hospitals should be coordinated jointly by medical and nursing directors for obstetric and pediatric services.

MEDICAL PROVIDERS

By virtue of their qualifications, individuals are granted privileges to practice by an institution's governing body. A hospital is responsible for granting privileges and verifying the applicant's credentials from the primary source. The credentials required and the privileges extended vary according to the level of care provided.

Basic Care Facility (Level I)

The perinatal care program at a hospital providing basic care should be coordinated jointly by the chiefs of the obstetric, pediatric, nursing, and midwifery services. This administrative approach requires close coordination and unified policy statements. The coordinators of perinatal care at a basic care hospital are responsible for developing policy, maintaining appropriate guidelines, and collaborating and consulting with the professional staff of hospitals providing specialty and subspecialty care in the region. In hospitals that do not separate these services, one person may be given the responsibility for coordinating perinatal care.

A qualified physician or certified nurse–midwife should attend all deliveries. Collaborative practice involving a multidisciplinary team is encouraged. This team may consist of obstetrician–gynecologists and certified nurse–midwives as well as other health care professionals who function within the context of their educational preparation and scope of practice. For example, certified nurse–midwives are educated in the disciplines of nursing and midwifery and possess evidence of certification meeting the requirements of the American College of Nurse–Midwives. Certified nurse–midwives may provide care for low-risk women in the antepartum, intrapartum, and postpartum periods; manage normal newborns; and provide primary gynecologic services in accordance with state law or regulations. Obstetrician–gynecologists' training, credentials, and responsibilities place them in the role of team leaders, but various other providers are needed for unique contributions that are valuable and important to the quality of patient outcomes. Clinical practice relationships between obstetrician–gynecologists and certified nurse–midwives should provide for mutually agreed on written medical guidelines and protocols for clinical practice that define the individual and shared responsibilities of certified nurse–midwives and obstetrician–gynecologists, or other physicians with obstetric hospital privileges, in the delivery of health care services and for ongoing communication that provides for and defines appropriate consultation between obstetrician–gynecologists and certified nurse–midwives. These guidelines also should provide for informed consent about the involvement of obstetrician–gynecologists, other physicians with obstetric hospital privileges, certified nurse–midwives, and other health care providers in the services offered. The obstetrician should be informed of the patient's condition and progress as appropriate for the situation.

Hospitals should ensure the availability of skilled personnel for perinatal emergencies. Anesthesia personnel with credentials to administer obstetric anesthesia should be available on a 24-hour basis. At least one person whose primary responsibility is for the newborn and who is capable of initiating neonatal resuscitation should be present at every delivery. Either that person or someone else who is immediately available should have the skills required to perform a complete resuscitation, including endotracheal intubation and administration of medications. This resuscitation should be performed according to the American Heart Association/ American Academy of Pediatrics Neonatal Resuscitation Program or an equivalent formal program. When required, one or two additional persons should be available to assist with neonatal resuscitation (see "Neonatal Resuscitation" in Chapter 7).

Specialty Care Facility (Level II)

A board-certified obstetrician–gynecologist with special interest, experience, and, in some situations, a subspecialty in maternal–fetal medicine should be chief of the obstetric service at a specialty care hospital. A board-certified pediatrician with special interest, experience, and, in some situations, subspecialty certification in neonatal–perinatal medicine should be chief of the neonatal care service. These physicians should coordinate the hospital's perinatal care services and, in conjunction with other medical, anesthesia, nursing, respiratory therapy, and hospital administration staff, develop policies concerning staffing, procedures, equipment, and supplies.

Care of high-risk neonates should be provided by appropriately qualified physicians. A general pediatrician should have the expertise to assume responsibility for acute, although less critical, care of newborns; understand the need for proper continuity of care and be capable of providing it; and share responsibility with a consulting neonatologist for the development and delivery of effective services for newborns at risk in the hospital and community. In collaboration with a physician, care may be provided by qualified advanced-practice nurses (APNs) who have formal education and training as well as supervised clinical experience in the care of newborns.

The director of obstetric anesthesia services should be board certified in anesthesia and should have training and experience in obstetric anesthesia. Anesthesia personnel with privileges to administer obstetric anesthesia should be available according to hospital policy. Policies regarding the provision of obstetric anesthesia, including the necessary qualifications of personnel who are to administer anesthesia and their availability for both routine and emergency deliveries, should be developed.

The hospital staff also should include a radiologist and a clinical pathologist who are available 24 hours per day. Specialized medical and surgical consultation also should be available.

Subspecialty Care Facility (Level III)

Ideally, the director of the maternal–fetal medicine service of a hospital providing subspecialty care should be a full-time, board-certified obstetrician with subspecialty certification in maternal–fetal medicine. The director of the newborn intensive care unit should be a full-time, board-certified pediatrician with subspecialty certification in neonatal–perinatal medicine. As co-directors of the perinatal service, these physicians are responsible for maintaining practice guidelines; developing the operating budget; evaluating and purchasing equipment; planning, developing, and coordinating in-hospital and outreach educational programs; and participating in the evaluation of perinatal care. If they are in a regional center, they should devote their time to patient care services, research, and teaching and should coordinate the services provided at their hospital with those provided at basic- and specialty-care hospitals in the region.

Other maternal–fetal medicine specialists and neonatologists who practice in the subspecialty care facility should have qualifications similar to those of the chief of their service. A maternal–fetal medicine specialist and a neonatologist should be readily available for consultation 24 hours per day. Personnel qualified to manage obstetric or neonatal emergencies should be in-house.

Obstetric and neonatal diagnostic imaging should be available 24 hours per day. Pediatric subspecialists, rather than adult subspecialists, in cardiology, neurology, hematology, and genetics should be available for consultation. Consultant services in pediatric nephrology, metabolism, endocrinology, gastroenterology–nutrition, infectious diseases, pulmonology, immunology, pathology, and pharmacology also are needed. In addition, pediatric surgeons and pediatric surgical subspecialists (eg, cardiovascular surgeons; neurosurgeons; and orthopedic, ophthalmologic, urologic, and otolaryngologic surgeons) should be available for consultation and care. Evidence indicates that management of neonates and young children by adult subspecialists rather than pediatric subspecialists results in greater costs, longer hospital stays, and potentially greater morbidity.

A board-certified anesthesiologist with special training or experience in maternal–fetal anesthesia should be in charge of obstetric anesthesia services at a subspecialty care hospital. Personnel with privileges in the administration of obstetric anesthesia should be available in the hospital 24 hours per day. Personnel with credentials in the administration of neonatal and pediatric anesthesia should be available as needed.

Nurse Providers

Delivery of safe and effective perinatal nursing care requires appropriately qualified registered nurses in adequate numbers to meet the needs of each patient in accordance with the care setting. The number of staff and level of skill required are influenced by the scope of nursing practice and the degree of nursing responsibilities within an institution. Nursing responsibilities in individual hospitals vary according to the level of care provided by the facility, practice procedures, number of professional registered nurses and ancillary staff, and professional nursing activities in continuing education and research. Intrapartum care requires the same labor intensiveness and expertise as any other intensive care and, accordingly, perinatal units should have the same adequately trained personnel and fiscal support.

Changing trends in medical management and technologic advances influence and may increase the nursing workload. Each hospital should determine the scope of nursing practice for each nursing unit and specialty department. The scope of practice should be based on national nursing guidelines for the specialty area of practice and should be in accordance with state law and regulations. A multidisciplinary committee, including representatives from hospital, medical, and nursing administration, should follow published professional guidelines, consult state nurse practice acts and any accompanying regulations, identify the types and numbers of procedures performed in each unit, delineate the direct and indirect nursing care activities performed, and identify the activities that are to be performed by nonnursing personnel.

Trends in neonatal care have resulted in an increased use of APNs. An advanced-practice neonatal nurse (APNN) must have completed an educational program of study and supervised practice beyond the level of basic nursing. Included in this category are the following nursing professionals (note that the term *neonatal nurse clinician* is imprecise and should no longer be used):

- A *neonatal clinical nurse specialist* is a registered nurse with a master's degree who, through study and supervised practice at the graduate level, has become expert in the theory and practice of neonatal nursing.

- A *neonatal nurse practitioner* (NNP) is a registered nurse with clinical expertise in neonatal nursing who has received a formal education with supervised clinical experience in the care of newborns. These nurses manage a caseload of neonatal patients with consultation, collaboration, and medical supervision. Using their acquired knowledge of pathophysiology, pharmacology, and physiology, NNPs exercise independent judgment in the assessment and diagnosis of newborns and in the performance of certain delegated procedures. Additionally, NNPs are involved in education, consultation, and research at various levels.

The spectrum of duties performed by an APNN will vary according to the institution and may be determined by state laws and regulations. Each of these duties requires advanced education. Nationally recognized certification examinations exist for each category of an APNN. The following guidelines are recommended:

1. Medical care provided by an APNN in a newborn intensive care unit should be supervised by a neonatologist. In basic and specialty nurs-

ery units, a board-certified pediatrician with special interest and experience in neonatal medicine may provide supervision.

2. Collaboration and consultation with other health professionals is an important aspect of the APNN's role.

3. Certification by a qualified national certification board or certification eligibility by completion of a recognized formal program of education with a supervised practice component meeting state practice requirements is recommended for entry level into practice.

4. An APNN is responsible for maintaining clinical expertise and knowledge of current therapy by participating in continuing education and scholarly activities.

Recommended nurse/patient ratios for perinatal services are shown in Table 2–1. Additional personnel are necessary for indirect patient care activities. Close evaluation of all factors involved in a specific case is essential for establishing an acceptable nurse/patient ratio. Variables such as birth weight, gestational age, and diagnosis of patients; patient turnover; acuity of patients' conditions; patient or parent education needs; bereavement care; mixture of skills of the staff; environment; types of delivery; and use of anesthesia must be taken into account in determining appropriate nurse/patient ratios. The efficiency of nursing care can be enhanced by a team approach.

Basic Care Facility (Level I)

Perinatal nursing care at a basic care facility should be under the direction of a registered nurse. The registered nurse's responsibilities include directing perinatal nursing services, guiding the development and implementation of perinatal policies and procedures, collaborating with medical staff, and consulting with hospitals that provide specialty and subspecialty care in the region.

For antepartum care, it is recommended that a registered nurse, whose responsibilities include the organization and supervision of antepartum, intrapartum, and neonatal nursing services, be on duty. The presence of one or more registered nurses or licensed practical nurses with demonstrated knowledge and clinical competence in the nursing care of women, fetuses, and newborns during labor, delivery, and the

Table 2–1. Recommended Registered Nurse/Patient Ratios for Perinatal Care Services

Registered Nurse/Patient Ratio	Care Provided
Intrapartum	
1:2	Patients in labor
1:1	Patients in second stage of labor
1:1	Patients with medical or obstetric complications
1:2	Oxytocin induction or augmentation of labor
1:1	Coverage for initiating epidural anesthesia
1:1	Circulation for cesarean delivery
Antepartum/Postpartum	
1:6	Antepartum and postpartum patients without complications
1:2	Patients in postoperative recovery
1:3	Antepartum and postpartum patients with complications but in stable condition
1:4	Newborns and those requiring close observation
Newborns	
1:6–8*	Newborns requiring only routine care
1:3–4	Normal mother–newborn couplet care
1:3–4	Newborns requiring continuing care
1:2–3	Newborns requiring intermediate care
1:1–2	Newborns requiring intensive care
1:1	Newborns requiring multisystem support
1:1 or greater	Unstable newborns requiring complex critical care

*This ratio reflects traditional well newborn nursery care. If breastfeeding or couplet care is provided, a registered nurse coordinates and administers care for the mother and newborn couple (1:3–4 couples). If it is necessary to separate the well mother and newborn couple, and return the newborn to a central nursery, the mother–newborn registered nurse is still responsible for the mother–newborn couple. Another registered nurse would provide care for the newborn in the central nursery. At least one registered nurse should be available at all times in each occupied basic care nursery when newborns are physically present in the nursery. In special care and subspecialty care nurseries, a minimum of two registered nurses, with training and expertise in neonatal nursing, should be in immediate attendance (National Association of Neonatal Nurses. Minimum staffing in NICUs. NANN Position Statement 3009. Glenview [IL]: NANN 1999. Available at www.nann.org/public/articles/309.doc. Retrieved June 10, 2002). Direct care of newborns in the nursery may be provided by ancillary personnel under the registered nurse's direct supervision. Adequate staff is needed to respond to acute and emergency situations at all times.

postpartum and neonatal periods is suggested. Ancillary personnel, supervised by a registered nurse, may provide support to the patient and attend to her personal comfort.

Intrapartum care should be under the direct supervision of a registered nurse. Responsibilities of the registered nurse include initial evaluation and admission of patients in labor; continuing assessment and evaluation of patients in labor, including checking the status of the fetus, recording vital signs, observing the fetal heart rate, performing obstetric examinations, observing uterine contractions, and supporting the patient; determining the presence or absence of complications; supervising the performance of nurses with less training and experience and of ancillary personnel; and staffing of the delivery room at the time of delivery. This registered nurse also should be capable of monitoring the fetal heart rate. A licensed practical nurse or nurse assistant, supervised by a registered nurse, may provide support to the patient and attend to her personal comfort.

Postpartum care of the woman and her newborn should be supervised by a registered nurse whose responsibilities include initial and ongoing assessment, newborn care education, support for the attachment process, preparation for healthy parenting, preparation for discharge, and follow-up of the woman and her newborn within the context of the family. This registered nurse should have training and experience in the recognition of normal and abnormal physical and emotional characteristics of the mother and her newborn. A licensed practical nurse or nurse assistant, supervised by a registered nurse, may provide support to the mother and attend to her personal comfort.

Specialty Care Facility (Level II)

Specialty care hospitals should have a director of perinatal and neonatal nursing services who has overall responsibility for inpatient activities in the respective obstetric and neonatal areas. This registered nurse should be an APN with specialized education in obstetric or neonatal care.

In addition to fulfilling nursing responsibilities in basic care hospitals, nursing staff in the labor, delivery, and recovery areas should be able to identify and respond to the obstetric and medical complications of pregnancy, labor, and delivery. A registered nurse with advanced training and experience in routine and high-risk obstetric care should be assigned to the labor and delivery area at all times. In the postpartum period, a registered nurse should be responsible for providing support for women and families with newborns who require intensive care and for facilitating visitation and communication with the neonatal intensive care unit (NICU).

Licensed practical nurses and unlicensed personnel with appropriate training in perinatal care and supervised by a registered nurse may provide assistance with the delivery of care, provide support to the patient, and attend to her personal comfort. All nurses caring for ill newborns must possess demonstrated knowledge in the observation and treatment of newborns, including cardiorespiratory monitoring. Furthermore, the registered nursing staff of an intermediate-care nursery in a specialty care hospital should be able to monitor and maintain the stability of cardiopulmonary, neurologic, metabolic, and thermal functions; assist with special procedures, such as lumbar puncture, endotracheal intubation, and umbilical vessel catheterization; and perform emergency resuscitation. They should be specially trained and able to initiate, modify, or stop treatment when appropriate, according to established protocols, even when a physician or APN is not present. In units where neonates receive mechanical ventilation, medical, nursing, or respiratory therapy staff who have demonstrated ability to intubate the trachea, manage mechanical ventilation, and decompress a pneumothorax should be continually available (see Table 2–1). The nursing staff should be formally trained and validated in neonatal resuscitation. The unit's medical director should define and supervise the delegated medical functions, processes, and procedures performed by various categories of personnel.

Subspecialty Care Facility (Level III)

The director of perinatal and neonatal nursing services at a subspecialty care hospital should have overall responsibility for inpatient activities in the maternity–newborn care units. This registered nurse should have experience and training in obstetric or neonatal nursing or both, as well as in the care of patients at high risk. Preferably, this individual has an advanced degree.

For antepartum care, a registered nurse should be responsible for the direction and supervision of nursing care. All nurses working with high-risk antepartum patients should have evidence of continuing education in maternal–fetal nursing. An APN who has been educated and prepared at the master's level should be on staff to coordinate education.

For intrapartum care, a registered nurse should be in attendance within the labor and delivery unit at all times. This registered nurse should be skilled in the recognition and nursing management of complications of labor and delivery.

For postpartum care, a registered nurse should be in attendance at all times. This registered nurse should be skilled in the recognition and nursing management of complications in women and newborns.

Registered nurses in the NICU should have specialty certification or advanced training and experience in the nursing management of high-risk neonates and their families. They also should be experienced in caring for unstable neonates with multiorgan system problems and in specialized care technology. An APN should be available to the staff for consultation and support on nursing care issues. Additional nurses with special training are required to fulfill regional center responsibilities, such as outreach and transport (see "Transport Procedure" and "Outreach Education" in Chapter 3).

The obstetric and neonatal areas may be staffed by a mix of professional and technical personnel. Assessment and monitoring activities should remain the responsibility of a registered nurse or an APN in obstetric–neonatal nursing, even when personnel with a mixture of skills are used.

SUPPORT PROVIDERS

All Facilities

Personnel who are capable of determining blood type, crossmatching blood, and performing antibody testing should be available on a 24-hour basis. The hospital's infection control personnel should be responsible for surveillance of infections in women and neonates, as well as for the development of an appropriate environmental control program (see "Infection Control" and "Environmental Control" in Chapter 10). A radiologic technician should be readily available 24 hours per day to perform portable X-rays. Availability of a postpartum care provider with expertise in lactation is strongly encouraged. The need for other support personnel depends on the intensity and level of sophistication of the other support services provided. An organized plan of action that includes personnel and equipment should be established for identification and immediate resuscitation (see "Neonatal Resuscitation" in Chapter 7).

Specialty (Level II) and Subspecialty (Level III) Care Facilities

The following support personnel should be available to the perinatal care service of specialty and subspecialty care hospitals:

- At least one full-time, master's degree-level, medical social worker (for every 30 beds) who has experience with the socioeconomic and psychosocial problems of high-risk women and fetuses, ill neonates, and their families. Additional medical social workers are required when there is a high volume of medical or psychosocial activity.
- At least one occupational or physical therapist with neonatal expertise
- At least one registered dietitian or nutritionist who has special training in perinatal nutrition and can plan diets that meet the special needs of high-risk women and neonates
- Qualified personnel for support services, such as laboratory studies, radiologic studies, and ultrasound examinations (these personnel should be available 24 hours per day)
- Respiratory therapists or nurses with special training who can supervise the assisted ventilation of neonates with cardiopulmonary disease
- Pharmacy personnel who can work to continually review their systems and process of medication administration to ensure that patient care policies are maintained

The hospital's engineering department should include air-conditioning, electrical, and mechanical engineers and biomedical technicians who are responsible for the safety and reliability of the equipment in all perinatal care areas.

EDUCATION

In-Service and Continuing Education

The medical and nursing staff of any hospital providing perinatal care at any level should be knowledgeable about current maternal and neonatal care through joint in-service sessions. These sessions should cover the diagnosis and management of perinatal emergencies, as well as the management of routine problems and family-centered care. The staff of each unit also should have regular multidisciplinary conferences at which the patient care problems are presented and discussed.

The staff of regional centers should be capable of assisting with the in-service programs of other hospitals in their region on a regular basis. Such assistance should include periodic visits to those hospitals, as well as periodic review of the quality of patient care provided by those hospitals. Regional center staff should be accessible for consultation at all times. The medical and nursing staff of hospitals providing specialty and subspecialty care should participate in formal courses or conferences. Regularly scheduled conferences may include the following subjects:

- Review of the major perinatal illnesses and their treatment and nursing care
- Review of perinatal statistics, the pathology related to all deaths, and significant surgical specimens
- Review of current X-ray films and ultrasound material
- Family-centered care
- Review of perinatal complications and outcomes

Perinatal Outreach Education

Design and coordination of a program for perinatal outreach education should be provided jointly by neonatal and obstetric physicians and APNs. Responsibilities should include assessing educational needs; planning curricula; teaching, implementing, and evaluating the program; collecting and using perinatal data; providing patient follow-up information to referring community personnel; writing reports; and maintaining informative working relationships with community personnel and outreach team members.

Ideally, a maternal–fetal medicine specialist, a certified nurse–midwife, an obstetric nurse, a neonatologist, and a neonatal nurse should be members of the perinatal outreach education team. Other professionals (eg, a social worker, respiratory therapist, occupational and physical therapist, and/or nutritionist) also may be assigned to the team. Each member should be responsible for teaching, consulting with community professionals as needed, and maintaining communication with the program coordinator and other team members.

Each subspecialty care center in a regional system is responsible for organizing an education program that is tailored to meet the needs of the perinatal health professionals and institutions within the network. The various educational strategies that have been found to be effective include a series of seminars, audiovisual and media programs, self-instruction booklets, and clinical practice rotations. Perinatal outreach education meetings should be held at a routine time and place to promote standardization and continuity of communication among community professionals and regional center personnel. As mandated by the subspecialty boards, a subspecialty care center that has a fellowship training program should have an active research program.

Physical Facilities

The physical facilities in which perinatal care is provided should be conducive to care that meets the unique physiologic and psychosocial needs of parents, neonates, and families (see "Family-Centered Care" in Chapter 1). Special facilities should be available when deviations from the norm require uninterrupted physiologic, biochemical, and clinical observation of patients throughout the perinatal period. Labor, delivery, and newborn care facilities should be located in close proximity to each other. When these facilities are distant from each other, provisions should be made for appropriate transitional areas.

The following recommendations are intended as general guidelines and should be interpreted with consideration given to local needs. It is recognized that individual limitations of physical facilities for perinatal care may impede strict adherence to these recommendations. Furthermore, every facility will not have each of the functional units described. Provisions for individual units should be consistent with a regional perinatal care system and state and local public health regulations.

Obstetric Functional Units

The patient's personal needs, as well as those of her newborn and family, should be considered when obstetric service units are planned. The service should be consolidated in a designated area that is physically arranged to prohibit unrelated traffic through the service units. The obstetric facility should incorporate the following components of maternity and newborn care:

- Antepartum care for patient stabilization or hospitalization before labor

- Fetal diagnostic testing (eg, nonstress and contraction stress testing, biophysical profile, amniocentesis, and ultrasound examinations)

- Labor observation and evaluation for patients who are not yet in active labor or who must be observed to determine whether labor has actually begun; hospital obstetric services should develop a casual, comfortable area ("false-labor lounge") for patients in prodromal labor

- Labor

- Delivery

- Postpartum maternal and newborn care

Where rooms are suitably sized, located, and equipped, some or all of the components of maternity care listed previously can be combined in one or more rooms. For example, to maximize economy and flexibility of staff and space, many hospitals have successfully combined functions into labor–delivery–recovery (LDR) rooms or labor–delivery–recovery–postpartum (LDRP) rooms. Single-room maternity care (SRMC) services use LDRP rooms for intrapartum care and also for postpartum care of both the woman and her neonate (breastfeeding).

In planning for antepartum, intrapartum, and postpartum beds, an analysis of the present patterns of care should be reviewed and consideration should be given to the following types of information:

- Projected birth rates

- Projected cesarean delivery rates

- Occupancy projections that address "peaks and valleys" in the census

- Present (and projected) number of women in the unit during peak periods, as well as the length of the peak periods

- Numbers and types of high-risk births
- Anticipated lengths of stay for women during labor, delivery, and recovery
- Anticipated changes in technology

The following facilities should be available to both antepartum and postpartum units and, in appropriate circumstances, may be shared:

- Unit director and head nurse's office
- Nurses' station
- Medical records area
- Conference room
- Patient education area
- Staff lounge, locker rooms, and on-call sleep rooms
- Examination and treatment room(s)
- Secure area for storage of medications
- Instrument cleanup area
- Area and equipment for bedpan cleansing
- Sitz bath facilities
- Kitchen and pantry
- Workroom and storage area
- Sibling visiting area

Nonobstetric Patients

The labor and delivery area should be used for nonobstetric patients only during periods of low occupancy. The obstetric department, in conjunction with the hospital administration, should establish written policies according to state and local regulations indicating which nonobstetric patients may be admitted to the labor and delivery suite. Under all circumstances, however, labor and delivery patients must take precedence over nonobstetric patients in this area. Clean gynecologic operations may be performed in the delivery rooms if patients are adequately screened to eliminate infectious cases and if enough personnel are present to prevent any compromise in the quality of obstetric care.

Labor

The room provided for a woman in labor should be private. Each room should be equipped with a comfortable chair. Each woman should have direct access to a private toilet and hand-washing in her room. Ideally, each room should have a shower or bathtub and a window. Ideally, the woman and her family should not have to be moved from one room to another for delivery or for postpartum and newborn care.

Areas used for women in labor should have the following equipment:

- Sterilization equipment (if there is no central sterilization equipment)
- X-ray view box
- Stretchers with side rails
- Equipment for pelvic examinations
- Emergency drugs
- Suction apparatus, either operated from a wall outlet or portable equipment
- Cardiopulmonary resuscitation cart (maternal and neonatal)
- Protective gear for personnel exposed to body fluids
- Warming cabinets for solutions and blankets
- A labor or birthing bed and a footstool
- A storage area for the patient's clothing and personal belongings
- Sufficient work space for information management systems
- One or more comfortable chairs
- Adjustable lighting that is pleasant for the patient and adequate for examinations
- An emergency signal and intercommunication system
- Adequate ventilation and temperature control
- A sphygmomanometer and stethoscope
- Mechanical infusion equipment

- Fetal monitoring equipment
- Oxygen outlets
- Access to at least one shower for use by patients in labor
- A writing surface for medical records
- Storage facilities for supplies and equipment

The room should have adequate space for support persons, personnel, equipment, and for the patient to ambulate in labor. Labor rooms should have a single bed and require a minimum of 100 net sq ft. Labor rooms used for intensive care of high-risk patients in hospitals with no designated high-risk units should be planned with a minimum of 160 net sq ft and should have at least two oxygen and two suction outlets. Design or renovation should include planning for information management systems at bedside and at workstations and for computer management of medical information.

Patients with significant medical or obstetric complications should be cared for in a room that is specially equipped with cardiopulmonary resuscitation equipment and other monitoring equipment necessary for observation and special care. This room is best located in the labor and delivery area and should meet the physical standards of any other intensive care room in the hospital. When patients with significant medical or obstetric complications receive care in the labor and delivery area, the capabilities of the unit should be identical to those of an intensive care unit.

Delivery

Delivery can be performed in a properly sized and equipped delivery room or LDR/LDRP room. Where delivery rooms are used, they should be close to the labor rooms to afford easy access and to provide privacy to women in labor. A comfortable waiting area for families should be adjacent to the delivery suite, and restrooms should be nearby.

Traditional delivery rooms and cesarean delivery rooms are similar in design to operating rooms. Vaginal deliveries can be performed in either room, whereas cesarean delivery rooms are designed especially for that purpose and, therefore, are larger. The traditional delivery room should be 350 net sq ft with a 9-ft ceiling. A cesarean delivery room should be 400 net sq ft. Each room should be well lighted and environmentally controlled to prevent chilling of the woman and the neonate. Cesarean deliveries should be performed in the obstetric unit, and postpartum sterilization capabilities should be available in that area when appropriate.

Each delivery room should be maintained as a separate unit that has the following equipment and supplies necessary for normal delivery and for the management of complications:

- Birthing bed that allows variations in position for delivery
- Instrument table and solution basin stand
- Instruments and equipment for vaginal delivery, repair of lacerations, cesarean delivery, and emergency laparotomy or hysterectomy
- Solutions and equipment for the intravenous administration of fluids
- Equipment for administration of all types of anesthesia, including equipment for emergency resuscitation of the patient
- Individual oxygen, air, and suction outlets for the mother and her neonate
- An emergency call system
- Mirrors for patients to observe the birth (optional)
- Wall clock with a second hand
- Equipment for fetal heart rate monitoring
- Neonatal resuscitation and stabilization unit (as defined in "Neonatal Functional Units" in this chapter)
- Scrub sinks strategically placed to allow observation of the patient

Trays containing drugs and equipment necessary for emergency treatment of both the patient and the neonate should be kept in the delivery room area. Equipment necessary for the treatment of cardiopulmonary resuscitation also should be easily accessible.

A workroom should be available for washing instruments. Instruments should be prepared and sterilized in a separate room; alternatively, these services may be performed in a separate area or by a central supply facility. There also should be a room for the storage and preparation of anesthetic equipment.

Postpartum and Newborn Care

The postpartum unit should be flexible enough to permit the comfortable accommodation of patients when the patient census is at its peak and allow the use of beds for alternate functions when the patient census is low. Postpartum rooms should ideally be occupied by a single family. Ideally, the room is equipped for newborn care, and the patient and her neonate are admitted to the room together. Each room in the postpartum unit should have a handwashing sink and, if possible, a toilet and shower. When this is not possible and it is necessary for patients to use common facilities, patients should be able to reach them without entering a general corridor. When the patient is breastfeeding, the room should have a handwashing sink, a mobile bassinet unit, and supplies necessary for the care of the newborn. Siblings may visit in the patient's room or in a designated space in the antepartum or postpartum area.

Larger services may have a specific recovery room for postpartum patients and a separate area for high-risk patients. The equipment needed is similar to that needed in any surgical recovery room and includes equipment for monitoring vital signs, suctioning, administering oxygen, and infusing fluids intravenously. Cardiopulmonary resuscitation equipment must be immediately available. Equipment for pelvic examinations also should be available.

Combined Units

Comprehensive obstetric and neonatal care can be provided for both low-risk and high-risk women and their newborns in a conventional obstetric unit that uses different rooms for labor, delivery, recovery, and newborn care; in an LDR unit that uses different rooms for intrapartum, postpartum, and newborn care; or in SRMC where an LDRP room is used for all stages of maternity and newborn care. Registered nurses who are cross-trained in antepartum care, labor and delivery, postpartum care, and neonatal care should staff this unit, increasing the continuity and quality of care.

Each LDR/LDRP room is a single-care room containing a toilet and shower with optional bathtub. A lavatory should be located in each room for scrubbing, handwashing, and neonate bathing. A window with an outside view is desirable in the LDR/LDRP room. Each room should contain a birthing bed that is comfortable during labor and can be readily converted to a delivery bed and transported to the cesarean delivery room when necessary. Separate oxygen, air, and suction facilities should be provided in two separate locations for the woman and the neonate. Gas outlets and wall-mounted equipment should be easily accessible but may be covered with a panel. Either a ceiling mount or a portable delivery light may be used, depending on the preference of the medical staff. An area within the room but distinct from the patient's area shall be provided for neonate stabilization and resuscitation.

Proper care of the patient requires sufficient space for a sphygmomanometer, stethoscope, fetal monitor, infusion pump, and regional anesthesia administration, as well as resuscitation equipment at the head of the bed. Proper care requires access to the newborn from three sides and quick transport to the nursery should the need arise. The family area should be farthest from the entry to the room, and there should be a comfortable area for the support person.

Equipment needed for labor, delivery, newborn resuscitation, and newborn care should be stored either in the room or in a nearby central storage or supply area, and should be immediately available to the LDR/LDRP room. For ease of movement, space below the foot of the bed should be adequate to accommodate equipment brought into the room as well as staff. Standard major equipment held in this area for delivery should include a fetal monitor, delivery case cart, linen hamper, and portable examination lights. A unit equipped for neonatal stabilization and resuscitation (described in "Neonatal Functional Units" in this chapter) should be available during delivery.

The workable size of an LDR/LDRP room is 256 net sq ft with room dimensions of 16 ft by 16 ft, excluding the toilet and shower. This room would be able to accommodate 6–8 people comfortably during the childbirth process. A minimum 5-ft clear space at the foot of the bed should be available for the providers to occupy during delivery.

Bed Need Analysis

Historically, the calculation of the number of patient rooms needed for all phases of the birth process was based on a simple ratio involving the number of births, the average lengths of stay, and the accepted occupancy levels. To best estimate patient room needs, each delivery service should thoroughly analyze functions, philosophies, and projections that will determine the types and quantities of rooms needed.

One planning method is to carefully analyze the activities that will occur in each type of room. For example, LDR/LDRP rooms should not routinely be used to accommodate care, such as outpatient testing, when another room would provide a more appropriate setting. Rooms that allow adequate privacy are recommended for the entire birth process, from labor through discharge.

In planning the number of LDR/LDRP rooms, the following questions should be addressed:

- Will patients scheduled for cesarean delivery use LDR/LDRP rooms or other types of patient rooms for their preoperative, recovery, and postpartum stays?

- What is the maximum projected number of annual births that will be accommodated?

- What is the length of stay for all antepartum, intrapartum, postpartum, and ambulatory patients?

- Are the LDR/LDRP rooms to be used for other purposes, such as triage or short-term observation for false labor or antepartum admission? If so, the length of stay and volume of all these activities must be used in the calculation of bed need.

- What are the current and projected rates for cesarean deliveries—both scheduled and unscheduled?

- What are the acceptable occupancy rates for all levels of patient rooms?

- What are the expected peak census and frequencies of peak occupancy?

Once the data have been accumulated, the following normative formula can be used to calculate the number of rooms needed by type of room (note that patient episodes—cases or activities—is used rather than the number of births):

$$\frac{\text{Number of patient episodes (considering all activities, such as admission, observation, and transitional care, in this room)}}{\text{365 days} \times \text{occupancy for the room type}} \times \text{Mean overall length of stay}$$

NEONATAL FUNCTIONAL UNITS

A neonatal service should have facilities available to perform the following functions:

- Resuscitation and stabilization
- Admission and observation
- Normal newborn nursery care
- Continuing care
- Intermediate care
- Intensive care
- Isolation
- Visitation
- Supporting service areas

Physically separate neonatal intensive, intermediate, and continuing care areas are a common alternative in nursery design. Consistency of nursing care provided and efficient staffing may be enhanced by having a mix of neonatal patients in a single area. Local circumstances should be considered in the design and management of these care areas.

Resuscitation and Stabilization

The resuscitation area should be illuminated to at least 100 foot-candles at the neonate's body surface and should contain the following items:

- Overhead source of radiant heat that can be regulated by the newborn's skin temperature

- Noncompressible resuscitation and examination mattress that allows access on three sides
- Wall clock
- Flat working surface for medical records
- Table or flat surface for trays and equipment
- Oxygen, compressed air, suction catheters, dry preferably warmed towels
- Resuscitation equipment, including bulb syringe, suction catheters, laryngoscope, endotracheal tubes and tape, meconium aspirator, ventilation bags and masks for term and preterm neonates, stethoscope, vascular access catheters
- Syringes, medications, solution(s) for volume expansion
- Equipment for examination, immediate care, and identification of the neonate
- Protective gear to prevent exposure to body fluids

The resuscitation area usually is within the delivery or LDR/LDRP room, although it may be in a designated, contiguous separate room. If resuscitation takes place in the delivery or LDR/LDRP room, the area should be large enough to allow for proper resuscitation of the newborn without interference with the care of the mother. Items contaminated with maternal blood, urine, and stool should be kept physically distant from the neonatal resuscitation area. The room temperature should be higher in the area for resuscitation or operating suites than is customary for patient rooms. After the neonate has been stabilized, if the mother wishes to hold her newborn, a radiant heater or prewarmed blankets should be available to keep the neonate warm. Although some newborns requiring resuscitation may remain with their mothers after stabilization, they will require increased vigilance for abnormal temperature, cardiorespiratory instability, hypoglycemia, apnea, and cyanosis. Nursing protocols addressing these issues are required. Qualified nursing staff should be available to monitor the newborn during this period.

A resuscitation area should be allotted a minimum of 40 net sq ft of floor space if it is within a delivery or LDR/LDRP room. A separate resuscitation room should have approximately 150 net sq ft of floor space. The area should have adequate suction, oxygen, and compressed-air outlets to accommodate simultaneous resuscitation of twins and should contain at least six electrical outlets. A separate resuscitation room also should have an electrical outlet to accommodate a portable X-ray machine, if needed. Electrical outlets should conform to regulations for areas in which anesthetic agents are administered.

Admission and Observation (Transitional and Stabilization Care)

The admission and observation area (for evaluating the neonate's condition in the first 4–8 hours of life) should be near or adjacent to the delivery and cesarean delivery room and preferably part of a recovery room, LDR/LDRP room, or other area for maternal recovery. Physical separation of the mother and her newborn during this period should be avoided. This evaluation may take place within one or more areas, including the room in which the mother is recovering, the LDR/LDRP room, or the newborn nursery. In some hospitals, the newborn nursery is the primary area for transitional care, both for neonates born within the hospital and for those born outside the hospital. No special or separate isolation facilities are required for neonates born at home or in transit to the hospital.

An estimated 40 net sq ft of floor space is needed for each neonate in the admission and observation area. The capacity required depends on the size of the delivery service and the duration of close observation. The number of observation stations required depends on the birth rate and the length of stay in the observation area. There should be a minimum of two observation stations. The admission and observation area should be well lighted and should contain a wall clock and emergency resuscitation equipment similar to that in the designated resuscitation area. Outlets also should be similar to those in the resuscitation area.

The physician's and nurse's assessment of the neonate's condition determines the subsequent level of care. When the admission and observation is in an LDR/LDRP room, the neonate remains in the room with the mother for breastfeeding. Neonates are never separated from their mothers, and are kept with their mothers in the LDR/LDRP rooms at all times. In services where the mother must be transferred from the room in which she delivers to a postpartum room, the newborn also is admitted to the postpartum room. Some neonates require transfer to an intermediate or intensive care area.

Newborn Nursery

Within each perinatal care facility there will be several types of units for newborn care. These units usually are defined by the content and complexity of care required by a specific group of infants.

Routine care of apparently normal term and some near-term neonates who have demonstrated successful adaptation to extrauterine life may be provided either in the newborn nursery or in the area where the woman is receiving postpartum care. The nursery should be close to the postpartum area. In a multifloor maternity unit, there should be a newborn nursery on each floor.

The number of bassinets in the newborn nursery should exceed the number of obstetric beds to accommodate multiple births, extended neonatal hospitalization, maternal illness, cesarean delivery, and fluctuations in demand. The bed requirement for the newborn nursery should be estimated by using data on the mean length of stay and annual number of liveborn, normal, term neonates. The use of combination LDR/LDRP rooms and rooming-in of newborns with mothers may substantially alter nursery bed requirements.

Because relatively few staff members are needed to provide care in the newborn nursery and because no bulky equipment is needed, 30 net sq ft of floor space for each neonate should be adequate. Bassinets should be at least 3 ft apart in all directions, measured from the edge of one bassinet to the edge of the neighboring bassinet. The newborn care area may be one room (in a small hospital) or one or more rooms (in larger hospitals). One registered nurse is recommended for every 6–8 neonates and should be available in each newborn-occupied area at all times (Table 2–1). Therefore, individual rooms should have accommodations for 6–8, 12–16, or 18–24 neonates. During decreased patient occupancy, central nurseries use nursing staff inefficiently. Direct care of those newborns remaining in the nursery may be provided by licensed practical nurses and unlicensed nursing personnel under the registered nurse's direct supervision.

The newborn nursery should be well lighted, have a large wall clock, and be equipped for emergency resuscitation. One pair of wall-mounted electrical outlets is recommended for each two neonatal stations. One oxygen outlet, one compressed-air outlet, and one suction outlet are recommended for every four neonatal stations. Cabinets and counters should be available within the newborn care area for storage of routinely used supplies, such as diapers, formula, and linens. If circumcisions are performed in the nursery, an appropriate table with adequate lighting is required. Electrical outlets to power portable X-ray machines are highly recommended.

Continuing Care

Several levels of care may be provided in the same nursery units or in different areas of the same hospital. It is important to distinguish between specific units and the levels of care provided in each unit. Recommendations regarding the intensity of care are made in the following paragraphs.

Low-birth-weight neonates, who are not ill but require frequent feeding, as well as those who require more hours of nursing than do normal neonates, should be taken to the continuing care area. This area should be close to the intermediate and intensive care areas so that neonates who have received intermediate or intensive care, but no longer require these levels of care, may be transferred to the continuing care area for convalescence. This area also is used for convalescing neonates who have returned to specialty facilities from an outside intensive care unit.

Because the care of neonates in this area requires appropriate equipment as well as more personnel than are needed in the newborn nursery, more space is needed per patient unit. There should be 50 net sq ft of floor space for each patient station, with approximately 4 ft between bassinets or incubators.

As in the resuscitation and stabilization area and the admission and observation area, equipment for emergency resuscitation is required in the neonatal continuing care area. It may be most conveniently kept on an emergency cart or in a cabinet, but it should be readily available. Each neonatal station should have six electrical outlets, one oxygen outlet, one compressed-air outlet, and one suction outlet. In addition, the equipment and supplies required in the newborn nursery should be available in the continuing care area. Provisions should be made for the comfort of parents or personnel who feed neonates in both incubators and bassinets.

Intermediate Care

Sick neonates who do not require intensive care but require 6–12 hours of nursing care each day should be taken to the intermediate care area. Newborns requiring complex care, such as assisted ventilation, for more than several hours should be moved to an intensive care area. The neonatal intermediate care area should be close to the delivery and cesarean delivery room and the intensive care area, and away from general hospital traffic. It should have radiant heaters or incubators for maintaining body temperature, as well as infusion pumps, cardiopulmonary monitors, and equipment for ventilatory assistance.

At least 100–120 net sq ft per newborn is suggested for subspecialty patients, but for intermediate care this space may be less. Space needed for other purposes (eg, for desks, counters, cabinets, corridors, and treatment rooms) should be added to the space needed for patients. There should be at least 4 ft between incubators, bassinets, or radiant heaters in intermediate care areas. Aisles should be 5 ft wide.

Neonates receiving intermediate care may be housed in a single large room or in two or more smaller rooms. In the latter case, each room should accommodate some multiple of 4–6 newborn stations because one registered nurse is required for every three to four neonates who require intermediate care. Large rooms allow greater flexibility in the use of equipment and assignment of personnel, but less privacy for parental involvement in newborn care.

Eight electrical outlets, two oxygen outlets, two compressed-air outlets, and two suction outlets should be provided for each patient station. In addition, the area should have a special outlet to power the neonatal unit's portable X-ray machine. All electrical outlets for each patient station should be connected to both regular and auxiliary power. An oxygen tank for emergency use should be stored but readily available for each newborn receiving wall-supplied oxygen.

All equipment and supplies for resuscitation should be immediately available within the intermediate care unit. These items may be conveniently placed on an emergency cart.

Intensive Care

Constant nursing and continuous cardiopulmonary and other support for severely ill newborns should be provided in the intensive care area.

Because emergency care is provided in this area, laboratory and radiologic services should be readily available 24 hours per day. The results of blood gas analyses should be available shortly after sample collection. In many centers, a laboratory adjacent to the intensive care unit provides this service.

The neonatal intensive care area should be near the delivery area and cesarean delivery room(s) and should be easily accessible from the hospital's ambulance entrance. It should be located away from routine hospital traffic. Intensive care may be provided in a single area or in two or more separate rooms.

The number of nursing, medical, and surgical personnel required in the neonatal intensive care area is greater than that required in less acute perinatal care areas. In addition, the amount and complexity of equipment required also are considerably greater. Therefore, incubators or overhead warmers should be separated by at least 6 ft, and aisles should be 8 ft wide. The area should have 150 net sq ft of floor space for each neonate, plus space for desks, cabinets, and corridors. In addition, the educational responsibilities of a subspecialty facility require that the design of its neonatal intensive care area include space for instructional activities and office space for files on the region's perinatal experience.

Each patient station needs 16–20 electrical outlets, 3–4 oxygen outlets, 3–4 compressed-air outlets, and 3–4 suction outlets. Like those in the intermediate care area, all electrical outlets for each patient station should be connected to both regular and auxiliary power. In addition, each room should have a special outlet to power the portable X-ray machine housed in the NICU. An oxygen tank for emergency use should be stored but readily available for each newborn receiving wall-supplied oxygen.

Equipment and supplies in the intensive care area should include all those needed in the resuscitation and intermediate care areas. Immediate availability of emergency oxygen is essential. In addition, equipment for long-term ventilatory support should be provided. Respirators should be equipped with nebulizers or humidifiers with heaters. Continuous on-line monitoring of oxygen concentrations, body temperature, heart rate, respiration, oxygen saturation, transcutaneous oxygen tension, transcutaneous carbon dioxide tension, and blood pressure levels should be available. Supplies should be kept close to the patient station so that nurses are not away from the neonate unnecessarily and may use their time and skills efficiently. A central modular supply system can enhance efficiency.

In some cases, certain surgical procedures (eg, ligation of a patent ductus arteriosus) are performed in an area in or adjacent to the NICU. Specific procedures addressing preparatory cleaning, physical preparation of the unit, presence of other newborns, venting of volatile anesthetics, and quality assessment should be documented in writing. Equipment, facilities, and supplies for this area, as well as procedures, must conform to or be comparable to those required for similar procedures in the surgical department of the hospital. The latter includes adequate air exchange (at least six air changes per hour).

Visitation

Parents should have access to their newborns 24 hours per day at all levels of care within all functional units and should be encouraged to participate in the care of their newborns (see "Visiting Policies" in Chapter 7). Generally, parents can be with their newborns in the woman's room.

Special provisions may be necessary when neonates are in special care units (ie, continuing, intermediate, or intensive care units). In these situations, women often are discharged from the hospital before their newborns and sometimes must travel long distances to be with them. Several systems have been developed to meet the needs of parents and their newborns under these circumstances (eg, rooms for parents in the hospital, adjacent facilities outside the hospital provided by the hospital, or other lodgings nearby). A period of mother–newborn rooming-in before discharge is highly desirable when special care is needed. In addition, intensive and intermediate care units require special areas that are appropriately furnished for the counseling of parents, the breastfeeding of newborns, and the support of grieving women and families.

Supporting Service Areas

Utility Rooms. Both clean and soiled utility rooms are needed in neonatal care areas. A separate clean utility room is used for storing breast milk and storing and preparing formulas, medications, and supplies frequently needed for the care of neonates in all functional units. The use of ready-mixed formulas, unit-dose medications, and disposable supplies and equipment has decreased the need for clean utility rooms; however, storage areas and clean working surfaces within each functional unit may replace them. Separate storage areas should be available for foodstuffs, medications, and clean supplies. Utility rooms should not have direct lighting because some of the formulas, medications, and supplies may be light sensitive.

A utility room for storing used and contaminated material before it is removed from the care area is highly desirable. It should have negative air pressure, with 100% of its air exhausted to the outside. There should be a two-door zone, one providing direct access from within the unit, and another from outside the unit. This room should contain a countertop and a sink with hot and cold running water that is turned on and off by knee or foot controls, soap and paper towel dispensers, and a covered waste receptacle with foot control. A separate deep sink with hot and cold running water should be available for cleaning equipment prior to its return to the central service department for resterilization.

Storage Areas. A three-level storage system is desirable. The first storage area should be the central supply department of the hospital. The second storage area should be adjacent to or within the patient care areas. In this area, routinely used supplies, such as diapers, formula, linen, cover gowns, medical records, and information booklets, may be stored. Generally, space is required in this area only for the amount of each item used between deliveries from the hospital's central supply department (eg, daily or three times weekly). The third area is needed for the storage of items frequently used at the neonate's bedside.

The bedside cabinet storage area should be approximately 8 net cu ft for each bed patient unit in the newborn nursery, 16 net cu ft for each bed patient unit in the intermediate care area, and 24 net cu ft for each bed patient unit in the intensive care area. The newborn nursery requires approximately 3 net cu ft per patient for secondary storage of items such as linen and formula. In the resuscitation and stabilization area, the admission and observation area, and the continuing, intermediate, and intensive care areas, there should be approximately 8 net cu ft per patient for secondary storage of syringes, needles, intravenous infusion sets, and sterile trays needed in procedures, such as umbilical vessel catheterization, lumbar puncture, and thoracotomy.

Large equipment items (eg, bassinets, warmers, radiant heaters, phototherapy units, and infusion pumps) should be stored in a clean, enclosed storage area in close proximity to, but not within, the immediate patient care area. Approximately 6 net sq ft of floor space for equipment is required for each patient in the newborn nursery, 18 net sq ft for each patient in the intermediate care area, and 30 net sq ft for each patient in the intensive care area. Easily accessible electrical outlets are desirable in this area.

Treatment Rooms. Many facilities have developed areas for resuscitation and stabilization, admission and observation, intermediate care, and intensive care in which each patient station constitutes a treatment area. This has largely eliminated the need for a separate treatment room for procedures, such as lumbar punctures, intravenous infusions, venipuncture, and minor surgical procedures. A separate treatment area may be necessary, however, if neonates in the newborn nursery or continuing care area or the postpartum new family unit are to undergo certain procedures (eg, circumcision). The facilities, outlets, equipment, and supplies in the treatment area should be similar to those of the resuscitation area. The amount of space required depends on the procedures performed.

Scrub Areas

At the entrance to each nursery, there should be a scrub area that can accommodate all personnel entering the area. It should have a sink that is large enough to prevent splashing, with faucets operated by foot or knee controls. A backsplash should be provided to prevent standing or retained water. Sinks for handwashing should not be built into counters used for other purposes. The scrub areas also should contain racks, hooks, or lockers for storing clothing and personal items, as well as cabinets for clean gowns, a receptacle for used gowns, and a large wall clock with a sweep second hand for timing handwashing.

Scrub sinks should have foot-operated, knee-operated, or photoelectric-operated faucets and should be large enough to control splashing and to prevent retained water. These sinks should be provided at a minimum ratio of one for at least every 6–8 patient stations in the newborn nursery and one for every 3–4 patient stations in the intermediate or intensive care area. In addition, one scrub sink is needed in the resuscitation and stabilization area, and one is needed for every 3–4 patient stations in the admission and observation area and in the continuing care area.

Nursing Areas

Space should be provided at the bedside, not only for patient care, but also for instructional and medical record activities. A flat writing surface (eg, a clipboard) is needed.

A nurses' medical record area or desk for tasks such as compiling more detailed records, completing requisitions, and handling specimens is useful. Physicians also may perform medical record and clerical activities in this area. Maintaining medical records should be considered an unclean procedure, and personnel who have been working in medical records should wash their hands before they have further contact with a neonate.

The unit director or head nurse should have an office close to the newborn care areas. Nurses' dressing rooms preferably should be adjacent to a lounge and should contain lockers, storage for clean and soiled scrub attire, toilets, and showers.

Education Areas

A conference room suitable for educational purposes is highly desirable, particularly for specialty and subspecialty facilities. It should be in or adjacent to the maternal–newborn areas.

Clerical Areas

The control point for patient care activities is the clerical area. It should be located near the entrance to the neonatal care areas so that personnel can supervise traffic and limit unnecessary entry into these areas. It should have telephones and communication devices that connect to the various neonatal care areas and the delivery suite. In addition, patients' medical records, computer terminals, and hospital forms may be located in the clerical area.

GENERAL CONSIDERATIONS

Newborn Security

Security devices should be part of an overall security program to protect the physical safety of newborns, families, and staff. Both the NICU and normal nurseries should be designed to minimize the risk of newborn abduction. Policies and procedures for visitation, transfer, and discharge of neonates should include identification and verification of the neonate and designated attendants.

Evacuation Plan

An evacuation plan should be developed for each perinatal care area (ie, antepartum care, labor and delivery, postpartum care, the normal newborn nursery, intermediate care, and intensive care). The policy should specify: 1) who orders the evacuation and destination, 2) who designates the assignments, 3) the roles and responsibilities of the staff, and 4) what equipment is needed. A floor plan that indicates designated evacuation routes should be posted in a conspicuous place in each unit. The policy and floor plan should be reviewed with the staff at least annually.

Safety and Environmental Control

Because of the complexities of environmental control and monitoring, a hospital environmental engineer must ensure that all electrical, lighting, air composition, and temperature systems function properly and safely. A regular maintenance program should be specified to ensure that systems continue to function as designed after initial occupancy.

The environmental temperature in newborn care areas should be independently adjustable, and control should be sufficient to prevent hot and cold spots, particularly when heat-generating equipment (eg, a radiant warmer) is in use. The air temperature should be kept at 23.8–26.1°C (75–79°F). Humidity should be kept between 30–60% and should be controlled through the heating and air-conditioning system of the hospital. Condensation on wall and window surfaces should be avoided.

A minimum of six air changes per hour is recommended, and a minimum of two changes should be outside air. The ventilation pattern should inhibit particulate matter from moving freely in the space, and intake and exhaust vents should be placed so as to minimize drafts on or near the patient beds. Ventilation air delivered to the NICU should be filtered at 90% efficiency.

Fresh-air intake should be located at least 25 ft from exhaust outlets of ventilating systems, combustion equipment stacks, medical or surgical vacuum systems, plumbing vents, or areas that may collect vehicular exhausts or other noxious fumes.

Radiation exposure to newborns, families, and staff is another safety concern. Radiation exposure to personnel is negligible at a distance of more than 1 ft lateral to the primary vertical roentgen beam. Care should be taken to ensure that only the patient being examined is in the primary beam. It is unnecessary for families or personnel to leave the area during the roentgen exposure.

Illumination

Ambient lighting levels in newborn intensive care rooms should be adjustable through a range of at least 10–600 lux (approximately 1–60 ft-c) as measured at each bedside. Both natural and artificial light sources should have controls that allow immediate darkening of any bed position sufficient for transillumination when necessary. Artificial light sources should have a visible spectral distribution similar to that of daylight but should avoid unnecessary ultraviolet or infrared radiation by the use of appropriate lamps, lenses, or filters.

Appropriate general lighting levels for NICUs have not been established. In the past, relatively high levels (60–100 ft-c) have been recommended to allow evaluation of a newborn's skin color and perfusion at any spot in the NICU.

Newly constructed or renovated NICUs also should be able to provide ambient lighting at levels recommended by the Illuminating Engineering Society (10–20 ft-c). In most cases, these levels are adequate.

Studies have demonstrated benefits to some NICU patients exposed to diurnal variation in ambient lighting that reduces nighttime levels to as low as 0.5 ft-c. If these preliminary studies are confirmed and problems surrounding the evaluation of skin color and perfusion under low-light conditions can be adequately resolved, newly designed units also should possess the capability to reduce general lighting to a similar degree.

Nurseries should have the capability for adjustable illumination. Multiple switching can be helpful in this regard, but unless a master switch also is provided, this method can pose serious difficulties when rapid darkening of a room is required to permit transillumination.

Because perception of skin tones is critical in the NICU, light sources must be as balanced and as free of glare or veiling reflections as possible. Although harmful in high doses, ultraviolet radiation might be useful in small doses because of photobiologic effects in the skin. The magnitude of both harmful and beneficial doses for the newborn has not yet been defined.

Until better data are available, the output of ultraviolet radiation by fluorescent fixtures (including phototherapy lights) in patient care areas should be minimized by plastic or glass shields that filter out most ultraviolet radiation. Separate procedure lighting that provides no more than 1,000–1,500 lux (100–150 ft-c) of illumination to the patient bed should be available at each patient care station.

Lighting should minimize shadows and glare, and it should be controlled with a rheostat so that it can be provided at less than maximal levels whenever possible. Light should be highly framed so that newborns at adjacent bed stations will not experience any increase in illumination. Temporary increases in illumination necessary to evaluate a newborn or to perform a procedure should be possible without increasing lighting levels for other newborns in the same room.

High levels of light necessary to perform a procedure may represent a danger to the developing retina. Given the lack of safety standards, it may be prudent to design directable lighting, where the procedure light can be framed away from the eyes of patients during use.

Illumination of support areas within the NICU, including medical records area, medication preparation area, reception desk, and handwashing areas, should conform to the specifications of the Illuminating Engineering Society. Illumination should be adequate in the areas of the NICU where staff perform important or critical tasks. In locations where these functions overlap with patient care areas (eg, close proximity of the nurse medical records area to patient beds), the design should permit separate light sources with independent controls so that the very different needs of sleeping newborns and working nurses can be accommodated to the greatest possible extent.

Windows

Windows provide an important psychologic benefit to staff and families in the NICU. Properly designed natural light is the most desirable illumination for nearly all nursing tasks, including updating medical records and evaluating newborn skin tone. However, placing newborns too close to external windows can cause serious problems with temperature control and glare, so providing windows in the NICU requires careful planning and design.

At least one source of natural light should be visible from each patient care area. External windows in patient care rooms should be glazed with insulating glass to minimize heat gain and loss. They should be situated at least 2 ft away from any part of a patient bed to minimize radiant heat loss from the newborn. All external windows should be equipped with shading devices that are easily controlled to allow flexibility at various times of day. These shading devices should be either contained within the window or easily cleanable.

Interior Finish

Off-white or pale-beige walls minimize distortion of staff's color perception in patient care areas. This advantage can be nullified by the use of inappropriate fluorescent lighting. Brighter colors may be used elsewhere. Windows in neonatal care areas should have opaque shades that make it possible to darken the area for procedures such as transillumination.

Oxygen and Compressed-Air Outlets

Newborn care areas should have oxygen and compressed air piped from a central source at a pressure of 50–60 psi. An alarm system that warns of any critical reduction in line pressure should be installed. Reduction valves and mixers should produce adjustable concentrations of 21–100% oxygen at atmospheric pressure for head hoods and 50–60 psi for mechanical ventilators.

Acoustic Characteristics

Newborn bed areas and the spaces opening onto them should be designed to produce minimal background noise and to contain and absorb much of the transient noise that arises within the nursery. The ventilation system, monitors, incubators, suction pumps, mechanical ventilators, and staff produce considerable noise, and the noise level should be monitored intermittently. The construction and redesign of neonatal care areas should include acoustic absorption units or other means to ensure that the peak sound intensity does not exceed 90 dB and preferably remains lower than that level. Background noise mean level should not exceed 70 dB. Staff members should take particular care to avoid noise pollution in enclosed patient spaces (eg, incubators). Care should be taken to avoid spaces shaped so as to focus or amplify sound levels, thus creating "hot spots" that exceed the maximum recommended noise levels.

Electrical Outlets and Electrical Equipment

All electrical outlets should be attached to a common ground. All electrical equipment should be checked for current leakage and grounding adequacy when first introduced into the neonatal care area, after any repair, and periodically while in service. Current leakage allowances, preventive maintenance standards, and equipment quality should meet the standards developed by the Joint Commission on Accreditation of Healthcare Organizations. Personnel should be thoroughly and repeatedly instructed on the potential electrical hazards within the neonatal care areas.

Bibliography

American Academy of Pediatrics Committee on Fetus and Newborn. Advanced practice in neonatal nursing. AAP News 1992;8:17 (reaffirmed 1995).

American Institute of Architects Academy of Architecture for Health. Guidelines for design and construction of hospital and health care facilities 1996–97. Washington, DC: The American Institute of Architects Press; 1996.

Facilities and equipment for care of pediatric patients in a community hospital. American Academy of Pediatrics Committee on Hospital Care. Pediatrics 1998;101:1089–90.

Graven SN, Bowen FW Jr, Brooten D, Eaton A, Graven MN, Hack M, et al. The high-risk infant environment. Part 1. The role of the neonatal intensive care unit in the outcome of high-risk infants. J Perinatol 1992;12:164–72.

Graven SN, Bowen FW Jr, Brooten D, Eaton A, Graven MN, Hack M, et al. The high-risk infant environment. Part 2. The role of caregiving and the social environment. J Perinatol 1992;12:267–75.

March of Dimes Birth Defects Foundation, Committee on Perinatal Health. Toward improving the outcome of pregnancy: the 90s and beyond. White Plains (NY): MDBDF; 1993.

National Association of Neonatal Nurses. Neonatal nursing standards, guidelines, and related documents: annotated bibliography. Petaluma (CA): NANN; 1993.

National Association of Neonatal Nurses. Standards of care for neonatal nursing practice. Petaluma (CA): NANN; 1993.

Noise: a hazard for the fetus and newborn. American Academy of Pediatrics Committee on Environment Health. Pediatrics 1997;100:724-7.

Smith JA. The family birthplace: planning and designing today's obstetric facilities. Chicago (IL): American Hospital Publishing; 1995.

White RD. Recommended standards for newborn ICU design. Committee to establish recommended standards for newborn ICU design. J Perinatol 1999; 19(8P + 2):S1-S12.

CHAPTER 3

Interhospital Care of the Perinatal Patient

Interhospital transport of pregnant women and neonates is an essential component of regional perinatal care. The goal is to care for high-risk women and neonates in facilities that provide the required level of specialized care. Women who are at risk for complications that pose significant risk for adverse outcome or whose neonates are likely to require intensive support should be considered candidates for referral during the antepartum period. Neonates born to women transported during the antepartum period have better survival rates and decreased risks of long-term sequelae than those who are transferred after birth.

Interhospital transport of a pregnant woman is recommended if appropriate services and staff are not available for either the woman or her neonate at the referring facility. Both the facilities and the professionals providing health care to pregnant women need to understand their obligations under the law for patient transfer.

Federal law requires all Medicare-participating hospitals to provide an appropriate medical screening examination for any individual seeking medical treatment at an emergency department to determine whether the patient has an emergency medical condition (see Appendix D). Some states have similar statutory requirements. These laws also place strict requirements on the transfer of these patients. A woman having contractions is not considered to be having an emergency medical condition if there is adequate time for her safe transfer before delivery or if the transfer will not pose a threat to the health or safety of the woman or the fetus.

Program Components

There are three types of perinatal patient transport. These types of transport are used for patients who have been transferred between facilities.

1. Maternal transport—A pregnant woman is transferred during the antepartum or intrapartum period for special care of the woman or the neonate or both.

2. Neonatal transport:

   • A team is sent from one hospital, often a regional center, to the referring hospital to evaluate and stabilize the neonate at the referring hospital and then transfer the neonate back to the first hospital.

   • A team is sent from the referring hospital with a neonate who is being transferred to another hospital for specialized or intensive care.

   • A team is sent from one hospital to the referring hospital to evaluate and stabilize the neonate and then transfer the neonate to a third hospital. Such a transfer may be necessary because of bed constraints or the need for specialized care only available at the third hospital.

3. Return transport—A woman or her neonate, after receiving intensive or specialized care at a referral center, is returned to the original referring hospital or to a local hospital for continuing care after the problems that required the transfer have been resolved. This should be done in consultation with the referring physician.

To ensure optimal care of high-risk patients, the following components should be part of a regional referral program:

• Formal transfer agreements between participating hospitals

• Risk identification and assessment of problems that are expected to benefit from consultation and transport

• Assessment of the perinatal capabilities and determination of conditions necessitating consultation, referral, or transfer by the medical staff of each participating hospital

• Resource management

• Adequate financial and personnel support

- A reliable, accurate, and comprehensive communication system between participating hospitals
- Determination of responsibility for each of these functions

An interhospital transport program should provide 24-hour service. It should include a receiving or program center responsible for ensuring that high-risk patients receive the appropriate level of care, a dispatching unit to coordinate the transport of patients between facilities, an appropriately equipped transport vehicle, and a specialized transport team. The program also should have a system for providing a continuum of care by various providers, including the personnel and equipment required for the level of care needed, as well as outreach education and program evaluation.

Responsibilities

Each of the functional components of an interhospital transport program has specific responsibilities. If the transport is done by the referring hospital, the referring physician and hospital retain responsibility until the transport team arrives with the patient at the receiving hospital. If the transport team is sent by the receiving hospital, the receiving physician or designee assumes responsibility for patient care from the time the patient leaves the referring hospital. It should be emphasized that during the preparation for transport by the transport team, the referring physician and hospital have retained responsibility for the patient unless there have been other prior agreements which determine this responsibility. Regardless of the site of origin of the transport team, qualified staff should accompany the patient to the receiving hospital.

Medical–Legal Aspects

Many legal details of perinatal transport are not well defined. However, all involved parties (eg, the referring hospital and personnel, the receiving hospital and personnel, and the transportation carriers or corporations) assume a number of responsibilities for which they are accountable:

- Each transport system must comply with the standards and regulations set forth by local, state, and federal agencies.

- Informed consent for transfer, transport, and admission to and care at the receiving hospital should be obtained before the transport team moves the patient. All federal and state laws regulating patient transfer must be followed. The completed consent form should be signed by the patient or parent or guardian and witnessed; a copy should be placed in the patient's medical record. If the neonatal patient requires an emergency procedure before the parents' arrival at the receiving facility, the informed consent for this procedure should be obtained before departure from the referring facility if this action will not adversely delay the transport.

- Consent for any surgical procedures should be obtained by surgical staff by telephone.

- Formal agreements between hospitals should be developed to outline procedures for transport and responsibilities for patient care.

- Hospital medical staff policies should delineate the level of capability of their perinatal units, which conditions should prompt consultation, and which patients should be considered for transfer.

- Relevant personal identification must be provided for the patient to wear during transport.

- Patient care guidelines, standing orders, and verbal communication with the designated transport physician are to be used to initiate and maintain patient care interventions during transport.

The professional qualifications and actions of the transport team are the responsibility of the institution that employs the team. Insurance must be adequate to protect both patients and transport team members.

Director

The director of the transport program should be either a subspecialist in maternal–fetal medicine or neonatology or an obstetrician–gynecologist or pediatrician with special expertise in these subspecialty areas. The program director's responsibilities include:

- Training and supervising staff
- Ensuring appropriate review of all transport records

- Developing and implementing patient care protocols
- Developing and maintaining standardized patient records and a database to track the program
- Identifying trends and effecting improvements in the transport system by regularly reviewing:
  — Operational aspects of the program, such as response times, effectiveness of communications, and equipment issues
  — Evaluation forms prepared by the referring and receiving hospitals soon after each transport
- Developing protocols for programs which use multiple modes of transportation (ground, helicopter, airplane)
- Determining which mode of transport should be used and conditions, such as weather, which would preclude the use of a particular form of transport
- Developing alternative plans for care of the patient if a transport cannot be accomplished
- Ensuring that proper safety standards are followed during transport
- Requiring the transportation services to follow established guidelines regarding maintenance and safety

The director may delegate specific responsibilities to other persons or groups, but retains the responsibility of ensuring that these functions are appropriately addressed.

Referring Hospital

Referring physicians should be familiar with the transport system, including how to gain access to and appropriately use its services. The referring physician is responsible for evaluating and stabilizing the patient's condition before transfer.

When being transferred, each patient should be accompanied by a maternal or neonatal transport form. This form should contain general information about the patient, including the reason for referral, the transport mode, and any additional information that may enhance understanding of the patient's needs. Also provided should be relevant neonatal medical information that maximizes the opportunity for appropriate and timely care and minimizes duplication of tests and diagnostic procedures at the receiving hospital. The newborn must have appropriate identification bands in place.

The following items should be sent with a neonate:

- Properly labeled, red-topped tubes of clotted maternal and umbilical cord blood with label identification consistent with the newborn identification bands

- Copies of all relevant maternal antepartum, intrapartum, and postpartum records

- All recent or new diagnostic or clinical information on the neonate, including imaging studies

Responsibility for care of the newborn should be delineated between the referring team and the transport team. Parental consent should be obtained for transfer to and treatment of the neonate at the receiving hospital. The referring physician should personally transfer care to the transport team or should designate another physician to transfer care. A report on the neonate's care should be provided by the referring hospital's nursing staff to the appropriate transport team member.

RECEIVING CENTER

The receiving center is responsible for the overall coordination of the regional program. It should ensure that interhospital transport is organized in a way that ensures that patients will receive the appropriate level of care.

Contingency plans should be in place to avoid a shortage of beds for patients needing tertiary care. These plans should include provisions for accepting or transferring patients among the cooperating centers or to an alternate receiving center, rather than only the receiving center affiliated with the referral center, when special circumstances warrant (eg, patient census or need for specialized services, such as extracorporeal membrane oxygenation).

The receiving center is responsible for providing referring physicians with:

- Access by telephone on a 24-hour basis to communicate with receiving obstetric and neonatal units

- Follow-up on the neonate by telephone, letter, or fax, provided all federal, state, and local requirements are met
- A complete summary, including diagnosis, an outline of the hospital course, and recommendations for ongoing care for each patient at discharge
- Ongoing communication and follow-up

DISPATCHING UNITS

Dispatching units are responsible for the following activities:

- Providing rapid coordination of vehicles and staff
- Serving as a communication link between the transport team and the referring and receiving hospitals
- Communicating the transport team's estimated time of arrival at the referring hospital to pick up the patient so that any planned therapeutic or diagnostic interventions can be completed in time
- Communicating the patient's estimated time of arrival at the receiving center so that all resources can be mobilized and ready
- Coordinating any connections that need to be made between air transport and ground ambulances

Personnel

The transport team collectively should have the expertise necessary to provide supportive care for a wide variety of emergency conditions that can arise with high-risk women and neonates. Team members may include physicians, neonatal nurse practitioners, registered nurses, respiratory therapists, and emergency medical technicians. The composition of the transport team should be consistent with the expected level of medical need of the patient being transported. Transport personnel also should be thoroughly familiar with the transport equipment to ensure that any malfunction en route can be handled without the assistance of hospital maintenance staff.

Equipment

Safe and successful patient transfer depends on the equipment available to the transport team. The kinds and amounts of equipment, medications, and supplies needed by the transport team depend on the type of transport (maternal or neonatal), the distance of the transfer, the type of transport vehicle used, and the resources available at the referring medical facility. The transport equipment and supplies should be based on the needs of the most seriously ill patients to be transported and should include essential medications and special supplies needed during stabilization and transfer.

The transport team generally needs the following items to perform its functions:

- Equipment for monitoring physiologic functions (heart rate, blood pressure levels [invasive or noninvasive], temperature [skin or axillary], respiratory rate, noninvasive pulse oximetry, and transcutaneous oxygen or carbon dioxide)
- Resuscitation and support equipment (intravenous pumps, suction apparatus, mechanical ventilators, and newborn incubators)
- Portable medical gas tanks attached to a flowmeter, with or without a blender that can be easily integrated with vehicle or building sources of pressurized gas during transport if patients dependent on ventilators are transported
- Electrical equipment that is capable of alternating current or extended direct-current operation or both and is compatible with the sources in the transport vehicle or medical facility

The performance characteristics of transport equipment should be tested for the most severe environmental conditions of air or ground transport that may be encountered. Equipment performance may be altered by a harsh electromagnetic environment, altitude changes, vibration, forces of acceleration, or extremes of temperature and humidity. Hospital-based equipment may cause electromagnetic interference with aircraft navigation or communication systems. Altered performance of medical or aircraft systems could affect the safety of the transport team and the patient.

All equipment should be tested to ensure accuracy and safety in flight. The Federal Aviation Administration and the U.S. Food and Drug Administration have no comprehensive testing guidelines. The comprehensive testing programs of the U.S. Department of Defense have discovered flaws in hospital-based medical equipment that could affect safety when used in air transport. The U.S. Army Aeromedical Research Laboratory at Fort Rucker in Alabama has tested medical equipment for helicopter use, and the Armstrong Laboratory at Brooks Air Force Base in Texas has tested equipment for airplanes. These laboratories can report on completed equipment tests or conduct new evaluations. The following organizations also can offer assistance in choosing medical equipment suitable for use in aircraft:

Association of Air Medical Services
110 North Royal Street, Suite 307
Alexandria, Virginia 22314-3234
(703) 836-8732; Fax: (703) 836-8920
www.aams.org

Emergency Care Research Institute
5200 Butler Pike
Plymouth Meeting, PA 19462-1298
(610) 825-6000; Fax: (610) 834-1275
www.ecri.org

Federal Aviation Administration
800 Independence Avenue, SW
Washington, DC 20591
(202) 366-4000
www.faa.gov

National Aeronautics and Space Administration
Washington, DC 20546-0001
(202) 358-0000; Fax: (202) 358-3251
www.nasa.gov

Professional Aeromedical Transport Association
A-11 Airport Road
Punta Gorda, FL 33982
800-541-7517; Fax: (941) 639-3945
schaeferamb.com/PATA/

Several factors should be considered in selecting vehicles for an interhospital transport system. Ground transportation is most appropriate for short-range transport. The use of airplanes allows for coverage of a large referral area but is more expensive, requires skilled operators and specially trained crews, and may actually prolong the time required for response and transport over relatively short distances because of the time needed to prepare for flight. Helicopters can shorten response and transport time over intermediate distances or in highly congested areas but are very expensive to maintain and operate.

The decision to use aircraft in a patient transport system requires special commitments from the director and members of the transport team. During air transport, the pilot should be considered an integral part of the transport team. Therefore, the pilot should be included in appropriate decision making and should have the authority to change, modify, or cancel the mission for safety reasons.

Transport Procedure

Interhospital transport should be considered if the necessary resources or personnel for optimal patient outcomes are not available at the facility currently providing care. The resources available at both the referring and the receiving hospitals should be considered. The risks and benefits of transport, as well as the risks and benefits associated with not transporting the patient, should be assessed. Transport may be undertaken if the physician determines that the well-being of either the woman or the fetus would not be adversely affected or that the benefits of transfer outweigh the foreseeable risks. The staff of the referring hospital should consult with the receiving hospital as soon as the need for transport of a woman or her neonate is considered.

Transportation of patients to an alternate receiving center solely because of third-party payer issues (eg, conflicts between managed care plans and referring and receiving hospital affiliations) should be strongly discouraged and may even be illegal in certain situations. All transfers should be based on medical need.

If the patient to be transferred is a neonate, the family should be given an opportunity to see and touch the neonate beforehand. A transport team member should meet with the family to explain what the team will be doing en route to the receiving hospital. The patient, personnel, and all equipment should be safely secured inside the transport vehicle.

PATIENT CARE AND INTERACTIONS

Where appropriate, the following important components of patient care during transport should be implemented:

- Patients should be observed continuously.
- Vital signs should be monitored and recorded.
- Ventilator pressures and inspired oxygen percentages should be monitored.
- Uterine activity of maternal patients and fetal heart rates should be monitored.
- Neonatal patients should be kept in a neutral thermal environment and should receive appropriate respiratory support and additional monitoring, such as assessment of blood gases, oxygen saturation, and blood glucose, as clinically indicated.
- Intravenous fluids and medications should be given, monitored, and recorded as required.
- The team should be prepared to perform lifesaving invasive procedures, such as placement of a chest tube and intubation, on neonatal patients.

On arrival at the receiving hospital, the following activities are recommended:

- The receiving staff should be prepared to address any unresolved problems or emergencies involving the transported patient.
- The transport team should report the patient's history and clinical status to the receiving staff.
- The receiving staff should inform the patient's family, as well as the referring physician and staff at the referring hospital, of the condition of the patient on arrival to the receiving hospital and periodically thereafter.
- On completion of the patient transfer, the transport team or other designated personnel should immediately restock and reequip the transport vehicle in anticipation of another call.

RETURN TRANSPORT

Patients whose condition has stabilized and who no longer require specialized services should be considered for return transport. Transporting the patient back to the referring hospital:

- Allows the family to return to their home, often permitting more frequent interactions between the family and the patient
- Involves the providers who will ultimately be responsible for the continuing care of the patient earlier in the care process
- Preserves specialized services for patients who require them and allows for a better distribution of resources
- Enhances the integrity of the regionalized care system and emphasizes the partnership between the hospitals in the system

Economic barriers, including those imposed by managed care organizations, which restrict or raise barriers to this movement of patients are detriments to optimal patient care. Every effort should be made to eliminate these artificial constraints.

Transfer is best accomplished after detailed communication between physicians and nursing services at both hospitals outlining the patient's care requirements and the anticipated course of the patient to ensure that the hospital receiving the return transport can provide the needed services. These services must not only be available, but they must be provided in a consistent fashion and be of the same quality as those that the patient is receiving in the regional center. Further, if special equipment or treatment is required at the hospital receiving the patient, arrangements for these should be made before the patient is transferred. Lastly, there also must be an understanding that if problems arise that cannot be cared for in an appropriate manner at the receiving hospital, the patient will be returned to the regional center or the regional center will participate in developing an alternative care plan.

It is important that parents consent to the return transfer of the newborn and understand the benefits to them and their neonate. Their comfort with this process will be enhanced if they realize that the regional center and the referring hospital are working together in a regionalized system of care, that there is frequent communication between the staffs of the two hospitals, that there will be continuing support after the return transport, and that the patient will be returned to the regional center if necessary. It also may be helpful if parents visit the facility to which the neonate will be transported before transfer.

A comprehensive plan for follow-up of the patient after return transfer and after discharge from the hospital should be developed. This plan should outline the required services and identify the party bearing the responsibility for follow-up.

To ensure optimal care during a return transfer, the following guidelines are recommended:

- The patient's (or parents') informed consent for return transfer should be obtained.

- Return transfer should be accomplished via an adequately equipped vehicle with trained personnel so that the level of care received by the patient remains the same during transport.

- Staffing at both hospitals should be adequate to ensure a safe transition of care.

- The family should be notified of the transfer so that they may be present at the accepting facility when transfer occurs.

- Appropriate records, including a summary of the hospital course, diagnosis, treatments, recommendations for ongoing care, and follow-up should accompany the patient.

- The transport team should call the referring hospital and the neonate's parents to inform them of the completion of the transport and to report the neonate's condition.

- The center that provided the higher level of care should provide easily accessible consultation on current or new problems to professional staff at the return transfer facility.

Outreach Education

Critical to the appropriate use of a regional referral program is a program to educate the public and users about its capabilities. The receiving center and receiving hospitals should participate in efforts to educate the public about the kinds of services available and their accessibility.

Outreach education should reinforce cooperation between all individuals involved in the interhospital care of perinatal patients. Receiving hospitals should provide all referring hospitals with information about their response times and clinical capabilities and should ensure that providers know about the specialized resources that are available through the perinatal care network. Primary physicians should be informed as changes occur in indications for consultation and referral of high-risk perinatal patients and for the stabilization of their conditions. Each receiving hospital also should provide continuing education and information to referring physicians about current treatment modalities for high-risk situations. Effective outreach programs will improve the care capabilities of referring hospitals and may allow for some patients to either be retained, or if transferred, to be return transferred earlier in their course.

Program Evaluation

Ideally, the director of a regional program should coordinate program evaluation based on patient outcome data and logistic information. Program monitoring should include the following information:

- Unexpected neonatal morbidity (eg, hypothermia or tension pneumothorax) or mortality during transport
- Morbidity or mortality of patients at the receiving hospital
- Frequency of failure to transfer patients generally considered to require tertiary care (eg, newborns born at <32 weeks of gestation)
- Availability of all the services that may be needed by the perinatal patient
- Accessibility of services, capability to connect the patient quickly and appropriately with the services needed, and programs to promote patient and community awareness of available and appropriate regional referral programs

These data should be tracked as part of the transport team's and the receiving hospital's ongoing quality improvement programs.

Bibliography

American Academy of Pediatrics, Task Force on Interhospital Transport. Guidelines for air and ground transport of neonatal and pediatric patients. 2nd ed. Elk Grove Village (IL): AAP; 1999.

American College of Obstetricians and Gynecologists. Guidelines for women's health care. 2nd ed. Washington, DC: ACOG; 2002.

Guidelines for the transfer of critically ill patients. Guidelines Committee of the American College of Critical Care Medicine; Society of Critical Care Medicine and American Association of Critical-Care Nurses Transfer Guidelines Task Force. Crit Care Med 1993;21:931–7.

March of Dimes Birth Defects Foundation, Committee on Perinatal Health. Toward improving the outcome of pregnancy: the 90s and beyond. White Plains (NY): MDBDF; 1993.

CHAPTER 4

Antepartum Care

A comprehensive antepartum care program involves a coordinated approach to medical care and psychosocial support that optimally begins before conception and extends throughout the antepartum period. Health care professionals should integrate the concept of family-centered care into antepartum care (see "Family-Centered Care" in Chapter 1). Care should include an assessment of the parents' attitudes toward the pregnancy, the support systems available, and the need for parenting education. Couples should be encouraged to participate in developing a birthing plan and in making well-informed decisions about pregnancy, labor, delivery, and the postpartum period.

Preconceptional Care

Preconceptional care consists of the identification of those conditions that could affect a future pregnancy or fetus and that may be amenable to intervention. For example, adverse effects on the fetus, including spontaneous abortion or congenital anomalies caused by maternal phenylketonuria or poorly controlled diabetes mellitus, can be reduced if strict metabolic control is achieved before conception and continued throughout pregnancy. Conversely, establishing metabolic control of these conditions later in pregnancy is believed to be of lesser benefit. Alternatively, prenatal diagnosis of fetal genetic abnormalities can provide parents with options regarding the continuation of the pregnancy and permit targeted prenatal and neonatal care to optimize outcomes.

All health encounters during a woman's reproductive years, particularly those that are a part of preconceptional care should include counseling on appropriate medical care and behavior to optimize pregnancy outcomes. The following maternal assessments may serve as the basis for such counseling:

- Family planning and pregnancy spacing
- Family history
- Genetic history (both maternal and paternal)
- Medical, surgical, pulmonary, and neurologic history
- Current medications (prescription and nonprescription)
- Substance use, including alcohol, tobacco, and illicit drugs
- Domestic abuse and violence
- Nutrition
- Environmental and occupational exposures
- Immunity and immunization status
- Risk factors for sexually transmitted diseases
- Obstetric history
- Gynecologic history
- General physical examination
- Assessment of socioeconomic, educational, and cultural context

Vaccination(s) should be offered to women found to be at risk for or susceptible to rubella, varicella, and hepatitis B. Screening for human immunodeficiency virus (HIV) infection should be strongly recommended (see Chapter 9 for further discussion of viral infections). A number of tests can be performed for specific indications:

- Screening for sexually transmitted diseases
- Testing to assess proven etiologies of recurrent pregnancy loss
- Testing for maternal diseases based on medical or reproductive history
- Mantoux skin test with purified protein derivative for tuberculosis
- Screening for genetic disorders based on racial and ethnic background:
  — Sickle hemoglobinopathies (African Americans)

— β-thalassemia (Mediterraneans, Southeast Asians, and African Americans)

— α-thalassemia (African Americans and Asians, especially from Thailand)

— Tay–Sachs disease (Ashkenazi Jews, French Canadians, and Cajuns)

— Gaucher's, Canavan, and Niemann-Pick disease (Ashkenazi Jews)

— Cystic fibrosis (CF) (Caucasians of European and Ashkenazi Jewish Descent)

• Screening for other genetic disorders on the basis of family history (eg, CF, fragile X syndrome for family history of nonspecific, predominantly male-affected, mental retardation; Duchenne muscular dystrophy)

Patients should be counseled regarding the benefits of the following activities:

• Exercising

• Reducing weight before pregnancy, if obese

• Increasing weight before pregnancy, if underweight

• Avoiding food faddism

• Preventing HIV infection

• Determining the time of conception by an accurate menstrual history

• Abstaining from tobacco, alcohol, and illicit drug use before and during pregnancy

• Consuming folic acid, 0.4 mg per day, while attempting pregnancy and during the first trimester of pregnancy for prevention of neural tube defects (NTDs); women who have had a prior NTD-affected pregnancy are at high risk of having a subsequent affected pregnancy (see "Preconceptional Nutritional Counseling" as follows)

• Maintaining good control of any preexisting medical conditions (eg, diabetes, hypertension, systemic lupus erythematosus, asthma, seizures, thyroid disorders, and inflammatory bowel disease)

Preconceptional Nutritional Counseling

Consumption of a balanced diet with the appropriate distribution of the basic food pyramid groups is especially important during pregnancy. Diet can be affected by food preferences, cultural beliefs, and eating patterns. A woman who is a complete vegan or food faddist or who has special dietary restrictions secondary to medical illnesses, such as phenylketonuria, diabetes mellitus, inflammatory bowel disease, or renal disease, may require special dietary measures as well as vitamin and mineral supplements. Women who frequently diet to lose weight, fast, skip meals, have eating disorders or unusual eating habits should be identified and counseled. The patient's access to food and the ability to purchase food can be pertinent. One way to evaluate nutritional status is to calculate the woman's body mass index at the preconceptional visit (Table 4-1). Additional risk factors for nutritional problems include adolescence, tobacco and substance abuse, history of pica during a previous pregnancy, high parity, and mental illness.

Neural tube defects, such as anencephaly and spina bifida, have multifactorial origins but their etiology often may involve abnormalities in homocysteine metabolism that are potentially remediable by folic acid dietary supplementation. Indeed, the first occurrence of NTDs may be reduced if women of reproductive age take 0.4 mg of folic acid daily both

Table 4–1. Recommended Ranges of Total Weight Gain for Pregnant Women by Prepregnancy Body Mass Index for Singleton Gestation*

Weight-for-Height Category		Recommended Total Weight Gain	
Category	Body Mass Index	kg	lb
Low	<19.8	12.5–18	28–40
Normal	19.8–26	11.5–16	25–35
High	26–29	7–11.5	15–25
Obese	>29	≥7	≥15

*The range for women carrying twins is 35 to 45 lb (16 to 20 kg). Young adolescents (<2 years after menarche) and African-American women should strive for gains at the upper end of the range. Short women (<62 in. or <157 cm) should strive for gains at the lower end of the range.

Reprinted and adapted with permission from Nutrition during pregnancy and lactation, an implementation guide. Copyright 1992 by the National Academy of Sciences. Courtesy of the National Academy Press, Washington, DC.

before conception and during the first trimester of pregnancy as recommended by the Centers for Disease Control and Prevention. A woman with a history of a prior NTD-affected pregnancy can reduce the 3% recurrence risk of NTDs by more than 70% if she supplements her daily diet with 4 mg of folic acid for the month before conception and for the first trimester of pregnancy. This dose should be consumed as a separate supplement, not as multiple multivitamin tablets, to avoid excessive intake of fat-soluble vitamins (see "Vitamin and Mineral Toxicity" in this chapter). The U.S. Food and Drug Administration has established rules under which specified grain products are required to be fortified with folic acid at levels ranging from 0.43–1.4 mg per pound of product. These amounts are designed to enable women to more easily consume 0.4 mg of folic acid daily. However, these amounts of fortified folic acid are intended to keep the daily intake of folic acid less than 1 mg. Because the amount of folic acid consumed in fortified grain products may be less than the amount recommended to prevent NTDs, supplementation is still recommended.

Routine Antepartum Care

Women who receive early and regular prenatal care are more likely to have healthier infants. The early diagnosis of pregnancy is important in establishing a management plan. This plan of care should take into consideration the medical, nutritional, psychosocial, and educational needs of the patient and her family, and it should be periodically reevaluated and revised in accordance with the progress of the pregnancy.

All pregnant women should have access in their community to readily available and regularly scheduled obstetric care, beginning in early pregnancy and continuing through the postpartum period. Pregnant women also should have access to unscheduled or emergency visits on a 24-hour basis. Timing of access varies dependent on the nature of the problem.

WOMEN WITH PHYSICAL DISABILITIES

Pregnancy and parenting for women with physical disabilities may have some unique medical and social aspects but are rarely precluded by the disability itself. Few, if any, physical disabilities directly limit fertility.

Health care professionals have the responsibility to provide appropriate reproductive health services to these women or arrange adequate consultation or referral. Nonbiased preconceptional counseling for couples in which one partner has a physical disability may decrease subsequent psychosocial and medical complications of pregnancy. Screening and provision of disability-specific information, such as folate supplementation for women who have spina bifida, is highly desirable.

Once pregnancy occurs, the patient should have early contact with an obstetrician. Counseling about prenatal testing and options should be comprehensive and nondirective. Regular consultation or referral may be required to achieve the optimum outcome, such as in cases of spinal cord injury or multiple sclerosis. Detailed pregnancy care plans should be developed in negotiation with managed care and other insurers to increase access to and use of prenatal care services, assure appropriate postpartum hospital length of stay, and arrange postpartum home care services, if necessary. Cesarean delivery should be done only for obstetric indications. Community resources for childbirth, breastfeeding, and parenting education should be identified early in the pregnancy, and timely referrals should be made for the pregnant woman and her family.

General Patient Education

Patient education is an essential element of prenatal care. The physician or other providers participating in antepartum care should discuss the following information with each patient:

- Scope of care that is provided in the office (see Appendix H)
- Laboratory studies that may be performed
- Expected course of the pregnancy
- Signs and symptoms to be reported to the physician (eg, vaginal bleeding, rupture of membranes, or decreased fetal movements)
- Anticipated schedule of visits
- Physician coverage of labor and delivery
- Cost to the patient of prenatal care and delivery (eg, insurance plan participation)

- Practices to promote health maintenance (eg, use of safety restraints, including lap and shoulder belts)
- Educational programs available
- Options for intrapartum care
- Planning for hospital discharge and child care
- Encouraging breastfeeding (see Chapter 7)
- Choosing the child's physician

SAUNA AND HOT TUB EXPOSURE

There is extensive animal data to indicate that hyperthermia induced during organogenesis is teratogenic. The major malformations most commonly thought to result from human maternal febrile illnesses are NTDs. Many early studies were troubled with methodologic problems of recall bias and most could not distinguish etiologically between the fever and the infectious agent that caused it or the medications that were used to treat it. Some prospective studies now suggest that it is the fever per se that is teratogenic. Studies in the late 1970s suggested that sauna and hot tub use also might cause hyperthermia and congenital malformations. The probability of significantly increasing core body temperature depends on the temperature of the sauna or hot tub, duration of exposure, and for hot tubs, the extent of submersion. Many women will not voluntarily remain in a hyperthermic environment long enough to increase their core temperatures, but some may. Pregnant women might reasonably be advised to remain in saunas for no more than 15 minutes and hot tubs for no more than 10 minutes. As an additional precaution, there is less surface area to absorb heat and more surface area to radiate it if the head, arms, shoulders and upper chest are not submerged in a hot tub.

SPECIALIZED COUNSELING

Nutrition in Pregnancy

Each pregnant woman should be provided with information about balanced nutrition, as well as ideal caloric intake and weight gain. Maternal nutrition can contribute positively to maintaining or improving the woman's health as well as to the delivery of a healthy term newborn of an appropriate weight. Nutrition counseling is an integral part of perinatal care for all patients. It should focus on a well-balanced, varied nutritional food plan that is consistent with the patient's access to food and food preferences. Patient educational materials on nutrition are available from the American College of Obstetricians and Gynecologists (ACOG) (www.acog.org), the U.S. Public Health Service (www.os. dhhs.gov/phs), and the March of Dimes Birth Defects Foundation (www.modimes.org). Dietary counseling and intervention based on special or individual needs usually are most effectively accomplished by referral to a nutritionist or registered dietitian. Each subspecialty care center should have counseling programs available for the wide range of nutritional disorders that can be encountered by practitioners.

The recommended dietary allowances for most vitamins and minerals increase during pregnancy (see Table 4–2).The National Academy of Sciences recommends 27 mg of ferrous iron supplementation (present in most prenatal vitamins) be given to pregnant women daily because the iron content of the standard American diet and the endogenous iron stores of many American women are not sufficient to provide for the increased iron requirements of pregnancy. The treatment of frank iron-deficiency anemia requires dosages of 60–120 mg of elemental iron each day. Iron absorption is facilitated by or with vitamin C supplement or ingestion between meals or at bedtime on an empty stomach. See Table 4–3 for examples of vitamin and mineral food sources. Women should supplement their diets with folic acid before and during pregnancy (see "Preconceptional Nutritional Counseling" in this chapter). Women should be cautioned to keep these supplements and any other medications out of the reach of children.

Women also should be instructed about appropriate weight gain. The Institute of Medicine (IOM) suggests that a weight gain of 25–35 lb is appropriate for the average weight woman. In contrast, the guidelines for significantly overweight women have not been well established, although the IOM also suggests that weight gains of 15–25 lb in these patients also are associated with optimal pregnancy outcomes. The IOM

Table 4–2. Recommended Daily Dietary Allowances for Adolescent and Adult Pregnant and Lactating Women

	Pregnant			Lactating		
	14–18 years	**19–30 years**	**31–50 years**	**14–18 years**	**19–30 years**	**31–50 years**
Fat-soluble vitamins						
Vitamin A	750 µg	770 µg	770 µg	1,200 µg	1,300 µg	1,300 µg
Vitamin D*	5 µg	5 µg	5 µg	5 µg	5 µg	5 µg
Vitamin E	15 mg	15 mg	15 mg	19 mg	19 mg	19 mg
Vitamin K	75 µg	90 µg	90 µg	75 µg	90 µg	90 µg
Water-soluble vitamins						
Vitamin C	80 mg	85 mg	85 mg	115 mg	120 mg	120 mg
Thiamin	1.4 mg	1.4 mg	1.4 mg	1.4 mg	1.4 mg	1.4 mg
Riboflavin	1.4 mg	1.4 mg	1.4 mg	1.6 mg	1.6 mg	1.6 mg
Niacin	18 mg	18 mg	18 mg	17 mg	17 mg	17 mg
Vitamin B_6	1.9 mg	1.9 mg	1.9 mg	2 mg	2 mg	2 mg
Folate	600 µg	600 µg	600 µg	500 µg	500 µg	500 µg
Vitamin B_{12}	2.6 µg	2.6 µg	2.6 µg	2.8 µg	2.8 µg	2.8 µg
Minerals						
Calcium*	1,300 mg	1,000 mg	1,000 mg	1,300 mg	1,000 mg	1,000 mg
Phosphorus	1,240 mg	700 mg	700 mg	1,250 mg	700 mg	700 mg
Iron	27 mg	27 mg	27 mg	10 mg	9 mg	9 mg
Zinc	13 mg	11 mg	11 mg	14 mg	12 mg	12 mg
Iodine	220 µg	220 µg	220 µg	290 µg	290 µg	290 µg
Selenium	60 µg	60 µg	60 µg	70 µg	70 µg	70 µg

*Recommendations measured as Adequate Intake (AI) instead of Recommended Daily Dietary Allowance (RDA). An AI is set instead of an RDA if insufficient evidence is available to determine an RDA. The AI is based on observed or experimentally determined estimates of average nutrient intake by a group (or groups) of healthy people.

Data from Institute of Medicine. Dietary reference intakes for calcium, phosphorus, magnesium, vitamin D, and fluoride. Washington, DC: National Academy Press; 1997. Institute of Medicine (US). Dietary reference intakes for thiamin, riboflavin, niacin, vitamin B6, folate, vitamin B12, pantothenic acid, biotin, and choline. Washington, DC: National Academy Press; 1998. Institute of Medicine (US). Dietary reference intakes for vitamin C, vitamin E, selenium, and carotenoids. Washington, DC: National Academy Press; 2000. Institute of Medicine (US). Dietary reference intakes for vitamin A, vitamin K, arsenic, boron, chromium, copper, iodine, iron, manganese, molybdenum, nickel, silicon, vanadium, and zinc. Washington, DC: National Academy Press; 2002.

Table 4–3. Vitamin and Mineral Food Sources

Nutrient	Food Source
Vitamin A	Green leafy vegetables; dark yellow vegetables (eg, carrots and sweet potatoes); whole, fortified skim and low-fat milks; liver
Vitamin C	Citrus fruits (eg, oranges, lemons, grapefruit), strawberries, broccoli, tomatoes
Vitamin D	Fortified milk, fish liver oils, exposure to sunlight
Vitamin E	Vegetable oils, whole-grain cereals, wheat germ, green leafy vegetables
Folate	Green leafy vegetables, orange juice, strawberries, liver, legumes, nuts
Calcium	Milk and milk products; sardines and salmon with bones; collard, kale, mustard, and turnip greens
Iron	Meat, liver, dried beans and peas, iron-fortified cereals, prune juice

suggests that for underweight women, a weight gain of 28–40 lb is appropriate. In general, caloric intake is calculated at 25–35 kcal/kg of optimal body weight. An additional 100–300 kcal per day is recommended during pregnancy. Because optimal outcome can occur over a relatively wide range of weight gain, the provider can be flexible. These recommendations can be adjusted to specific subgroups of patients, such as adolescents and women who are obese, of lower socioeconomic status, or short. Following the IOM weight gain guidelines for singleton gestations improves the likelihood of delivering a normal-weight newborn (Table 4–1). Assessment of weight gain during pregnancy is important and should be documented appropriately, preferably on a form specifically designed for that purpose. If a patient is economically unable to meet nutritional needs, she should be referred to federal food and nutrition programs, such as the Special Supplemental Food Program for Women, Infants, and Children.

Vitamin and Mineral Toxicity

Although vitamin A is essential, excessive vitamin A (>10,000 IU per day) may be associated with fetal malformations. The amount of vitamin A in standard prenatal vitamins (4,000–5,000 IU) is well below this toxic level. The use of beta carotene, the precursor of vitamin A found in fruits and vegetables, has not been shown to produce vitamin A toxicity.

Dietary intake of vitamin A in the United States appears to be adequate to meet the needs of most pregnant women throughout gestation. Therefore, routine supplementation during pregnancy is not recommended. In cases in which the dietary intake of vitamin A may not be adequate (for example, in strict vegetarians), dietary intake should be supplemented. Supplementation with 5,000 IU of vitamin A per day should be considered the maximum intake before and during pregnancy. This is well below the probable minimum human teratogenic dose. Prenatal multivitamins in common use contain 5,000 IU or less of vitamin A, but vitamin tablets containing 25,000 IU or more of vitamin A are available as over-the-counter preparations. Pregnant women or those planning to become pregnant who use high doses of vitamin A supplements (and retinol) should be cautioned about the potential teratogenicity.

Excessive vitamin and mineral intake (ie, more than twice the recommended dietary allowances) should be avoided during pregnancy. For example, excess iodine is associated with congenital goiter, and excess vitamin A is associated with anomalies of bones, the urinary tract, and the central nervous system. There also may be toxicity of other fat-soluble vitamins (D, E, and K).

Exercise in Pregnancy

In the absence of either medical or obstetric complications, 30 minutes or more of moderate exercise per day on most if not all days of the week is recommended for pregnant women. Generally, participation in a wide range of recreational activities appears to be safe during pregnancy; however, each sport should be reviewed individually for its potential risk, and activities with a high risk of falling or those with a high risk for abdominal trauma should be avoided. Pregnant women should avoid supine positions during exercise as much as possible.

Recreational and competitive athletes with uncomplicated pregnancies can remain active during pregnancy and should modify their usual exercise routines as medically indicated. The pregnant, competitive athlete may require close obstetric supervision. Women should not take up a new, strenuous sport during pregnancy, and previously inactive women and those with medical or obstetric complications should be evaluated before recommendations for physical activity participation during pregnancy are made. Additionally, a physically active woman with a history of or risk for preterm labor or fetal growth restriction should be advised to reduce her activity in the second and third trimesters. Warning signs to terminate exercise while pregnant include:

- Chest pain
- Vaginal bleeding
- Dizziness
- Headache
- Decreased fetal movement
- Amniotic fluid leakage
- Muscle weakness
- Calf pain or swelling
- Preterm labor
- Regular uterine contractions

Tobacco Use

Inquiry into tobacco use and smoke exposure should be a routine part of the prenatal visit. Patients should be strongly discouraged from smoking. Multiple studies have demonstrated a clear association between maternal smoking and perinatal morbidity and mortality. Placenta previa, abruptio placentae, and preterm rupture of membranes are factors in many pregnancy losses in smokers. It is estimated that there would be a 10% reduction in perinatal mortality and an 11% reduction in the incidence of low birth weight if smoking during pregnancy were eliminated. Infant health risks include sudden infant death syndrome, hospitalization, and neurodevelopmental abnormalities. For pregnant women who smoke fewer than 20 cigarettes per day, the provision of a 5–15-minute five-step counseling session and pregnancy-specific educational materials increases cessation by 30–70%. Physicians should refer to the following smoking cessation guidelines:

- Ask all patients about smoking status and document the response in the medical record to remind providers to ask patients about smoking status at follow-up visits.

- Advise patients who smoke to stop.
- Assess the willingness of the patient to attempt to quit within 30 days.
- Assist patients who are interested in quitting by providing pregnancy-specific, self-help smoking cessation materials.
- Arrange during regular follow-up visits to track the progress of the patient's attempt to quit smoking.

Although nicotine replacement products or other pharmaceuticals as smoking cessation aids are effective for reducing smoking in nonpregnant women, they have not been sufficiently evaluated to determine their effectiveness and safety in pregnancy. Nicotine gum and patches should be considered in pregnant women only after nonpharmacologic treatments (eg, counseling) have failed, and if the increased likelihood of smoking cessation, with its potential benefits, outweighs the unknown risk of nicotine replacement and potential concomitant smoking.

Substance Use and Abuse

All pregnant women should be questioned at their first prenatal visit about their past and present use of alcohol, nicotine, and other drugs. Use of specific screening questionnaires may improve detection rates. A woman who acknowledges the use of alcohol, nicotine, cocaine, or other mood-altering drugs should be counseled about the perinatal implications of their use during pregnancy and offered referral to an appropriate drug-treatment program if chemical dependence is suspected. Large numbers of women of childbearing age abuse potentially addictive and mood-altering drugs. Use of cocaine, marijuana, diazepam, other prescription drugs, and approximately 150 other substances can lead to chemical dependency. Depending on geographic location, it is estimated that 1–40% of pregnant women have used one of these substances during pregnancy. Data suggest that approximately 1 in 10 neonates is exposed to one or more mood-altering drugs during pregnancy; the number varies only slightly for publicly versus privately insured patients.

Women should be dissuaded from alcohol consumption during pregnancy because there is no known safe amount. Patients should be informed that prenatal alcohol abuse is a preventable cause of birth defects, including mental retardation and neurodevelopmental deficits. Fetal alcohol syndrome is characterized by three findings: 1) growth restriction, 2) facial abnormalities, and 3) central nervous system dysfunction. Although fetal alcohol syndrome is more prevalent among chronic alcoholics (prevalence 6–50%), it has been reported with lesser amounts of alcohol use.

Chemical dependency is likely to be a chronic, relapsing, and progressive disease. Many drug-dependent pregnant women do not seek early prenatal care and therefore are at increased risk for medical and obstetric complications. Drug-exposed neonates often go unrecognized and are discharged from the newborn nursery to homes where they are at increased risk for a complex of medical and social problems, including abuse and neglect.

To reinforce and encourage continued abstinence, periodic questioning or drug or metabolite testing may be desirable for a pregnant woman who reports substance use before or during pregnancy. Testing of the mother or the neonate or both also may be useful in some clinical situations, even when substance use has not been suspected previously. Such circumstances include the presence of unexplained intrauterine growth restriction, third-trimester stillbirth, unexpected preterm birth, or abruptio placentae in a woman not known to have hypertensive disease. Because positive test results have implications for patients that transcend their health, patients should give informed consent before testing. The requirements for consent to test vary from state to state, and practitioners should be familiar with the testing and the reporting requirements in their states.

Warning signs of drug abuse include noncompliance with prenatal care (eg, late entry to care, multiple missed appointments, or no prenatal care), evidence of poor nutrition, encounters with law enforcement, and marital and family disputes during the pregnancy. Screening of all patients at delivery is not recommended. Screens are likely to be negative when drugs were used early in pregnancy, and a urine screen can be negative even when women have taken some drugs during the 48 hours before delivery. Toxicologic analysis of hair and meconium have been reported to be more sensitive methods of identifying illicit drug use, although urine remains the most frequently used specimen for screening. Because the components of urine toxicology screens vary among laboratories, physicians should verify with their laboratory which metabolites are included in its screen.

To identify drug-exposed neonates, the child's physician should obtain a thorough maternal history from all pregnant women in a nonthreatening, organized manner. Practitioners also should be aware that laws in some states consider in utero drug exposure to be a form of child abuse or neglect and require reporting of positive drug tests in pregnant women or their newborns to the state's child protection agency. Finally, patients also should be advised to consult with their health care providers before using nonprescription drugs or herbal remedies.

Domestic Violence

Risk assessment during pregnancy should universally include identification of women who are victims of domestic violence. Domestic violence, also known as intimate partner violence, has been identified as a significant public health problem affecting millions of American women each year. There is no single profile of an abused woman. Victims come from all racial, economic, educational, religious, ethnic, and social backgrounds. Victims are both adolescents and adults.

Research indicates that the majority of abused women continue to be victimized during pregnancy. Violence against women also may begin or escalate during pregnancy and affects both maternal and fetal wellbeing. The prevalence of violence during pregnancy ranges from 1% to 20% with most studies identifying rates between 4% and 8%. The presence of violence between intimate partners also affects the children in the household. Studies demonstrate that child abuse occurs in 33–77% of families in which there is abuse of adults. Among women who are being abused, 27% have demonstrated abusive behavior toward their children while living in the violent environment.

Abuse may involve threatened and/or actual physical, sexual, verbal, or psychologic abuse. The fundamental issues at play are power, control, and coercion. There is no clearly established set of symptoms that signal abuse. However, listed as follows are some of the obstetric presentations of abused women:

- Unwanted pregnancy
- Late entry into prenatal care, missed appointments
- Substance abuse or use
- Poor weight gain and nutrition
- Multiple, repeated somatic complaints

With the possible exception of preeclampsia, domestic violence is more prevalent than any major medical condition detected through routine prenatal screening. Detection may be possible by discussing with the patient that pregnancy sometimes places increased stress on a relationship and then by asking how the woman and her partner resolve their differences. In many cases, however, women will not disclose their abuse unless asked directly. Abused women usually are forthright when asked directly in a caring, nonjudgmental manner. The likelihood of disclosure increases with successive inquiries.

Screening should be conducted in private with only the patient present. Translation services may be helpful in inquiring about these issues. Screening can be accomplished by prefacing the following questions with the simple statement that "because violence against women is so common, I ask all of my patients the following questions:"

- Within the past year, have you been threatened or actually hit, slapped, kicked, or otherwise physically hurt by anyone?
- Since you have been pregnant, have you been threatened or actually hit, slapped, kicked, or otherwise physically injured by anyone?
- Within the past year, has anyone forced you into sexual relations when you were not willing?

If a patient confides that she is being abused, verbatim accounts of the abuse should be recorded in the patient's medical record. The clinician should inquire about her immediate safety and the safety of her children. Clinicians should become familiar with local resources, and referrals to appropriate counseling, legal, and social service advocacy programs should be made. Additionally, physicians should be familiar with state laws that may require reporting of domestic violence. In any case, child abuse is always reportable. When the clinician suspects abuse, whether or not it is corroborated by the woman, supportive statements should be offered, and the need for follow-up should be addressed. It is important to encourage abused women, with the assistance of social services, to begin to create an "escape" plan, with a reliable safe haven for retreat, particularly if they believe the violence is escalating.

ANTEPARTUM SURVEILLANCE

Antepartum surveillance begins with the first prenatal visit, at which time the physician or nurse begins to compile an obstetric database. Appendix A contains a format for documenting information and the database recommended by ACOG.

The frequency of follow-up visits is determined by the individual needs of the woman and an assessment of her risks. The frequency and regularity of scheduled prenatal visits should be sufficient to enable providers to accomplish the following activities:

- Monitor the progression of the pregnancy
- Provide education and recommended screening and interventions
- Reassure the woman
- Assess the well-being of the woman and her fetus
- Detect medical and psychosocial complications and institute indicated interventions

Generally, a woman with an uncomplicated pregnancy is examined every 4 weeks for the first 28 weeks of pregnancy, every 2–3 weeks until 36 weeks of gestation, and weekly thereafter. Women with medical or obstetric problems, as well as younger adolescents, may require closer surveillance; the appropriate intervals between scheduled visits are determined by the nature and severity of the problems (see Appendix H).

During each regularly scheduled visit, the health care provider should evaluate the woman's blood pressure, weight, urine for the presence of protein and glucose levels, uterine size for progressive growth and consistency with the estimated date of delivery, and fetal heart rate. After the patient reports quickening and at each subsequent visit, she should be asked about fetal movement, contractions, leakage of fluid, or vaginal bleeding.

Estimated Date of Delivery

Management of pregnancy requires establishing an estimated date of delivery. Problems such as intrauterine growth restriction, preterm labor, and postterm pregnancy are managed most effectively when an accurate estimated date of delivery is known. In addition, accurate gestational dating is important for the application and interpretation of certain antepartum tests (eg, maternal serum screening for trisomy 21 and NTDs or assessment of fetal maturity). If there is a size-date discrepancy or if menstrual dates are uncertain, an ultrasound examination is indicated for the purpose of dating. Such an examination is most accurate when performed before 20 weeks of gestation. Ultrasound is considered to be consistent with menstrual dates if there is gestational age agreement to within 1 week by crown–rump measurement obtained at 6–11 weeks, or within 10 days by the average of multiple biometric measurements obtained at 12–20 weeks.

Routine Testing

Certain laboratory tests should be performed routinely in pregnant women. The following tests are performed early in pregnancy, as appropriate, and the results are made available to the physician responsible for care of the newborn:

- Hematocrit or hemoglobin levels
- Urinalysis, including microscopic examination
- Urine testing to detect asymptomatic bacteriuria (eg, urine culture)
- Determination of blood group and CDE (Rh) type
- Antibody screen
- Determination of immunity to rubella virus
- Syphilis screen
- Cervical cytology (as needed)

- Hepatitis B virus surface antigen
- Human immunodeficiency virus antibody testing

All pregnant women should receive education and counseling about preventing HIV infection as part of their regular prenatal care, as long as it is not a prerequisite for or barrier to prenatal HIV testing. Testing for HIV with notification is recommended for all pregnant women, as permitted by local and state regulations. Refusal of testing should be documented. In some states, it is necessary to obtain the woman's written authorization before disclosing her HIV status to health care providers who are not members of her health care team (see Chapter 9).

For couples planning pregnancy or seeking prenatal care, it is recommended that screening should be offered to those at higher risk of having children with CF (Caucasians, including Ashkenazi Jews) and in whom the testing is most sensitive in identifying carriers of a CF mutation. It is further recommended that screening should be made available to couples in other racial and ethnic groups who are at lower risk and in whom the test may be less sensitive. For those couples to whom screening will be offered, it is recommended that this be done when they seek preconceptional counseling or infertility care, or during the first and early second trimester of pregnancy.

Recommended intervals for additional tests that are indicated after the first prenatal visit are detailed on the ACOG Antepartum Record (see Appendix A). Additional laboratory evaluations, such as testing for sexually transmitted diseases, genetic disorders (see "Preconceptional Care" in this chapter), and tuberculosis, are recommended or offered on the basis of the patient's history and physical examination or in response to public health guidelines. Pregnancy is not a contraindication for Mantoux skin test with purified protein derivative for tuberculosis and may be indicated in high-risk areas or for health care workers. Tests for sexually transmitted diseases may be repeated in the third trimester if the woman has specific risk factors for these diseases. These tests may be mandated by local and state regulations. Early in the third trimester, measurement of hemoglobin or hematocrit levels should be repeated.

Although prenatal ultrasonography is not recommended routinely, specific purposes for its use include assessment of fetal age, growth, and anatomy. In some instances, repeated or planned serial ultrasound examinations may be indicated, such as for women with D (Rh) isoimmunization or other causes of fetal hydrops.

Influenza Vaccination

All women who will be in the second and third trimesters of pregnancy during the influenza season should be offered influenza vaccine. The influenza vaccine is strongly recommended for women at high risk for influenza complications. Pregnant women with medical conditions that increase their risk for complications from influenza should be offered the vaccine before the influenza season, regardless of the stage of pregnancy. Administration of the influenza vaccine is considered safe at any stage of pregnancy.

Ongoing Risk Assessment and Management

Identification of risk factors for poor outcomes is critical to minimize maternal and neonatal morbidity and mortality. Appendixes B and C provide essential data important for early and ongoing risk assessment. Although a correlation can be seen between antenatal risk factors and the development of problems, a significant percentage of intrapartum and neonatal problems occur among patients without identified antenatal risk factors. In many instances, special obstetric problems require a multidisciplinary approach to antepartum care. Some conditions may require the involvement of a maternal–fetal medicine subspecialist, geneticist, pediatrician, neonatologist, anesthesiologist, or other medical specialist in the evaluation, counseling, and care of the patient.

Antibody Testing

Antibody tests can be repeated in an unsensitized, D-negative patient at 26–28 weeks of gestation (see also "Isoimmunization in Pregnancy" in this chapter). She also should receive anti-D immune globulin prophylactically at that time. In addition, any unsensitized, D-negative patient should receive anti-D immune globulin if she has had one of the following conditions or procedures:

- Ectopic gestation
- Abortion (either threatened, spontaneous, or induced)
- Procedure associated with possible fetal-to-maternal bleeding, such as chorionic villus sampling (CVS) or amniocentesis
- Condition associated with fetal–maternal hemorrhage (eg, abdominal trauma, abruptio placentae)
- Delivery of a D-positive newborn

Diabetes Screening

All pregnant patients should be screened for gestational diabetes mellitus (GDM) whether by patient's history, clinical risk factors, or a laboratory screening test to determine blood glucose levels. Although universal glucose challenge screening for GDM is the most sensitive approach, there may be pregnant women at low risk who are less likely to benefit from testing. Such low-risk women should have all of the following characteristics:

- Age younger than 25 years
- Not a member of a racial or ethnic group with a high prevalence of diabetes mellitus (eg, Hispanic, African, Native American, South or East Asian, or Pacific Islands ancestry)
- Body mass index of 25 or less
- No history of abnormal glucose tolerance
- No previous history of adverse pregnancy outcomes usually associated with GDM
- No known diabetes mellitus in first-degree relative

Teratogens

Major birth defects are apparent at birth in 2–3% of the general population, and their possible occurrence is a frequent cause of anxiety among pregnant women. Many patient inquiries concern the teratogenic potential of environmental exposures. Unfortunately, there often is little scientifically valid information on which a risk estimate in human pregnancy can be based. Patients should be counseled that relatively few agents have been identified that are known to cause malformations in exposed pregnancies. Relatively few patients will have been exposed to agents that are known to be associated with increased risk for fetal malformations or mental retardation. The health care provider may wish to consult with or refer such a patient to a health professional with special knowledge or experience in teratology and birth defects.

Many patients raise questions about the methods of detecting birth defects related to drug exposure. Amniocentesis or CVS for chromosome analysis is not helpful for the diagnosis of birth defects caused by teratogens. Although obstetric ultrasonography has been the mainstay of surveillance for teratogen-induced congenital anomalies, its sensitivity varies with the experience and skill of the imager as well as the specific anatomic abnormality. However, even in expert hands the overall sensitivity of ultrasonography in the detection of fetal anatomic anomalies is in the range of 50–70%.

Concerns are frequently expressed over the teratogenic potential of diagnostic imaging modalities used during pregnancy including X-ray, ultrasonography, and magnetic resonance imaging. The imaging modality that causes the most anxiety for both obstetrician and patient is X-ray or ionizing radiation. Much of this anxiety is secondary to a general misperception that any radiation exposure is harmful and may result in injury to or anomaly of the fetus. This anxiety may lead to inappropriate therapeutic abortion. In fact, most diagnostic X-ray procedures are associated with few, if any, risks to the fetus. Moreover, according to the American College of Radiology, no single diagnostic X-ray procedure results in radiation exposure to a degree that would threaten the well-being of a developing preembryo, embryo, or fetus. Therefore, diagnostic X-ray during pregnancy is not an indication for therapeutic abortion.

Some women are exposed to X-rays before pregnancy is diagnosed. Occasionally, X-ray procedures are indicated during pregnancy for significant medical problems or trauma. Concern about radiation exposure during pregnancy should not prevent medically indicated diagnostic X-ray studies when these are important for the care of the woman. When such a study is indicated, the radiologist should be consulted to minimize the extent of exposure of the fetus. There is no contraindication to a diagnostic X-ray that is likely to be beneficial in the diagnosis and treatment of a pregnant woman. Patients concerned about previously performed or planned diagnostic studies should have counseling to allay these concerns.

Ultrasonography and magnetic resonance imaging do not involve radiation exposure. These types of imaging studies are increasingly being used to provide diagnostic information and to avoid the use of X-ray studies. Although the safety of ultrasonography has been established, comparatively few studies have analyzed the teratogenic potential of magnetic resonance imaging in the first trimester.

Most diagnostic studies in which radioisotopes are used are not hazardous to the fetus and incur low levels of radiation exposure. A typical technetium Tc 99m scan results in a fetal dose of less than 0.5 rads, and a thallium 201 scan also results in a small dose. Many of these isotopes are excreted in the urine. Therefore, women should be advised to drink plenty of fluids and to void frequently after a radionuclide study.

One important exception is the use of iodine 131 for the treatment of hyperthyroidism. The fetal thyroid gland begins to incorporate iodine actively by the end of the first trimester. Administration of iodine 131 after this time can result in concentration of the radiation within, and destruction of, the fetal thyroid gland. Iodine 131 is therefore contraindicated for therapeutic use during pregnancy. By comparison, there are few reports on the safety of radioisotope imaging of the maternal thyroid during pregnancy and such studies should be undertaken only after careful consideration of the risks and benefits of the procedure.

Maternal Serum Screening

Women who are younger than 35 years as of the estimated delivery date should be offered multiple marker serum screening to assess the risk of trisomy 21, ideally between 16 and 18 weeks of gestation by menstrual dating. In women aged 35 years or older as of the estimated delivery date, multiple marker testing cannot be recommended as an equivalent alternative to cytogenetic diagnosis for detection of trisomy 21. Women with singleton pregnancies who will be age 35 years or older at delivery should be offered prenatal diagnosis for fetal aneuploidy. Serum screening for NTDs by maternal serum alpha-fetoprotein (MSAFP) testing also should be offered to all pregnant women not undergoing amniocentesis for assessment of amniotic fluid alpha-fetoprotein values, ideally between 16 and 18 weeks of gestation. Samples should be submitted to a clinical laboratory that has a quality improvement program, has normative data specific to each week of gestational age, and provides interpretations and risk assessment that take into account maternal weight, race, diabetic status, and, for trisomy 21 screening, maternal age. The laboratory should be able to confirm that the specific combination of tests and the particular assays performed will yield a detection rate of trisomy 21 of at least 60% and a positive rate of screening of 5% or less after ultrasound correction of gestational age.

Trisomy 21

A screening result that indicates a midtrimester risk of trisomy 21 that is equal to or greater than that of a 35-year-old woman as of the estimated delivery date usually is considered positive. This usually is a 1:270 midtrimester risk for the occurrence of trisomy 21. If ultrasonography does not reveal an error in gestational dating—or diagnose a fetal disorder—amniocentesis should be offered to analyze fetal karyotype.

Neural Tube Defects

The results of MSAFP testing may be used to screen for NTDs. The use of a standard screening cutoff (2.5 multiples of the median) will detect approximately 80% of cases of open spina bifida and 90% of cases of anencephaly. Patients with elevated MSAFP levels are evaluated by ultrasonography to detect identifiable causes of false-positive results (eg, fetal death, multiple gestation, underestimation of gestational age) and for targeted study of fetal anatomy for NTDs and other defects (eg, omphalocele, gastroschisis, cystic hygroma). Amniocentesis may be recommended to confirm the presence of open defects and to obtain a fetal karyotype. Amniocentesis may be offered even when ultrasonography does not reveal an identifiable defect or cause for the elevated MSAFP level.

Prenatal Diagnosis of Genetic Disorders in Patients at Increased Risk

Prenatal genetic diagnosis should be offered in circumstances in which there is a definable increased risk for a fetal genetic disorder that may be diagnosed by one or more methods. Prenatal genetic screening or diagnosis should be voluntary and informed. In most circumstances, test results are normal and provide patients with a high degree of reassurance that a particular disorder does not affect a fetus. Early prenatal genetic diagnosis also affords patients the option to terminate affected pregnancies. Alternatively, a positive diagnosis may allow a patient to prepare for the birth of an affected child and, in some circumstances, may be important in establishing a plan for care during pregnancy, labor, delivery, and the immediate neonatal period.

GENETIC RISK ASSESSMENT AND COUNSELING

Many couples at increased risk for having children with genetic disorders can benefit from genetic counseling (see "Preconceptional Care" in this chapter). An example of current screening criteria is listed in the ACOG Antepartum Record in Appendix A. Health care providers should be aware that many single-gene disorders are discovered each year and may be tracked using Internet databases, such as "Online Mendelian Inheritance in Man" (www.ncbi.nlm.nih.gov/entrez/query.fcqi?db = OMIM).

Sometimes the problem is relatively straightforward. For example, the health care provider can readily explain the well-known relationship between advanced maternal age and autosomal trisomies. The maternal age-adjusted risks for chromosome abnormalities are shown in Table 4-4. In other cases, referral to a geneticist may be necessitated by the complexities of determining risks, evaluating a family history of such abnormalities, interpreting laboratory tests, or providing counseling. Regardless of the indication, counseling is essential before genetic screening or antenatal diagnostic tests are performed.

Prenatal genetic counseling addresses the risk of occurrence of a genetic disorder in a family. In this process, the primary health care provider, a medical geneticist, or other trained professional attempts to help the individual or family:

- Comprehend the medical facts, including the diagnosis, probable course of the disorder, and available management
- Appreciate the way in which heredity contributes to the disorder and the risk of occurrence or recurrence in specific relatives

Table 4–4. Chromosome Abnormalities in Term, Liveborn Neonates*

Maternal Age	Risk of Trisomy 21 at Delivery	Risk of Chromosomal Abnormalities[†]
20	1/1,667	1/526
21	1/1,667	1/526
22	1/1,667	1/526
23	1/1,429	1/500
24	1/1,250	1/476
25	1/1,250	1/476
26	1/1,176	1/476
27	1/1,111	1/455
28	1/1,053	1/435
29	1/1,000	1/417
30	1/952	1/385
31	1/909	1/385
32	1/769	1/322
33	1/602	1/286
34	1/485	1/238
35	1/378	1/192
36	1/289	1/156
37	1/224	1/127
38	1/173	1/102
39	1/136	1/83
40	1/106	1/66
41	1/82	1/53
42	1/63	1/42
43	1/49	1/33
44	1/38	1/26
45	1/30	1/21
46	1/23	1/16
47	1/18	1/13
48	1/14	1/10
49	1/11	1/8

*Because sample sizes for some intervals are relatively small, 95% confidence limits are sometimes relatively large. Nonetheless, these figures are suitable for genetic counseling.

[†]47,XXX excluded for ages 20–32 years (data not available).

Modified from Hook EB, Cross PK, Schreinemachers DM. Chromosomal abnormality rates at amniocentesis and in live-born infants. JAMA 1983;249:2034–2038. Copyrighted 1983, American Medical Association; Hook EB. Rates of chromosome abnormalities at different maternal ages. Obstet Gynecol 1981;58:282–85.

- Understand the options for dealing with the risk of recurrence, including prenatal genetic diagnosis
- Choose the course of action that seems appropriate in view of the risk and the family's goals and act in accordance with that decision
- Make the best possible adjustment to the disorder in an affected family member and to the risk of recurrence in another family member

Therefore, the key elements in genetic counseling are accurate diagnosis, communication, and nondirective presentation of options. The counselor's function is not to dictate a particular course of action but to provide information that will allow couples to make informed decisions.

DIAGNOSTIC TESTING

Amniocentesis

Transabdominal amniocentesis is the technique most commonly used for obtaining fetal cells for genetic studies. This well-established, safe, and reliable procedure usually is performed at approximately 16 weeks of gestation. The cells obtained via amniocentesis can be used for blood typing or cytogenetic, metabolic, or other DNA testing. Alpha-fetoprotein and acetylcholinesterase can be measured in the supernatant fluid to detect open fetal NTDs. Significant maternal injury from amniocentesis is rare, and the estimated risk of spontaneous abortion caused by amniocentesis at 15 weeks of gestation or later is less than 1%. Increased loss rates are associated with more than three needle insertions. Amniocenteses performed at 11–13 weeks of gestation have been associated with relatively high postprocedure loss rates of 2–5%, an increased occurrence of talipes equinovarus (1.4%), and increased cell culture failure rates.

Chorionic Villus Sampling

Chorionic villus sampling is a technique for removing a small sample (5–40 mg) of placental tissue (chorionic villi) for performing chromosomal, metabolic, or DNA studies. It generally is performed between 10 and 12 weeks of gestation, either by a transabdominal or a transcervical approach. Chorionic villi, however, cannot be used for the prenatal diagnosis of NTDs. Therefore, women who have undergone cytogenetic testing by CVS should be offered MSAFP screening for the detection of NTDs. Although CVS offers the advantage of first-trimester prenatal diagnosis, the procedure-related risk of pregnancy loss is approximately 0.5–1% higher than that for amniocentesis. The possibility that CVS performed before 10 weeks of gestation may cause limb reduction defects remains controversial but should be discussed in counseling. Until further information is available, CVS should not be performed before 10 weeks of gestation.

Invasive Diagnostic Testing in Rh D-Negative Women

Because both amniocentesis and CVS can result in fetal-to-maternal bleeding, the administration of anti-D immune globulin is indicated for D-negative, unsensitized women who undergo either of these procedures. Fetal-to-maternal bleeding is more frequent with CVS, and because of the possibility of enhanced sensitization early in gestation, this procedure is not advisable in D-negative women who are already sensitized.

Tests of Fetal Well-Being

The goals of antepartum fetal surveillance include:
- Identifying patients at increased risk for stillbirth
- Reducing the risk of fetal demise after 24 weeks of gestation
- Avoiding unnecessary intervention

Although there have been no randomized clinical trials that clearly demonstrate improved perinatal outcome with the use of antepartum testing, or that determine the optimal time to initiate testing, these tests have become an integral part of clinical care of pregnancies suspected to be at increased risk of fetal demise. Indications for initiating such testing typically include the following conditions:
- Maternal conditions:
  - Antiphospholipid syndrome

— Hyperthyroidism (poorly controlled)
— Hemoglobinopathies (hemoglobin SS, SC, or S-thalassemia)
— Cyanotic heart disease
— Systemic lupus erythematosus
— Chronic renal disease
— Insulin-treated diabetes mellitus
— Hypertensive disorders

- Pregnancy-related conditions:
  — Pregnancy-induced hypertension
  — Decreased fetal movement
  — Oligohydramnios
  — Polyhydramnios
  — Intrauterine growth restriction
  — Postterm pregnancy
  — Isoimmunization (moderate to severe)
  — Previous fetal demise (unexplained or recurrent risk)
  — Multiple gestation (with significant growth discrepancy)

There are several tests used in clinical practice to assess fetal status. Commonly available tests (which are described in more detail in the following section) include:

- Assessment of fetal movement (eg, kick counts)
- Nonstress test (NST)
- Biophysical profile (BPP)
- Modified biophysical profile (NST plus amniotic fluid index)
- Contraction stress test (CST) or oxytocin challenge test (OCT)
- Doppler ultrasound of umbilical artery blood flow velocity

An important consideration in deciding when to begin antepartum testing is the prognosis for neonatal survival if intervention is undertaken for abnormal test results. Initiating testing at 32–34 weeks of gestation is appropriate for most pregnancies at increased risk of stillbirth, although in pregnancies with multiple or particularly worrisome high-risk conditions, testing may be initiated as early as 26–28 weeks of gestation. However, because the potential for iatrogenic harm to pregnancies is highest in preterm gestations, the low specificity of these tests needs to be considered. The implications of a nonreassuring fetal heart rate tracing at these early gestational ages are still unclear.

When the clinical condition that has prompted testing persists, a reassuring test (reactive NST, negative CST, or normal BPP) should be repeated periodically (either weekly or, depending on the test used and the presence of certain high-risk conditions, twice weekly) until delivery to monitor continued fetal well-being. In most clinical situations, a normal test result indicates that intrauterine fetal death is highly unlikely in the next 7 days. The risk of fetal death within 7 days of a reactive NST is approximately 3 per 1,000 fetuses. The risk of fetal death within 7 days of a BPP of 8–10 or a negative OCT or CST is 0.6–0.8 per 1,000 fetuses. In contrast, an abnormal test result or nonreassuring fetal assessment is frequently (50–90%) falsely worrisome and, therefore, should be corroborated whenever possible before potentially harmful interventions are undertaken. In the presence of certain high-risk conditions, such as prolonged pregnancy, insulin-treated diabetes mellitus beyond 36 weeks of gestation, intrauterine growth restriction, or pregnancy-induced hypertension, twice weekly testing may be appropriate.

The sequence of tests to determine fetal well-being may vary by practice and protocol. Each test has advantages and disadvantages, and no single test has been shown to be superior to the others in any specific clinical situation. The NST is the most commonly used screening test for antepartum fetal evaluation. It is easily performed in an outpatient setting with minimal staffing, there are no contraindications to performance of the test, and it can be easily archived for review. The BPP requires a trained ultrasonographer and ultrasonographic equipment. However, unless the study is videotaped, it cannot be reviewed. The BPP does have a lower false positive rate (20%) than NST alone (75–90%), and is supplanting the CST as a supplemental test following a nonreactive NST because of its ease of performance. Regardless of which antepartum surveillance test is used, the results and interpretation should be noted in the patient's medical record.

Assessment of Fetal Movement

A decrease in the maternal perception of fetal movement often but not invariably precedes fetal death, in some cases by several days. This observation provides the rationale for fetal movement assessment by the mother (kick counts) as a means of antepartum fetal surveillance. Whether programs of fetal movement assessment actually can reduce the risk of stillbirth is unclear. Neither the ideal number of kicks nor the ideal duration of daily movement count assessment has been defined. Perhaps more important than any single quantitative guideline is the mother's perception of a decrease in fetal activity in relation to a previous level. One approach to assessing fetal movement is to have the woman count distinct fetal movements on a daily basis after 28 weeks of gestation. The perception of 10 distinct movements in a period of up to 2 hours is considered reassuring. After 10 movements have been perceived, the count can be discontinued for that day. In the absence of a reassuring count, a biophysical means of fetal assessment should be used.

Nonstress Test

For the NST, the fetal heart rate is monitored with an external transducer for at least 20 minutes. The tracing is observed for fetal heart rate accelerations peaking at least 15 beats per minute higher than the baseline and lasting 15 seconds from baseline to baseline. The testing can be continued for an additional 40 minutes or longer to take into account the typical fetal sleep-wake cycle. Because fetal heart rate reactivity is a function of fetal maturity, more than 15% of NSTs performed before 32 weeks of gestation may be nonreactive in the absence of fetal compromise. The results of an NST are considered reactive (reassuring) if two or more fetal heart rate accelerations are detected within a 20-minute period, with or without fetal movement discernible by the mother. A nonreactive tracing is one without sufficient fetal heart rate accelerations in a 40-minute period. Acoustic stimulation (lasting 1 second) of a fetus that elicits fetal heart rate accelerations also is reassuring. The use of such stimulation can safely reduce overall testing time.

Contraction Stress Test

For a CST, the fetal heart rate is obtained using an external transducer, and uterine contraction activity is monitored with a tocodynamometer. A baseline tracing is obtained for 10–20 minutes. If at least three contractions of 40 seconds or more are present in a 10-minute period, uterine stimulation is not necessary. If not, contractions are induced with either nipple stimulation or intravenously administered oxytocin. With nipple stimulation, the patient is instructed to rub one nipple gently through her clothing for 2 minutes or until a contraction begins. Stimulation is then stopped and restarted after 5 minutes if an adequate contraction frequency has not been attained. The cycle is repeated until an adequate contraction pattern is obtained. If the use of oxytocin is preferred by the patient or if nipple stimulation is unsuccessful, an intravenous infusion of low-dose oxytocin can be initiated, usually at a rate of 0.5–1.0 mU/min, and increased every 15–20 minutes until an adequate contraction pattern occurs (ie, three contractions in 10 minutes). The results of the contraction stress test can be categorized as:

- Negative—No late or significant variable decelerations
- Positive—Late decelerations following 50% or more of contractions, even if the frequency of contractions is less than three in 10 minutes
- Equivocal-suspicious—Intermittent late or significant variable decelerations
- Equivocal-hyperstimulatory—Fetal heart rate decelerations that occur in the presence of contractions more frequent than every 2 minutes or lasting longer than 90 seconds
- Unsatisfactory—Fewer than three contractions within 10 minutes or a tracing that cannot be interpreted

Both oxytocin and nipple stimulation can produce hyperstimulation (contractions that occur more frequently than every 2 minutes or exceed 90 seconds in duration). If fetal heart rate decelerations occur in the presence of hyperstimulation, retesting is appropriate to ensure correct interpretation. Relative contraindications to inducing contractions for contraction stress testing generally include the following conditions:

- Preterm labor or certain patients at high risk for preterm delivery
- Preterm rupture of membranes
- Classical uterine incision scar or history of extensive uterine surgery
- Known placenta previa

BIOPHYSICAL PROFILE

Biophysical profile testing consists of an NST with the addition of four observations using real-time ultrasonography. The five components of a reassuring BPP are:

1. Nonstress test (which, if all of ultrasound components are normal, may be omitted without compromising the validity of the test results)

2. Fetal breathing movements—One or more episodes of rhythmic fetal breathing movements of 30 seconds or more within 30 minutes

3. Fetal movement—Three or more discrete body or limb movements within 30 minutes

4. Fetal tone—One or more episodes of fetal extremity extension with return to flexion, or opening or closing of a hand

5. Quantification of amniotic fluid volume—A pocket of amniotic fluid that measures at least 2 cm in two planes perpendicular to each other

   With BPP testing, a score of 2 (present) or 0 (absent) is assigned to each of the five observations. A score of 8 or 10 is reassuring. A score of 6 is equivocal and generally should lead to delivery at term, whereas retesting within 12–24 hours may be appropriate for a preterm fetus. A score of 4 or less is nonreassuring and warrants further evaluation and consideration of delivery. Irrespective of the score, more frequent BPP testing or consideration of delivery may be warranted when oligohydramnios is present.

MODIFIED BIOPHYSICAL PROFILE

As another approach to fetal surveillance, the modified BPP combines the use of an NST as a short-term indicator of fetal status with the assessment of amniotic fluid index as an indicator of long-term placental function. The amniotic fluid index is a semiquantitative, four-quadrant assessment of amniotic fluid depth. A value of less than or equal to five is considered indicative of significant oligohydramnios. The modified BPP is less cumbersome than complete BPP assessment and appears to be as predictive of fetal well-being as other approaches of biophysical fetal surveillance. Another approach is use of the ultrasound component of the BPP alone, without the use of the NST.

Doppler Ultrasound of Umbilical Artery

Umbilical artery Doppler flow ultrasound is a noninvasive technique to assess resistance to blood flow in the placenta. It is not a screening test for detecting fetal compromise in the general population, but can be used in conjunction with other biophysical tests in high-risk pregnancies associated with suspected intrauterine growth restriction. Umbilical artery Doppler flow velocimetry is based on the characteristics of the systolic blood flow and the diastolic blood flow. The most commonly used index to quantify the flow velocity waveform is the peak systolic to diastolic ratio, the systolic/diastolic ratio. As peripheral resistance increases, diastolic flow decreases, and the systolic/diastolic ratio increases. Reversed end-diastolic flow can be seen with severe cases of intrauterine growth restriction secondary to uteroplacental insufficiency and may suggest impending fetal demise.

Assessment of Fetal Pulmonary Maturation

Fetal pulmonary maturity should always be taken into consideration when delivering a fetus electively or preterm in high-risk pregnancies. Fetal lung maturity should be confirmed before all non-HIV infected elective deliveries at less than 39 weeks of gestation. All efforts should be made to administer a course of antenatal glucocorticoids to pregnancies at high risk for preterm delivery between 24–34 weeks of gestation to promote fetal lung maturation (see Chapter 5). The following fetal maturity tests are available:

- Lecithin/sphingomyelin ratio
- Phosphatidylglycerol
- Foam stability index
- Fluorescence polarization
- Optical density at 650 nm
- Lamellar body counts
- Saturated phosphatidylcholine

Although the lecithin/sphingomyelin ratio as first used is the "gold standard" for determining fetal lung maturity, the other tests are rapidly replacing the lecithin/sphingomyelin ratio in clinical practice because of their technical ease. Regardless of the test used, the probability of respiratory distress syndrome after a mature test result beyond 34 weeks of gestation is less than 5%. In contrast, all available tests that show immature results are relatively poor in predicting respiratory distress syndrome. However, because no test indicating maturity can completely eliminate the risk of respiratory distress syndrome or other neonatal complications, the risk of adverse neonatal outcome following delivery must be weighed against the potential risk of allowing the pregnancy to remain in utero.

Issues to Discuss with Patients Before Delivery

WORKING

A woman with an uncomplicated pregnancy usually can continue to work until the onset of labor. Women with medical or obstetric complications of pregnancy may need to make adjustments based on the nature of their activities, occupation, and specific complications. It also has been reported that pregnant women whose occupations require standing or repetitive, strenuous, physical lifting have a tendency to deliver earlier and have smaller for gestational age infants. Most women can plan to return to work several weeks after an uncomplicated vaginal delivery. Although a period of 4–6 weeks generally is required for a woman's physiologic condition to return to normal, the patient's individual circumstances should be considered when recommending resumption of full activity. It also is important for the development of children and the family unit that adequate family leave be available for parents to be able to participate in early childrearing. The federal Family and Medical Leave Act and state law should be consulted for information on family and medical leave.

AIR TRAVEL DURING PREGNANCY

In the absence of obstetric or medical complications, pregnant women can observe the same general precautions for air travel as the general population and can fly safely up to 36 weeks of gestation. However, most airlines restrict the working air travel of flight attendants after 20 weeks of gestation and restrict commercial airline pilots from flying once pregnancy is diagnosed. Air travel is not recommended at any time during pregnancy for women who have medical or obstetric complications for which likely emergencies cannot be predicted. Such complications may include increased risks for, or evidence of, preterm delivery, pregnancy-induced hypertension, poorly controlled diabetes mellitus, or sickle cell disease or trait, which may be exacerbated by high altitude.

In-craft environmental conditions, such as low cabin humidity and changes in cabin pressure, coupled with the physiologic changes of pregnancy, do result in maternal adaptations that could have transient effects on the fetus. These changes should not affect normal pregnant women; however, pregnant women with medical problems that may be exacerbated by a hypoxic environment, but who must travel by air, should be prescribed supplemental oxygen during air travel.

The risks of lower extremity edema and venous thrombotic events are increased by long hours of air travel immobilization and may be minimized by the use of support stockings and periodic movement of the lower extremities. Pregnant air travelers may help minimize in-flight discomfort by avoiding gas-producing foods and drinks before and during flight. Additionally, preventive antiemetic medication should be considered for pregnant women with increased nausea. Because air turbulence cannot be predicted and the risk for trauma is significant, pregnant women, as well as all air travelers, should be instructed to continuously use their seat belts while seated. The seatbelt should be belted low on the hipbones, between the protuberant abdomen and pelvis.

Childbirth Education Classes

Couples should be referred to appropriate educational literature and urged to attend childbirth education classes. Studies have shown that prepared childbirth education programs can have a beneficial effect on performance in labor and delivery. The prenatal period should be used to expose the prospective parents to information about labor and delivery, pain relief, obstetric complications and procedures, breastfeeding, normal newborn care, and postpartum adjustment. Other family members also should be encouraged to participate in childbirth education programs. Adequate preparation of family members may benefit the mother, the neonate, and, ultimately, the family unit. Many hospitals, community agencies, and other groups offer such educational programs. The participation of physicians, certified nurse–midwives, and hospital obstetric nurses in educational programs is desirable to ensure continuity of care and consistency of instruction. National organizations such as The Childbirth Education Association are available for assistance as well. Integration of parenting education in prenatal education is beneficial in facilitating transition to parenthood.

ANTICIPATING LABOR

As pregnancy progresses into the third trimester, all women should be informed of what to do if contractions become regular, if membrane rupture is suspected, or vaginal bleeding occurs. Patients should be given a telephone number to call where assistance is available 24 hours per day. Patients should be encouraged to refrain from consumption of solid food when active labor ensues. Pregnant women are at highest risk of aspiration pneumonitis when stomach contents are greater than 25 mL and when the pH of those contents is less than 2.5. Pregnancy slows gastric emptying and labor can delay it further. The type of aspiration pneumonitis that produces the most severe physiologic and histologic alteration is partially digested food. A detailed discussion of the analgesic and anesthetic options available for labor and delivery should be held during the third trimester. The physician's policy regarding episiotomy also may be reviewed at this time.

BREECH PRESENTATION AT TERM

If the fetus persists in a breech presentation at 36–38 weeks of gestation, women should be offered an external cephalic version. Contraindications to the procedure include multifetal gestation, nonreassuring fetal testing, suspected placental abruption or previa, fetal growth restriction, oligohydramnios, and serious maternal medical conditions. The success rate of the procedure ranges from 35–86% with an average success rate of approximately 58%. Patients with a persistent breech presentation at term in a singleton gestation should undergo a planned cesarean delivery. If the patient refuses a planned cesarean delivery, informed consent for vaginal delivery should be obtained and should be documented. In those instances in which breech vaginal deliveries are pursued, great caution should be used. A planned cesarean delivery does not apply to patients in advanced labor and likely to have an imminent delivery of a fetus in a breech presentation or to patients whose second twin is in a nonvertex presentation.

Vaginal Birth After Cesarean Delivery

If the patient has had a prior cesarean delivery, the risks and benefits of a trial of labor versus repeat cesarean delivery should be discussed with the patient. Advantages of a successful vaginal delivery include decreased risks for hemorrhage and infection, a shorter postpartum hospital stay, and a less painful more rapid recovery. The patient should be informed of contraindications to a trial of labor (eg, prior classical cesarean delivery, placenta previa, unstable fetal presentation). She also should be informed that the risk of uterine rupture is approximately 1% and that in the event of a rupture, there is a 10–25% risk of significant adverse fetal sequelae. Although catastrophic uterine rupture leading to perinatal death or permanent injury to the newborn is rare, occurring less often than 1 per 1,000 vaginal birth after cesarean delivery attempts, it does occur and may occur no matter what resources are available to deal with it. Such risks increase with more than one uterine surgery, use of cervical ripening or induction, macrosomia, and oxytocin augmentation. No woman should be mandated to undergo a trial of labor. The ultimate decision to attempt vaginal delivery after cesarean delivery or to undergo a repeat cesarean delivery should be made by the informed patient and her physician.

Umbilical Cord Blood Banking

Prospective parents may seek information regarding the new modality of umbilical cord blood banking. Health care providers should dispense the following information:

- Preliminary data show encouraging results in umbilical cord blood stem cell transplantation for a variety of diseases, although at this time the procedure remains investigational.
- The indications for autologous transplantation are limited.
- Banking should be considered if there is a family member with a current or potential need to undergo a stem cell transplantation.
- Philanthropic donation of umbilical cord blood for banking is encouraged.

SUPPORT OF BREASTFEEDING

During prenatal visits, the patient should be counseled regarding the nutritional advantages of human breast milk. Human milk is the most appropriate nutrient for newborns and provides significant immunologic protection against infection. Newborns who are breastfed have a decreased incidence of infection and require fewer hospitalizations than formula fed neonates. Women should be provided with information regarding available lactation consultation services and organizations (see "Breastfeeding" in Chapter 7).

CIRCUMCISION

The topic of newborn male circumcision should be discussed. Newborn circumcision is an elective procedure to be performed, at the request of the parents, on newborn boys who are physiologically and clinically stable. The American Academy of Pediatrics 1999 Task Force suggests that existing scientific evidence demonstrates potential medical benefits of newborn male circumcision (eg, reduced incidences of phimosis, urinary tract infection, and penile cancer). However, the data are not sufficient to recommend routine neonatal circumcision. Appropriate anesthesia should be provided for the procedure (see "Circumcision" in Chapter 7).

POSTPARTUM TUBAL STERILIZATION

For many women, postpartum tubal ligation offers a convenient and appropriate method of sterilization. Assuming maternal and neonatal well-being as well as adequate medical and nursing resources, it is reasonable to proceed with tubal sterilization following a vaginal delivery (see "Postpartum Tubal Sterilization" in Chapter 5). Postpartum sterilization is an elective procedure, and physicians should not proceed unless conditions are safe.

Physicians should follow hospital policy and adhere to any pertinent state or federal laws or regulations when performing a postpartum tubal sterilization. Appropriate counseling regarding risks of failure, permanence of the procedure, physical risks, and potential psychosocial reactions to the procedure should take place before delivery.

PREPARATION FOR DISCHARGE

Prospective parents should be aware of the timing of hospital discharge after delivery. The couple should be encouraged to prepare for discharge by setting up required resources for home health services, acquiring a newborn car seat, newborn clothing, and a crib that meets standard safety guidelines. The prospective parents should be apprised of proper newborn positioning during sleep. Reports have shown a significant reduction in the incidence of sudden infant death syndrome among newborns that are placed on their backs (as opposed to the prone position) during sleep. At some time during the prenatal period, parents should identify a pediatrician and would benefit from a consultation regarding newborn and pediatric care. The patient should be informed of the various options of pregnancy prevention and birth control. This may be done by individual instruction, reading material, or a variety of films or videotapes.

PSYCHOSOCIAL SERVICES

Confronting psychosocial issues, such as providing appropriate childcare, the need for simultaneous employment, guilt associated with unintended pregnancy, and other family conflicts, may be the most distressing aspect of a woman's pregnancy and postpartum recovery. A woman with ambivalent feelings about her pregnancy may benefit from additional support from the health care team. Patients should be informed that postpartum blues are a normal phenomenon which occur in more than 70% of women. Women may manifest a wide range of symptoms, including weeping, depression, restlessness, mood lability, and negative feeling toward their newborns. Although the syndrome generally is transient, patients should be followed for the development of more severe postpartum depression. Women with a history of depression are at increased risk for postpartum depression. Tools for predicting the incidence of postpartum depression would be valuable.

A woman with negative feelings about her pregnancy should receive additional support from the health care team, and she may need professional advice on the alternatives to completing the pregnancy and keeping the newborn. Family members and their interactions with the pregnant woman should be considered in whatever recommendations are made to the woman. Physicians should be aware of individuals and community agencies to which patients can be referred for additional counseling and assistance when necessary.

Conditions of Special Concern

ADOLESCENT PREGNANCY

One million pregnancies occur annually among American adolescents. Of these, approximately 40,000 occur in minors younger than 15 years; 41% of these pregnancies are terminated by elective abortion. Approximately 80% of births to minors younger than 18 years are to unmarried adolescents. Approximately 2–4% of unmarried adolescents relinquish their newborns for adoption.

The status of laws requiring mandatory parental involvement in a minor's abortion decision currently is in flux. Most states have statutes addressing this issue, although the content and degree of enforcement of these laws vary considerably. Minors typically have legal rights protecting their privacy regarding the diagnosis and treatment of pregnancy. The clinician should assess the adolescent's ability to understand the implications of the diagnosis of pregnancy and the options available. The duration of the pregnancy should be determined and documented. The following three options are available:

1. Continuation of the pregnancy with the intent of raising the child

2. Continuation of the pregnancy with the intent of relinquishing the newborn for adoption

3. Termination of the pregnancy

The patient should be informed about the options available, return for visits as needed, and understand the importance of a timely decision. She should be encouraged to include her parents (or a surrogate parent) and the father of the fetus. The patient's right to decide should be respected regarding who should be involved and what the outcome of the pregnancy will be. Many states have laws regarding adolescent rights, and the physician should be aware of these state laws when making health care decisions.

If the adolescent chooses to continue the pregnancy, she should be referred for psychosocial support. There is an increased incidence of delivery of low-birth-weight neonates, neonatal death, preterm delivery, preeclampsia, anemia, and sexually transmitted disease among pregnant adolescents, necessitating increased surveillance at times and appropriate medical management.

Postterm Gestation

Between 3% and 12% of pregnancies extend beyond the start of the 43rd week of gestation (294 days or more from the first day of the last menstrual period) and are considered postterm. Although many apparent cases of postterm pregnancy are the result of an inability to define the time of conception accurately, some patients clearly progress to excessively long gestations that can represent a significant risk to the fetus. Accurate assessment of gestational age may reduce the likelihood of misdiagnosis of postterm gestation.

Antepartum assessments by cervical examination, fetal heart rate testing (NST or CST), ultrasound evaluation of amniotic fluid volume, BPP, or a combination of these tests should be initiated between 41 and 42 weeks of gestation. Assessment should be repeated weekly or more often, depending on the clinical situation. If fetal testing is not reassuring, delivery usually is indicated. Even when fetal testing is reassuring but reliable dating establishes a gestational age of 42 weeks, induction of labor is an acceptable management strategy and may be associated with decreased cesarean delivery rates. In most instances, a patient is a candidate for induction of labor if the pregnancy is at greater than 41 weeks of gestation and the condition of the cervix is favorable.

ANTEPARTUM HOSPITALIZATION

Pregnant patients with complications who require hospitalization before the onset of labor should be admitted to a designated antepartum area, either inside or near the labor and delivery area. Obstetric patients with serious and acute complications should be assigned to an area where more intensive care and surveillance are available, such as the labor and delivery area or an intensive care unit. An obstetrician–gynecologist or a specialist in maternal–fetal medicine should be involved, either as the primary or the consulting physician, in the care of an obstetric patient with complications. When sufficiently recovered, the pregnant patient should be returned to the obstetric service, provided that her return does not jeopardize her own care or that of other obstetric patients.

Acutely ill obstetric patients who are likely to deliver neonates requiring intensive care should be cared for in specialty or subspecialty perinatal care centers depending on the medical needs of the mater-nal–fetal dyad. When feasible, antepartum transfer to specialty or sub-specialty perinatal care centers should be encouraged for these women.

Written policies and procedures for the management of pregnant patients seen in the emergency department or admitted to nonobstetric services should be established and approved by the medical staff and must comply with the requirements of federal and state transfer laws. When warranted by patient volume, a high-risk antepartum care unit should be developed to provide specialized nursing care and facilities for the mother and the fetus at risk. When this is not feasible, written poli-cies are recommended that specify how the care and transfer of pregnant patients with obstetric, medical, or surgical complications will be han-dled and where these patients will be assigned.

Whether an obstetric patient is admitted to the antepartum unit or to a nonobstetric unit, her condition should be evaluated soon thereafter by the primary physician or appropriate consultants. The evaluation should encompass a complete review of current illnesses as well as a medical, family, and social history. The condition of the patient and the reason for admission should determine the extent of the physical exam-ination performed and the laboratory studies obtained. A copy of the patient's current prenatal record should become part of the hospital medical record as soon as possible after admission. These policies also must comply with the requirements of federal and state transfer laws.

Isoimmunization in Pregnancy

The pathogenesis of blood group isoimmunization resulting in hemolytic disease of the newborn has been well described. Rational methods of assessing the extent of the disease and of treating the fetus have been developed. Since 1967, preventive therapy has been available for Rh D isoimmunization in the form of anti-D immune globulin. Despite this preventative measure, Rh D isoimmunization remains the most common cause of serious hemolytic disease of the fetus and newborn. Among the etiologies of residual Rh isoimmunization cases are failure to accurately type the patient's blood, transfusion of mismatched blood, early or severe fetal-to-maternal hemorrhage, and failure to administer a sufficient amount of anti-D immune globulin at delivery. Other common and relatively uncommon RBC antigens associated with hemolytic disease of the fetus and newborn include c, Kell, E, e, C^w, C, Ce, Kp^a, Kp^b, cE, k, Jk^a, s, Wr^a, and Fy^a.

If isoimmunization is noted during routine prenatal testing, the genotype of the father can be determined, or in the case of anti-D, estimated. In the case of paternal heterozygosity for the offending antigen, the fetal blood type often can be determined by DNA analysis of fetal cells obtained at amniocentesis. Should such a study reveal the absence of the target gene, the fetus is not at risk. If the fetus is affected, the patient should be referred for consultation with a maternal–fetal medicine specialist with experience in the management of such cases (see also "Antibody Testing" in this chapter).

Pregnancy Outcomes in Women Older than 35 Years as of the Estimated Delivery Date

In 1999, the birth rates for women in their 30s were the highest in more than three decades (89.6 per 1,000 for ages 30–34; 38.3 per 1,000 for ages 35–39). The birth rate for women aged 40–44 years increased to 7.4 per 1,000 births in 1999, a 95% increase since 1981 (at 3.8 per 1,000). Several factors have contributed to this increase in older pregnant women, including delayed childbearing because of career, aging of the baby boom generation, and assisted reproductive technologies (ARTs). With increasing maternal age, there is an increase in the presence of underlying medical conditions. It is important to review the potential additional risks advanced maternal age may pose and counsel the patient accordingly:

1. Cesarean delivery—Nearly all studies have noted an increase in the prevalence of cesarean delivery in older pregnant women. This increase persists despite similar labor management of older nulliparous women compared with nulliparous women aged 20–29 years.

2. Stillbirth and growth restriction—After correcting for the higher prevalence of aneuploidy in older pregnant women, the preponderance of published reports fail to demonstrate an increase in perinatal morbidity or mortality in previously healthy women.

3. Assisted reproductive technology and multiple gestation—Women older than 35 years are more likely to conceive via some form of ART than women younger than 35 years. With ART, there is a well-reported increase in multiple gestations. However, multipregnancy outcomes are similar among women older than 35 years compared with younger women.

4. Aneuploidy—Women older than 35 years who have children are at increased risk of fetal aneuploidy. This increased risk has been well reported. Advanced paternal age is implicated in an increased risk of autosomal dominant disorders, such as neurofibromatosis, achondroplasia, Apert's syndrome, and Marfan's syndrome. However, it is unclear what age constitutes advanced paternal age.

5. Medical conditions—There is no consensus in the literature as to whether older patients without preexisting medical conditions have a higher prevalence of preeclampsia, placenta previa, breech presentation, preterm delivery, or operative vaginal delivery. In general, increases in perinatal and maternal morbidity are likely because of the increased risk of developing medical disorders with advancing age.

Multifetal Gestations

The incidence of twin and higher-order multiple gestations has increased significantly over the past 20 years primarily because of the availability and increased use of ovulation-inducing drugs and newly developed ARTs, such as in vitro fertilization. Between 1971 and 1999, the number of triplet births more than quadrupled, increasing from 1,034 to 6,742.

ANTEPARTUM MANAGEMENT

Counseling

Ideal antepartum care requires recognition of the following four issues in management and a frank discussion with the patient regarding how these issues may affect her pregnancy:

1. Nutritional considerations—It is recommended that maternal dietary intake in a multiple gestation be increased by approximately 300 kcal per day higher than that for a singleton pregnancy. Supplementation should include iron and folic acid. Although optimal weight gain for women with multiple gestations has not been determined, it has been suggested that women with twin gestations gain 35–45 lb.

2. Prenatal diagnosis—The usual indications for prenatal diagnosis and counseling in a singleton pregnancy apply to twin and higher-order gestations. Because the incidence of twin gestation increases with maternal age, women with multiple gestations often are candidates for prenatal genetic diagnosis. Genetic counseling should make clear to the patient the need to obtain a sample from each fetus, the risk of chromosomal abnormalities, potential complications of the procedure, the possibility of discordant results, and the ethical and technical concerns when one fetus is found to be abnormal. There is evidence that the combined risk of fetal chromosome abnormality is higher in dizygotic twin gestations than a singleton gestation.

   Maternal serum alpha-fetoprotein screening programs contribute to the early detection of multiple gestations. Depending on the laboratory, a value greater than 4.5 multiples of the median in an uncomplicated twin gestation is abnormal, requiring further comprehensive ultrasound evaluation by an experienced ultrasonographer and possible amniocentesis for the detection of amniotic fluid alpha-fetoprotein and acetylcholinesterase. Although maternal serum screening for NTDs can be useful in twin pregnancies, its effectiveness, as well as that of multiple markers (ie, MSAFP, human chorionic gonadotropin, and estriol) for trisomy 21 is not well established.

There is no clear evidence of an increased risk of amniocentesis in twin versus singleton gestations. Chorionic villus sampling is an appropriate method of first-trimester prenatal diagnosis in multiple gestations. Difficulties that can arise with CVS in twin gestations include the inability to obtain an adequate sample and contamination of one sample with tissue from the second. In approximately 1% of patients, tissue can be obtained from only one placenta. When CVS is performed at centers with experienced operators, twin–twin contamination occurs in approximately 4–6% of samples, causing prenatal diagnostic errors.

3. Multifetal reduction—The greater the number of fetuses within the uterus, the greater the risk of preterm delivery and adverse perinatal outcome. Multifetal pregnancy reduction may be performed to decrease the risk of serious perinatal morbidity and mortality associated with preterm delivery by reducing the number of fetuses. Pregnancy loss is the main risk of multifetal pregnancy reduction and ranges from 6% to 26%. The benefit of this procedure is most clear in quadruplet and higher-order gestations because it increases the length of gestation of the surviving fetuses. It remains to be determined whether multifetal pregnancy reduction improves long-term neonatal outcomes of triplet gestations reduced to twin gestations.

4. Management of other complications—The patient carrying a multiple gestation should be informed that she is at risk for a number of other potential complications including, but not limited to, preterm labor, preterm rupture of membranes, discordant fetal growth and intrauterine growth restriction, abnormal fluid volumes, preeclampsia, death of one fetus, and discordancy for fetal anomalies. Twin–twin transfusion syndrome, monoamniotic twinning, conjoined twins, and acardia (or twin reversed arterial perfusion sequence) are complications of monochorionic gestations. The most significant and common complication of multiple pregnancy is preterm labor resulting in preterm delivery. Women pregnant with multiple gestations are at a higher risk for complications of tocolysis, such as the development of pulmonary edema, because of higher blood volume, lower colloid osmotic pressure, and anemia. No ben-

efit has been shown from the use of oral tocolysis in multiple gestations to prevent the onset of preterm labor or preterm birth.
Antenatal corticosteroids should be administered for induction of
fetal lung maturation to women with multiple pregnancies who
experience preterm labor or preterm membrane rupture at less than
34 weeks of gestation.

Antepartum Surveillance

When intrauterine growth restriction, abnormal fluid volumes, growth
discordance, pregnancy-induced hypertension, fetal anomalies, mono-
amnionicity, or other pregnancy complications occur, fetal surveillance,
including nonstress testing or the modified or standard BPP, is indicated. The BPP is as reliable in multiple gestations as in singleton gestations. Although some patients may find it difficult to distinguish fetal
movements between twins, fetal movement counting can be an adjunct
to these antepartum surveillance techniques. Umbilical cord velocimetry
may be helpful in evaluating the severely growth-restricted fetus, but its
role in antepartum fetal surveillance of the singleton or multiple gestation is yet to be determined.

CONTROVERSIES IN MANAGEMENT

There are many diagnostic or therapeutic modalities used in the care of
multiple gestations that are of unclear or unproven benefit. Among these
are:

- Ultrasonography—Ultrasonography can be useful in both prenatal
  diagnosis and surveillance. Although the value of routine screening in the general population to promote early diagnosis of multiple gestations is subject to debate, ultrasonography has a role in
  evaluating fetal growth and amniotic fluid volume once the diagnosis is established. Beginning at viability, serial estimations of
  fetal growth by ultrasonography are a prudent measure, because
  physical examination may be less reliable.

- Vaginal ultrasonography—This procedure has been used to measure cervical width, length, and funneling and to examine the relationship of these measurements to the risk of preterm birth.

Although this is a promising technique, further evaluation of transvaginal ultrasonography by a prospective randomized study is necessary to determine its role in the prevention of preterm birth.

- Cervical cerclage—This procedure is not recommended as a routine prophylactic measure in multiple gestations.

- Bed rest—Not only is hospital bed rest costly, stressful, and disruptive, there is no clear consensus that it is of any benefit. Numerous studies have failed to show that bed rest decreases the incidence of preterm delivery, lengthens gestation, or reduces neonatal morbidity in multiple gestations.

- Home uterine activity monitoring—Home uterine activity monitoring has been shown in a large randomized controlled trial not to improve perinatal outcome in multiple gestations.

SUMMARY

The incidence of twins, triplets, and higher-order multiple gestations has increased dramatically because of widespread use of ovulation-inducing drugs and advanced assisted reproductive techniques. There is increased perinatal and maternal morbidity and mortality associated with multifetal gestations. The practicing obstetrician managing these high-risk patients should be familiar with their special antepartum and intrapartum problems, but may need to consult with maternal–fetal medicine specialists.

Bibliography

Adashek JA, Peaceman AM, Lopez-Zeno JA, Minogue JP, Socol ML. Factors contributing to the increased cesarean birth rate in older parturient women. Am J Obstet Gynecol 1993;169:936–40.

The adolescent's right to confidential care when considering abortion. American Academy of Pediatrics. Committee on Adolescence. Pediatrics 1996;97:746–51.

Air travel during pregnancy. ACOG Committee Opinion 264. The American College of Obstetricians and Gynecologists. Obstet Gynecol 2001;98:1187–8.

Alfirevic Z, Neilson JP. Biophysical profile for fetal assessment in high risk pregnancies (Cochrane Review). In: The Cochrane Library 2, 2002. Oxford: Update Software.

American College of Obstetricians and Gynecologists. Advanced paternal age: risks to the fetus. ACOG Committee Opinion 189. Washington, DC: ACOG; 1997.

American College of Obstetricians and Gynecologists. Antepartum fetal surveillance. ACOG Practice Bulletin 9. Washington, DC: ACOG; 1999.

American College of Obstetricians and Gynecologists. Assessment of fetal lung maturity. ACOG Educational Bulletin 230. Washington, DC: ACOG; 1996.

American College of Obstetricians and Gynecologists. Domestic violence. ACOG Educational Bulletin 257. Washington, DC: ACOG; 1999.

American College of Obstetricians and Gynecologists. External cephalic version. ACOG Practice Bulletin 13. Washington, DC: ACOG; 2000.

American College of Obstetricians and Gynecologists. Gestational diabetes. ACOG Practice Bulletin 30. Washington, DC: ACOG; 2001.

American College of Obstetricians and Gynecologists. Management of isoimmunization in pregnancy. ACOG Educational Bulletin 227. Washington, DC: ACOG; 1996.

American College of Obstetricians and Gynecologists. Management of postterm pregnancy. ACOG Practice Patterns 6. Washington, DC: ACOG; 1997.

American College of Obstetricians and Gynecologists. Preconception and prenatal carrier screening for cystic fibrocis. ACOG Clinical and Laboratory Guidelines. Washington, DC: ACOG; 2001.

American College of Obstetricians and Gynecologists. Prenatal diagnosis of fetal chromosomal abnormalities. ACOG Practice Bulletin 27. Washington, DC: ACOG; 2001.

American College of Obstetricians and Gynecologists. Prevention of Rh D alloimmunization. ACOG Practice Bulletin 4. Washington, DC: ACOG; 1999.

American College of Obstetricians and Gynecologists. Psychosocial risk factors: perinatal screening and intervention. ACOG Educational Bulletin 255. Washington, DC: ACOG; 1999.

American College of Obstetricians and Gynecologists. Sexual assault. ACOG Educational Bulletin 242. Washington, DC: ACOG; 1997.

American College of Obstetricians and Gynecologists. Smoking cessation during pregnancy. ACOG Educational Bulletin 260. Washington, DC: ACOG; 2000.

American Medical Association. Report 9 of the Council on Scientific Affairs (A-99). Effects of work on pregnancy. Available at http://www.ama-assn.org/ama/pub/article/2036-2338.html. Retrieved June 17, 2002.

Bianco A, Stone J, Lynch L, Lapinski R, Berkowitz G, Berkowitz RL. Pregnancy outcome at age 40 and older. Obstet Gynecol 1996;87:917–22.

Briggs GG, Freeman RK, Yaffe SJ. Drugs in pregnancy and lactation: a reference guide to fetal and neonatal risk. 6th ed. Philadelphia (PA): Lippincott Williams & Wilkins; 2002.

Chasnoff IJ, Landress HJ, Barrett ME. The prevalence of illicit-drug or alcohol use during pregnancy and discrepancies in mandatory reporting in Pinellas County, Florida. N Engl J Med 1990;322:1202–06.

Chiarotti M, Strano-Ross S, Offidani C, Fiori A. Evaluation of cocaine use during pregnancy though toxicological analysis of hair. J Anal Toxicol 1996; 20:555–8.

Circumcision. ACOG Committee Opinion 260. The American College of Obstetricians and Gynecologists. Obstet Gynecol 2001;98:707–8.

Counseling the adolescent about pregnancy options. American Academy of Pediatrics. Committee on Adolescence. Pediatrics 1998;101:938–40.

Dildy GA, Jackson GM, Fowers GK, Oshiro BT, Varner MW, Clark SL. Very advanced maternal age: pregnancy after age 45. Am J Obstet Gynecol 1996; 175:668–74.

Drug-exposed infants. American Academy of Pediatrics. Committee on Substance Abuse. Pediatrics 1995;96:364–67.

Exercise during pregnancy. ACOG Committee Opinion 267. The American College of Obstetricians and Gynecologists. Obstet Gynecol 2002;98:171–3.

Felice ME, Feinstein RA, Fisher MM, Kaplan DW, Olmedo LF, Rome ES, et al. Adolescent pregnancy—current trends and issues: 1998 American Academy of Pediatrics Committee on Adolescence. Pediatrics 1999;103:516–20.

Graham JM Jr, Edwards MJ, Edwards MJ. Teratogen update: gestational effects of maternal hyperthermia due to febrile illnesses and resultant patterns of defects in humans. Teratology 1998;58:209–21.

Joint Commission on Accreditation of Healthcare Organizations. Comprehensive accreditation manual for hospitals. Oakbrook Terrace (IL): JCAHO; 2000.

Landry SH, Whitney JA. The impact of prenatal cocaine exposure: studies of the developing infant. Semin Perinatol 1996;20:99–106.

March of Dimes Birth Defects Foundation, Committee on Perinatal Health. Toward improving the outcome of pregnancy: the 90s and beyond. White Plains (NY): MDBDF; 1993.

Martin JA, MacDorman MF, Mathews TJ. Triplet births: trends and outcomes, 1971–94. Vital Health Stat 21 1997(55):1–20.

Metzger BE, Coustan DR. Summary and recommendations of the Fourth International Workshop-Conference on Gestational Diabetes Mellitus. The Organizing Committee. Diabetes Care 1998;21:B161–7.

Mode of term singleton breech delivery. ACOG Committee Opinion 265. Obstet Gynecol 2001;98:1189–90.

Peipert JF, Bracken MB. Maternal age: an independent risk factor for cesarean delivery. The American College of Obstetricians and Gynecologists. Obstet Gynecol 1993;81:200–5.

Prenatal genetic diagnosis for pediatricians. American Academy of Pediatrics. Committee on Genetics. Pediatrics 1994;93:1010–5.

Recommendations to prevent and control iron deficiency in the United States. Centers for Disease Control and Prevention MMWR Recomm Rep 1998;47 (RR-3):1–29.

Rodis JF, Egan JF, Craffey A, Ciarleglio L, Greenstein RM, Scorza WE. Calculated risk of chromosomal abnormalities in twin gestations. Obstet Gynecol 1990; 76:1037–41.

Spohr HL, Willms J, Steinhausen HC. Prenatal alcohol exposure and long-term developmental consequences. Lancet 1993;341:907–10.

Tan KH, Smyth R. Fetal vibroacoustic stimulation for facilitation of tests of fetal well being (Cochrane Review). In: The Cochrane Library, Issue 2, 2002. Oxford: Update Software.

Wald N, Cuckle H, Wu TS, George L. Maternal serum unconjugated oestriol and human chorionic gonadotrophin levels in twin pregnancies: implications for screening for Down's syndrome. Br J Obstet Gynaecol 1991;98:905–08.

CHAPTER 5

Intrapartum and Postpartum Care of the Mother

The goal of all labor and delivery units is a safe birth for mothers and their newborns. At the same time, staff should attempt to make the patient feel welcome, comfortable, and informed throughout the labor and delivery process. Ongoing risk assessment should determine appropriate care for the woman. The father, partner, or other primary support person should be made to feel welcome and encouraged to participate throughout the labor and delivery experience.

Labor and delivery is a normal physiologic process that most women experience without complications. Obstetric staff can greatly enhance this experience for the woman and her family by exhibiting a caring attitude and helping them understand the process. Efforts to promote healthy behaviors can be as effective during labor and delivery as they are during antepartum care. Physical contact between the newborn and the parents in the delivery room should be encouraged. Every effort should be made to foster family interaction and to support the desire of the family to be together.

Because intrapartum complications can arise, sometimes quickly and without warning, ongoing risk assessment and surveillance of the mother and the fetus are essential. The hospital, including a birthing center within a hospital complex, provides the safest setting for labor, delivery, and the postpartum period. This setting ensures accepted standards of safety that cannot be matched in a home birthing situation. The collection and analysis of data on the safety and outcome of deliveries in other settings, such as freestanding centers, have been problematic. The development of approved, well-designed research protocols, prepared in consultation with obstetric departments and their related institutional review boards, is appropriate to assess safety, feasibility, and birth outcomes in such settings. Until such data are available, the use of other settings is not encouraged. There may be exceptional situations, however, such as geographically isolated areas in which special programs are required.

Admission

Pregnant women may come to a hospital's labor and delivery area not only for obstetric care but also for evaluation and treatment of nonobstetric signs or symptoms of illness. However, a nonobstetric condition, such as various infectious diseases (eg, varicella) may be best treated in another area of the hospital. The obstetric department should establish policies in consultation with other hospital units or personnel, such as the emergency department or infectious disease coordinator, for coordinated care of pregnant women. Departments should agree on the conditions that are best treated in the labor and delivery area and those that should be treated in other hospital care units. Patients with medical or surgical conditions that could reasonably be expected to result in obstetric consequences should be evaluated by qualified obstetric care providers. The priority of that evaluation and the site where it is best performed should be determined by the patient's needs (including gestational age) and the care unit's ability to provide for those needs. The obstetric department also should establish policies for the admission of nonobstetric patients according to state regulations (see "Nonobstetric Patients" in Chapter 2). Federal and state regulations address the management and treatment of patients in hospital acute care areas, including labor and delivery (see Appendix D).

Written departmental policies regarding triage of patients who come to a labor and delivery area should be reviewed periodically for compliance with appropriate regulations. A pregnant woman who comes to the labor and delivery area should be evaluated in a timely fashion. Obstetric nursing staff may perform this initial evaluation, which should minimally include assessment of:

- Maternal vital signs
- Fetal heart rate
- Uterine contractions

The responsible obstetric provider should be informed promptly if any of the following findings are present or suspected:

- Vaginal bleeding
- Acute abdominal pain
- Temperature of 100.4°F or higher
- Preterm labor
- Preterm rupture of membranes (PROM)
- Hypertension
- Nonreassuring fetal heart rate

Any patient who is suspected to be in labor or who has rupture of the membranes or vaginal bleeding should be evaluated promptly in an obstetric service area. Whenever a pregnant woman is evaluated for labor, the following factors should be assessed and recorded in the patient's permanent medical record:

- Maternal vital signs
- Frequency and duration of uterine contractions
- Documentation of fetal well-being
- Urinary protein and glucose concentration
- Cervical dilatation and effacement, unless contraindicated (eg, placenta previa)
- Fetal presentation and station of the presenting part
- Status of the membranes
- Date and time of the patient's arrival and of notification of the provider
- Estimation of fetal weight and assessment of maternal pelvis

If the patient is in prodromal or early labor, and has no complications, admission to the labor and delivery area may be deferred after initial evaluation and documentation of fetal well-being. A patient with a transmissible infection should be admitted to a site where isolation techniques may be followed according to hospital policy.

If a woman has received prenatal care and a recent examination has confirmed the normal progress of pregnancy, her admission evaluation may be limited to an interval history and physical examination directed at the presenting complaint. Previously identified risk factors should be recorded in the medical record. If no new risk factors are found, attention may be focused on the following historic factors:

- Time of onset and frequency of contractions
- Status of the membranes
- Presence or absence of bleeding
- Fetal movement
- History of allergies
- Time, content, and amount of the most recent food or fluid ingestion
- Use of any medication

Serologic testing for hepatitis B virus surface antigen may be necessary as described in Chapter 9. Women who have not received prenatal care or who received care late in pregnancy are more likely to have sexually transmitted diseases and substance abuse problems. Social problems, such as poverty and family conflict, also may affect patients' health. A shortened obstetric hospital stay poses even greater problems for patients who have had no prenatal care. Routine obstetric screening tests (eg, hemoglobin, type and Rh), social intervention, and additional education may be needed within this limited period.

If no complications are detected during initial assessment in the labor and delivery area and if contraindications have been ruled out, qualified nursing personnel may perform the initial pelvic examination. Once the results of the examination have been obtained and documented, the provider responsible for the woman's care in the labor and delivery area should be informed of her status. The provider can make a decision regarding her management. The timing of the provider's arrival in the labor area should be based on this information and hospital policy. If epidural, spinal, or general anesthesia is anticipated, or if conditions exist that place the patient at risk for requiring rapid institution of an anesthetic, anesthesia personnel should be informed of the patient's presence soon after her admission. If a preterm delivery, infected or depressed newborn, or a prenatally diagnosed congenital anomaly is expected, the provider who will assume responsibility for the newborn's care should be informed. When the patient has been examined and instructions regarding her management have been given and noted on her medical record, all necessary consent forms should be signed and incorporated into the medical record.

By 36 weeks of gestation, preregistration for labor and delivery at the hospital should be confirmed. By 36 weeks of gestation, a copy of the prenatal medical record (see "ACOG Antepartum Record" in Appendix A) should be on file in the hospital's labor registration area, including information pertaining to the patient's antepartum course. Consideration should be given to providing periodic updates to the prenatal medical record on file.

At the time of a patient's admission to the labor and delivery area, pertinent information from the prenatal record should be noted in the admission records. Because labor and delivery is a dynamic process, all entries into a patient's medical record should include the date and time of occurrence. Blood typing and screening tests need not be repeated if they were performed during the antepartum period and no antibodies were present, provided that the report is in the hospital records. If results of the woman's laboratory evaluation are not known and cannot be obtained, blood typing, Rh D type determination, hepatitis B virus antigen, and a serologic test for syphilis should be drawn from the woman and performed on umbilical cord blood before discharge. Serologic testing for human immunodeficiency virus (HIV) infection should be encouraged and performed according to state law. Collection of umbilical cord blood may be useful for subsequent evaluation of ABO incompatibility if the mother is type O. Policies should be developed to ensure expeditious preparation of blood products for transfusion if the patient is at increased risk of hemorrhage or if the need arises.

At all times in the hospital labor and delivery area, the safety and well-being of the mother and the fetus are the primary concern and responsibility of the obstetric staff. This concern, however, should not unnecessarily restrict the activity of women with uncomplicated labor and delivery or exclude people who are supportive of her. The woman should have the option to stay out of bed during the early stages of labor, to ambulate, and to rest in a comfortable chair as long as the fetal status is reassuring. Concerns such as showers during labor, placement of intravenous lines, use of fetal heart rate monitoring, and restrictions on ambulation should be reviewed in departmental policies, taking into consideration physicians' preferences as well as patients' desires, comfort, privacy, and sense of participation. Likewise, the use of drugs for relief of pain during labor and delivery should depend on the needs and desires of the woman. The development of a birth plan that has been discussed previously with a woman's provider and placed in her medical record may promote her participation in and satisfaction with her care.

The woman's health care team should communicate regarding all factors that may pose a risk to her, her fetus, or her newborn. Obstetric departmental policies should include recommendations for transmitting to the nursery those maternal and fetal historical and laboratory data that may affect the care of the newborn. Information on conditions that may influence neonatal care also should be communicated. The lack of such data, perhaps through a lack of prenatal care, also should be made known to the nursery personnel. The physician who will care for the newborn should be identified on the maternal medical record (see Appendix A). Health care professionals who provide anesthesia should be notified of women who may be at significant risk of complications from anesthetic procedures (eg, women with hypertension, morbid obesity).

Labor

The onset of true labor is established by observing progressive change in a woman's cervix. This may require two or more cervical examinations that are separated by an adequate period to observe change. Even a well-prepared woman may arrive at the hospital labor and delivery area before true labor has begun. A policy that allows for adequate evaluation of patients for labor and that prevents unnecessary admissions to the labor and delivery unit is advisable.

FALSE LABOR AT TERM

Uterine contractions in the absence of cervical change are commonly called false labor. Treatment for this condition should be based on individual circumstances. Patients in prodromal labor, or patients who are not yet in active labor and must be observed to determine whether labor has begun, may be admitted to a casual, comfortable area. After observation and evaluation by appropriate hospital-designated personnel and assurance of fetal well-being, the patient may be discharged.

PREMATURE RUPTURE OF MEMBRANES AT TERM

Premature rupture of membranes is considered to be present when there is leakage of amniotic fluid before the onset of labor. Preparations for labor and delivery should begin when PROM occurs, whether at or before term, because labor frequently ensues. Management of PROM is not uniform, and several acceptable strategies exist for the care of patients with PROM. Each hospital's department of obstetrics and gynecology, in consultation with the department of pediatrics, should establish guidelines for the care of patients with PROM. These guidelines should address methods of diagnosis, induction of labor, timing and use of antibiotics for both prophylaxis and treatment of the mother and the fetus, and consideration of location of the delivery (see Chapter 6 for a discussion of the management of preterm PROM).

The diagnosis of PROM depends on history, physical examination, and laboratory confirmation. Diagnosis based on history alone is correct in more than 90% of patients. Nevertheless, all patients reporting symptoms that suggest ruptured membranes should be examined with a sterile speculum as soon as possible to confirm this diagnosis. Gross pooling of amniotic fluid in the vagina is nearly 100% diagnostic of PROM. Supportive laboratory testing includes vaginal pH, fern testing, and ultrasonographic estimation of amniotic fluid volume. Management is determined by the presence or absence of PROM.

The obstetric providers who perform the examination to confirm or rule out PROM should be aware of the causes of false-positive and false-negative test results that occur with the use of pH and fern testing. These causes include leakage of alkaline urine, cervical mucus, bacterial vaginosis, and blood.

If chorioamnionitis is diagnosed at any gestational age, labor should be induced. The diagnosis of chorioamnionitis alone is not an indication for cesarean delivery. In the presence of chorioamnionitis, the duration of PROM does not correlate with the risk of neonatal sepsis. In any labor occurring after rupture of membranes, vaginal examinations should be limited in number and attention paid to clean technique.

MANAGEMENT OF LABOR

Ideally, every woman admitted to the labor and delivery area should know who her principal designated health care provider will be. Members of the obstetric team should observe the patient to follow the progress of labor, record her vital signs and the fetal heart rate in her medical record at regular intervals, and make an effort to ensure her understanding of the events taking place. The provider principally responsible for the patient's care should be kept informed of her progress and notified promptly of any abnormality. When the patient is in active labor, that provider should be readily available (see "Preface," and "Cesarean Delivery" in this chapter).

Patients in active labor should avoid oral ingestion of anything except sips of clear liquids, occasional ice chips, or preparations for moistening the mouth and lips. When significant hydration is needed during a long labor, it should be given by intravenous infusion.

The progress of labor should be evaluated by periodic vaginal examinations. Attention to perineal hygiene may help reduce infection of the upper genital tract. If the membranes are ruptured, attention to clean technique is even more important. Sterile, water-soluble lubricants may be used to reduce discomfort during vaginal examinations. Antiseptics, such as povidone-iodine and hexachlorophene, have not been shown to decrease infections acquired during the intrapartum period. Furthermore, these agents may produce local irritation and are absorbed through maternal mucous membranes. Therefore, lubricants containing these agents, and sprays or liquids delivering them directly to the introitus, are not recommended for use during labor.

For women who are at no increased risk of complications, evaluation of the quality of the uterine contractions and pelvic examinations should be sufficient to detect abnormalities in the progress of labor. Vital signs should be recorded at regular intervals, at least every 4 hours. This frequency may be increased, particularly as active labor progresses according to clinical signs and symptoms. Documentation of the course of a woman's labor may include, but need not be limited to, the presence of physicians or nurses, position changes, cervical status, oxygen and drug administration, blood pressure levels, temperature, amniotomy or spontaneous rupture of membranes, color of amniotic fluid, and Valsalva's maneuver.

FETAL HEART RATE MONITORING

Either electronic fetal heart rate monitoring or intermittent auscultation may be used to determine fetal status during labor. Obstetric unit guidelines should clearly delineate the procedures to be followed for using these techniques according to the phase and stage of labor.

The method of fetal heart rate monitoring for fetal surveillance during labor may vary, depending on the risk assessment at admission, the preferences of the patient and obstetric staff, and departmental policy. If no risk factors are present at the time of the patient's admission, a standard approach to fetal surveillance is to determine and record the auscultated fetal heart rate just after a contraction at least every 30 minutes in the active phase of the first stage of labor and at least every 15 minutes in the second stage of labor.

If risk factors are present at admission or appear during labor, there is no difference in perinatal outcome between intermittent auscultation and continuous fetal monitoring if one of the following methods for fetal heart rate monitoring is used:

- During the active phase of the first stage of labor, the fetal heart rate should be determined and recorded at least every 15 minutes, preferably just after a uterine contraction, when intermittent auscultation is used. If continuous electronic fetal heart rate monitoring is used, the heart rate tracing should be evaluated at least every 15 minutes.

- During the second stage of labor, the fetal heart rate should be determined and recorded at least every 5 minutes if auscultation is used. If continuous electronic fetal heart rate monitoring is used, the tracing should be evaluated at least every 5 minutes.

The appropriate use of electronic fetal heart rate monitoring includes recording and interpreting the tracings. Nonreassuring findings should be noted and communicated to the physician or certified nurse–midwife so that appropriate intervention can occur. When a change in the rate or pattern has been noted, it also is important to document a subsequent return to reassuring findings. Terms that describe the fetal heart rate patterns (eg, early, late, or variable decelerations; accelerations; and beat-to-beat variability) should be used in both medical record entries and verbal communication among obstetric personnel.

Internal fetal heart rate monitoring and internal uterine pressure monitoring may be used to gain further information about fetal status and uterine contractility, respectively. Relative contraindications to internal fetal monitoring include maternal HIV infection and other high-risk factors for fetal infection, including herpes simplex virus and hepatitis B or hepatitis C virus.

Fetal scalp or acoustic stimulation that results in acceleration of the fetal heart rate is reassuring when the fetal heart rate pattern is difficult to interpret. A fetal scalp blood sample may be used to obtain information about fetal acid-base status during labor if the fetal heart rate pattern is nonreassuring or difficult to interpret.

If electronic fetal monitoring is used, all fetal heart rate tracings should be identified with the patient's name, hospital number, and the date and time of admission. All fetal heart rate tracings should be easily retrievable from storage so that the events of labor can be studied in proper relationship to the tracings.

Induction and Augmentation of Labor

Each hospital's department of obstetrics and gynecology should develop written protocols for preparing and administering oxytocin solution or other agents for labor induction or stimulation. Indications for induction and augmentation of labor should be stated. The qualifications of personnel authorized to administer oxytocic agents for this purpose should be described. The methods for assessment of the woman and the fetus before and during administration of these agents should be specified. Fetal heart rate monitoring should be performed as delineated for high-risk patients in active labor (see "Fetal Heart Rate Monitoring" in this chapter). Labor is induced when the benefits to either the woman or the fetus outweigh those of continuing the pregnancy. If oxytocin is used, the infusion should be administered by a device that permits precise control of the flow rate to ensure accurate, minute-to-minute control. Oxytocin also is used to augment labor and enhance inadequate uterine contractions in women in whom an assessment of the relationship between the maternal pelvis and fetal size is otherwise normal. Buccal, nasal, or intramuscular administration of oxytocin should not be used to induce or augment labor.

Various regimens exist for the administration of varying techniques and agents to stimulate uterine contractions. These regimens vary in initial dose, amount of incremental dose increase, and interval between dose increases. Each hospital's department of obstetrics and gynecology should determine which regimens will be standard for that hospital so that obstetric staff in the labor and delivery area may develop further guidelines for their application to individual patients. Regimens described as low-dose and with a less frequent increase are associated with a lower incidence of uterine hyperstimulation. Higher and more frequent dosage increases are credited with shortening time in labor and reducing the incidence of chorioamnionitis and the number of cesarean deliveries performed for dystocia, but increased rates of uterine hyperstimulation.

CERVICAL RIPENING

Cervical ripening may be beneficial if the cervix is unfavorable for induction. Acceptable interventions for preparing an unfavorable cervix for induction include mechanical dilation with laminaria or a 30 cc Foley catheter placed in the cervical canal, misoprostol as detailed below, and intravaginal or intracervical administration of prostaglandin E_2 (PGE_2) in doses appropriate for cervical ripening. If the fetus's estimated gestational age is near term, routine intravenous oxytocin induction or misoprostol administration usually is effective. Prostaglandin E_2 suppositories and more concentrated intravenous oxytocin regimens are both effective for terminating a pregnancy complicated by fetal death, especially at a gestational age of 28 weeks or less. Because of the risk of uterine rupture, the use of prostaglandins after 28 weeks of gestation should be discouraged if the woman has had prior major uterine surgery. Contraindications to the induction of labor or cervical ripening with prostaglandins include maternal cyanotic or ischemic cardiac disease and severe asthma.

Misoprostol, a prostaglandin E_1 analog, has been demonstrated to be an effective agent for the induction of labor. When compared with placebo, misoprostol decreased overall cesarean delivery rates, decreased oxytocin requirements, and achieved higher rates of vaginal delivery within 24 hours of induction. Misoprostol also compared favorably with intracervical and intravaginal PGE_2 preparations, with many studies demonstrating shorter times to delivery and reduced oxytocin requirements. Misoprostol use is not recommended for cervical ripening or induction of labor in patients with prior cesarean delivery or major uterine surgery.

When given in doses of 50 μg or more, misoprostol use has been associated with an increased rate of uterine hyperstimulation, uterine tachysystole, and meconium passage. These problems have not been seen with a dose of 25 μg misoprostol administered intravaginally as frequently as every 3 hours.

Misoprostol is currently available in 100-μg and 200-μg tablets, and the 100-μg tablet is not scored. If misoprostol is used for cervical ripening and induction, one quarter of a 100-μg tablet (ie, approximately 25 μg) should be considered for the initial dose. Doses should not be administered more frequently than every 3–6 hours. Both fetal heart rate and uterine activity should be monitored carefully in these patients. Doses should be held in the presence of a nonreassuring fetal heart rate or regular and frequent uterine contractions of moderate intensity.

When labor is induced, a physician who has privileges to perform cesarean deliveries should be readily available (see "Preface," and "Cesarean Delivery" in this chapter). The patient's medical record should document who is the responsible physician. A qualified member of the obstetric team should perform a vaginal examination for evaluation of the cervix before the induction is initiated. Personnel who are familiar with the effects of the agents used and who are able to identify both maternal and fetal complications should be in attendance during administration of the agent(s).

Hyperstimulation can occur with any of the available chemical techniques of cervical ripening or labor induction or augmentation. When the continuous administration of PGE_2 via vaginal insert is the technique used, the fetal heart rate and uterine activity should be monitored continuously as long as the device is in place and for at least 15 minutes after it is removed.

Induction of labor by "stripping" or "sweeping" the amniotic membranes is a relatively common practice. Risks associated with this procedure include infection, bleeding from an undiagnosed placenta previa or low-lying placenta, and accidental rupture of membranes. Membrane stripping may be associated with a higher frequency of spontaneous labor and with a decreased incidence of postterm gestation.

Artificial rupture of membranes is another nonpharmacologic method of labor induction that may be used, particularly when the cervix is favorable. Routine early amniotomy results in a modest reduction in the duration of labor. Care should be taken to palpate for an umbilical cord and to avoid dislodging the fetal head when artificially rupturing membranes. The fetal heart rate should be recorded before and immediately after the procedure.

When induction is necessary, it is reasonable to perform an amniotomy as an adjunct to oxytocin infusion, even with minimal cervical dilatation, if the presenting part is well applied to the cervix and the minimal risk of umbilical cord prolapse is outweighed by the perceived benefits of rapid induction. When the situation is less urgent, it is reasonable to wait to perform an amniotomy until cervical dilatation is more advanced. Rupture of membranes may reduce the efficacy of misoprostol or vaginal PGE_2 preparations although these preparations have been shown to work despite ruptured membranes.

AMNIOINFUSION

The transcervical infusion of sterile, balanced salt solutions during labor (amnioinfusion) may be used to ameliorate variable decelerations in the fetal heart rate tracing that are suspected to be caused by umbilical cord compression. This technique also has been used to dilute thick meconium. Amnioinfusion has been shown to reduce the risks of cesarean delivery and meconium aspiration. Because it is possible to introduce fluid into the uterus at too rapid a rate, each obstetric unit should establish a protocol for intrauterine pressure monitoring during amnioinfusion or limitations of the volume and infusion rate when the technique is used.

Analgesia and Anesthesia

Management of discomfort and pain during labor and delivery is an essential part of good obstetric practice. It is the responsibility of the obstetrician or certified nurse–midwife, in consultation with the anesthesiologist, if appropriate, to develop the most appropriate response to the woman's request for analgesia or anesthesia. In the absence of a medical contraindication, maternal request is a sufficient medical indication for pain relief during labor.

Some patients tolerate the pain of labor by using techniques learned in childbirth preparation programs. Although specific techniques vary, classes usually seek to relieve pain through the general principles of education, support, relaxation, paced breathing, focusing, and touch. The staff at the bedside should be knowledgeable about these pain management techniques and should be supportive of the patient's decision to use them.

Unless contraindicated, pharmacologic analgesics to ameliorate the pain of contractions should be made available on request to women in labor. The choice and availability of analgesic and anesthetic techniques depend on the experience and judgment of the obstetrician and anesthesiologist, the physical condition of the patient, the circumstances of labor and delivery, and the personal preferences of the obstetrician and the patient. Parenteral pain medications for labor pain decrease fetal heart rate variability and may limit the obstetrician's ability to interpret the fetal heart rate tracing. Considerations should be given to other agents in the setting of diminished short- or long-term fetal heart rate variability. High doses of narcotics are potentially depressing to both the woman and the fetus, and both patients should be carefully monitored. Barbiturates, tranquilizers, and narcotics can be administered during prodromal and early labor to allow the patient to rest.

Of the various pharmacologic methods used for pain relief during labor and delivery, regional analgesia techniques—epidural, spinal, and combined spinal epidural block—are the most flexible, effective, and least depressing to the central nervous system, allowing for an alert participating woman and an alert neonate. Unless contraindications are present, women who request regional analgesia should be able to receive it. It also should be noted that a low-grade maternal fever may be associated with a normally functioning epidural in the absence of infection.

Spinal analgesia alone, or in combination with epidural analgesia, may be used to provide pain relief during labor and delivery. This technique typically involves intermittent or continuous intrathecal administration of an opioid with or without a dilute solution of a local anesthetic. Some physicians perform a combined spinal-epidural technique. Depending on the technique used, the experience of the anesthesiologist, and the patient's response, ambulation to some extent may be possible during regional analgesia.

Paracervical block, when used for pain relief during labor, may result in fetal bradycardia. The fetal heart rate should be monitored closely before, during, and after the administration of paracervical block. Bupivacaine is contraindicated for use in paracervical block.

At the time of delivery, local infiltration of the perineum and pudendal block are safe anesthesia techniques to control the discomfort of delivery without impairing the woman's expulsive efforts. Spinal analgesia using dilute concentrations of local anesthetics with opioids may provide excellent analgesia with rapid onset for the second stage of labor. Spinal anesthesia with more concentrated local anesthetics can provide profound sensory and motor blockade if needed for maternal indications or to facilitate instrumented vaginal delivery. Although spinal anesthesia can provide adequate pain relief and muscle relaxation for nearly all vaginal deliveries, it typically results in profound sensory and motor blockade, which impairs maternal expulsive efforts. Therefore, spinal anesthesia typically is not administered until delivery is imminent or the physician has made a decision to perform an operative delivery. General anesthesia is rarely necessary for vaginal delivery and should be used only for specific indications.

For most cesarean deliveries, properly administered regional or general anesthesia is effective and has little adverse effect on the newborn. Because of the maternal risks associated with intubation and the possibility of aspiration during induction of general anesthesia, regional anesthesia may be the preferred technique and should be available in all hospitals that provide obstetric care. The advantages and disadvantages of both techniques should be discussed with the patient as completely as possible. Examples of circumstances in which rapid induction of general anesthesia may be indicated include a prolapsed umbilical cord with severe fetal bradycardia and acute hemorrhage in a hemodynamically unstable mother.

If properly chosen and administered, analgesia or anesthesia during labor and delivery has little or no lasting effect on the physiologic status of the neonate. At present, no evidence exists that the administration of analgesia or anesthesia during childbirth per se has a significant effect on the child's later mental and neurologic development.

Regional anesthesia in obstetrics should be initiated and maintained only by health care providers who are approved through the institutional credentialing process to administer or supervise the administration of obstetric anesthesia. These individuals must be qualified to manage anesthetic complications. An obstetrician may administer the anesthesia if granted privileges for these procedures. However, having an anesthesiologist or anesthetist provide this care permits the obstetrician to give undivided attention to the delivery.

It is the responsibility of the director of anesthesia services to make recommendations regarding the clinical privileges of all anesthesia service personnel. If obstetric anesthesia is provided by obstetricians, the director of anesthesia services should participate with a representative of the obstetric department in the formulation of procedures designed to ensure the uniform quality of anesthesia services throughout the hospital. Specific recommendations regarding these procedures are provided in the *Accreditation Manual for Hospitals* published by the Joint Commission on Accreditation of Healthcare Organizations. The directors of departments providing anesthesia services are responsible for implementing processes to monitor and evaluate the quality and appropriateness of these services in their respective departments.

Regional anesthesia should be administered only after the patient has been examined and the fetal status and progress of labor have been evaluated by a qualified individual. A physician with obstetric privileges who has knowledge of the maternal and fetal status and the progress of labor and who approves initiation of labor anesthesia should be readily available to deal with any obstetric complications that may arise. When regional anesthesia is administered during labor, the patient's vital signs should be monitored at regular intervals by a qualified member of the health care team.

When any of the following risk factors are present, anesthetic consultation in advance of delivery may be considered to permit formulation of a management plan:

• Marked obesity

• Severe edema or anatomic abnormalities of the face, neck, or spine, including trauma or surgery

• Abnormal dentition, small mandible, or difficulty opening the mouth

• Extremely short stature, short neck, or arthritis of the neck

• Goiter

• Serious maternal medical problems, such as cardiac, pulmonary, or neurologic disease

• Bleeding disorders

• Severe preeclampsia

• Previous history of anesthetic complications

• Obstetric complications likely to lead to operative delivery (eg, placenta previa or high-order multiple gestation)

When such risk factors are identified, a physician who is credentialed to provide general and regional anesthesia should be consulted in the antepartum period to allow for joint development of a plan of management including optimal location for delivery. Strategies thereby can be developed to minimize the need for emergency induction or general anesthesia in women for whom this would be especially hazardous. For those patients at risk, consideration should be given to the planned placement in early labor of an intravenous line and an epidural or spinal catheter with confirmation that the catheter is functional. If a patient at unusual risk of complications from anesthesia is identified (eg, prior failed intubation), strong consideration should be given to antepartum referral of the patient to allow for delivery at a hospital which can manage such anesthesia on a 24-hour basis.

Aspiration is a significant cause of anesthetic-related maternal morbidity and mortality, and the more acidic the aspirate, the greater the harm done. Therefore, prophylactic administration of an antacid before induction of a major regional or general anesthesia is appropriate. Particulate antacids may be harmful if aspirated; a clear antacid, such as a solution of 0.3 mol/L of sodium citrate or a similar preparation, may be a safer choice.

On rare occasions, it may be impossible to intubate an obstetric patient after the induction of general anesthesia. Equipment for emergency airway management, such as the laryngeal mask airway, combi tube, and fiberoptic laryngoscope, should be available whenever general anesthesia is administered.

Delivery

VAGINAL DELIVERY

Vaginal delivery is associated with less risk of operative and postoperative complications than cesarean delivery and results in shorter hospital stays. Vaginal delivery requires consideration of:

- The availability of professionals with special skills in neonatal resuscitation
- The availability of anesthesia personnel
- Obstetric attendants for the delivery
- The potential need to move a patient from a labor–delivery–recovery (LDR) room to an operative suite

The risk assessment performed on the patient's admission, the course of the patient's labor, the fetal presentation, any abnormalities encountered during the labor process, and the anesthetic technique in use or anticipated for delivery will all have an impact on the need for other professionals. At least one obstetric nurse, preferably the woman's designated primary nurse for the labor, should be present in the delivery room throughout the delivery. Under no circumstances should an attempt be made to delay birth by physical restraint or anesthetic means.

Episiotomy may be used to aid in the management of delivery in some situations. The routine use of episiotomy is not necessary and may lead to an increase in the risk of third- and fourth-degree perineal lacerations and to a delay in the patient's resumption of sexual activity.

Vaginal Birth After Cesarean Delivery

Despite extensive data regarding the risks and success rates of vaginal birth after cesarean delivery (VBAC), there is relatively little information regarding how labor should be conducted (see "Vaginal Birth After Cesarean Delivery" in Chapter 4):

- Limited data suggest that external cephalic version for breech presentation may be as successful for VBAC candidates as for women who have not undergone previous cesarean delivery.

- The use of prostaglandins for cervical ripening or labor induction in VBAC candidates is discouraged, as noted previously (see "Cervical Ripening" in this chapter). If induction of labor is necessary for a clear and compelling clinical indication, the potential increased risk of uterine rupture with the use of prostaglandins should be discussed with the patient and documented in the medical record.

- Oxytocin may be used for both labor induction and augmentation with close patient monitoring in VBAC candidates.

- Once labor has begun, the patient should be evaluated promptly. Most authorities recommend continuous electronic monitoring of both fetal heart rate and uterine contractions. The most common sign of uterine rupture is a nonreassuring fetal heart rate pattern with variable decelerations that may evolve into late decelerations, bradycardia, and undetectable fetal heart rate. Personnel familiar with the potential complications of VBAC should be vigilant for nonreassuring fetal heart rate patterns and inadequate progress in labor. Because uterine rupture may be catastrophic and evolve rapidly, VBAC should be attempted in institutions equipped to respond to emergencies with physicians immediately available to provide emergency care.

- Epidural analgesia and anesthesia may safely be used during a trial of labor and planned VBAC. Assurance of adequate pain relief during labor may encourage more women to choose a trial of labor. Success rates for VBAC are similar in women who do and those who do not receive epidural analgesia, as well as in those women who receive other types of pain relief. Epidural analgesia rarely masks the signs or symptoms of uterine rupture. The anesthesia service should be notified whenever there is a patient attempting VBAC in active labor on the labor floor.

There is nothing unique about delivering a newborn with a successful VBAC. The need to explore the uterus after a successful VBAC is controversial. Most asymptomatic scar dehiscences heal well, and there is no data to suggest that future pregnancy outcome is improved if the dehiscence is surgically repaired. Excessive vaginal bleeding or signs of hypovolemia at delivery require prompt and complete assessment of the previous scar and the entire genital tract.

Operative Vaginal Delivery

Forceps and vacuum extraction are valuable tools to effect operative vaginal delivery. Operator experience should determine which instrument should be used in a particular situation. The vacuum extractor is associated with an increased incidence of neonatal cephalohematomata, retinal hemorrhages, and jaundice when compared with forceps delivery. Neonatal care providers should be made aware of the mode of delivery to observe for potential complications associated with operative vaginal delivery. The following definitions and indications relate to both techniques.

Station. The relationship of the estimated distances, in centimeters, between the leading bony portion of the fetal head and the level of the maternal ischial spines. In classifying forceps and vacuum extraction procedures, the station of the fetal head must be stated as precisely as possible. Engagement of the head occurs when the biparietal diameter has passed through the pelvic inlet. It is clinically diagnosed when the leading bony portion of the fetal head is at or below the level of the ischial spines (station 0 or more). Although the preferred method to describe station beyond the level of the ischial spines is to estimate centimeters below the spines, some continue to find it useful to refer to station in estimated thirds of the maternal pelvis below the spines. An approximate correlation of these two methods of describing station would be:

- 2 cm = +1/3
- 4 cm = +2/3
- 6 cm = +3/3

Outlet Operative Vaginal Delivery. The application of forceps or vacuum when 1) the fetal scalp is visible at the introitus without separating the labia, 2) the fetal skull has reached the pelvic floor, 3) the fetal sagittal suture is in the anterior-posterior diameter or in the right or left occiput anterior or posterior position, and 4) the fetal head is at or on the perineum. According to this definition, rotation cannot exceed 45 degrees. There is no difference in perinatal outcome when deliveries involving the use of outlet operative vaginal deliveries are compared with similar spontaneous deliveries, and no data support the concept that rotating the head on the pelvic floor 45 degrees or less increases morbidity.

Low Operative Vaginal Delivery. The application of forceps or vacuum when the leading point of the fetal skull is at station +2 or more and is not on the pelvic floor. Low operative vaginal delivery applications have two subdivisions: 1) rotation 45 degrees or less (eg, left or right occipitoanterior to occiput anterior, or left or right occipitoposterior to occiput posterior) and 2) rotation more than 45 degrees. Although rotation of the fetal head often accompanies the use of the vacuum extractor, the vacuum should never be used to provide a direct rotational force to the fetal scalp.

Midpelvis Operative Vaginal Delivery. The application of forceps or vacuum when the fetal head is engaged but the leading point of the skull is above station +2. Under very unusual circumstances, such as the sudden onset of severe fetal or maternal compromise, application of forceps or vacuum above station +2 may be attempted while simultaneously initiating preparations for a cesarean delivery in the event that the operative vaginal delivery maneuver is unsuccessful. Neither forceps nor vacuum should be applied to an unengaged fetal presenting part or when the cervix is not completely dilated.

Indications for a forceps or vacuum extraction operation, including the position and station of the vertex at the time of application of the forceps or vacuum apparatus, should be identified in a detailed operative description in the patient's medical record. These indications include:

- Shortening the second stage of labor—Outlet forceps or vacuum extraction may be used to shorten the second stage of labor in the best interests of the woman or the fetus.

- Ending a prolonged second stage—The following periods are approximate; when these intervals are exceeded without continuing progress, the risks and benefits of allowing labor to continue should be assessed and documented:
  - Nulliparous patients—More than 3 hours with a regional anesthetic or more than 2 hours without a regional anesthetic
  - Parous patients—More than 2 hours with a regional anesthetic or more than 1 hour without a regional anesthetic

- Nonreassuring fetal heart rate

- Maternal indications (eg, cardiac disease, exhaustion)

The following conditions are required for forceps or vacuum extraction operations:

- A person with privileges for such procedures
- Assessment of maternal pelvis-fetal size relationship
- Adequate anesthesia
- Willingness to abandon attempted operative vaginal delivery
- Ability to perform emergency cesarean delivery (see "readily available" in the "Preface" and in "Cesarean Delivery" in this chapter)

CESAREAN DELIVERY

All hospitals offering labor and delivery services should be equipped to perform emergency cesarean delivery. The required personnel, including nurses, anesthesia personnel, neonatal resuscitation team members, and obstetric attendants, should be in the hospital or readily available (also see "Preface"). Any hospital providing an obstetric service should have the capability of responding to an obstetric emergency. No data correlate the timing of intervention with outcome, and there is little likelihood that any will be obtained. However, in general, the consensus has been that hospitals should have the capability of beginning a cesarean delivery within 30 minutes of the decision to operate. Some indications for cesarean delivery can be appropriately accommodated in greater than 30 minutes. Conversely, examples of indications that may mandate more expeditious delivery include hemorrhage from placenta previa, abruptio placentae, prolapse of the umbilical cord, and uterine rupture. Sterile materials and supplies needed for emergency cesarean delivery should be kept sealed but properly arranged so that the instrument table can be made ready at once for an obstetric emergency.

In-house obstetric and anesthesia coverage should be available in subspecialty care units. The anesthesia and pediatric staff responsible for covering the labor and delivery unit should be informed in advance when a complicated delivery is anticipated and when a patient with risk factors requiring a high-acuity level of care is admitted.

Elective repeat cesarean delivery is not a high-risk situation for the neonate. However, a qualified person who is skilled in neonatal resuscitation should be in the operative delivery room, with all equipment needed for neonatal resuscitation, to care for the neonate. The duties of the surgical and anesthetic teams may prevent them from performing immediate care of the newborn.

Before elective repeat cesarean delivery, the maturity of the fetus should be established. For patients with an indication for an elective repeat cesarean delivery, fetal maturity may be assumed if one of the following criteria is met:

- Fetal heart tones have been documented for 20 weeks by non-electronic fetoscope or for 30 weeks by Doppler ultrasound.

- Thirty-six weeks have elapsed since positive results were obtained from a serum or urine human chorionic gonadotropin pregnancy test performed by a reliable laboratory.

- An ultrasound measurement of the crown-rump length obtained at 6–11 weeks of gestation supports a current gestational age of 39 weeks or more.
- Clinical history and physical and ultrasound examinations performed at 12–20 weeks of gestation support a current gestational age of 39 weeks or more.

These criteria are not intended to preclude the use of menstrual dating. If any one criterion confirms gestational age assessment in a patient who has normal menstrual cycles and no immediate antecedent use of oral contraceptives, it is appropriate to schedule delivery at 39 weeks of gestation or later on the basis of menstrual dates. Another option is to await the onset of spontaneous labor.

In women requiring cesarean delivery, fetal surveillance should continue until abdominal sterile preparation has begun. If internal fetal heart rate monitoring is in use, it should be continued until the abdominal sterile preparation is complete.

MULTIPLE GESTATION

The following factors should be considered in the delivery of multiple gestations:

- Labor and delivery—Confirmation of fetal presentations by ultrasound is indicated on admission. Both twins should be monitored continuously during labor. Pediatric and anesthesia personnel should be immediately available, as well as blood bank services.
- Route of delivery—Controversy surrounds the preferred route of delivery for some multiple gestations, especially twins. Although cesarean delivery is frequently used for three or more fetuses, there are reports suggesting that vaginal delivery of triplet gestations, in appropriately monitored patients, is safe. Delivery should be based on individual needs and may depend on the clinician's practice and experience. In general, twins presenting as vertex–vertex should be anticipated to deliver vaginally. If the presenting twin is nonvertex, cesarean delivery is preferred by most physicians. In vertex–nonvertex presentations, cesarean delivery is not always necessary; vaginal delivery of twin B in the nonvertex presentation is a reasonable option for a neonate with an estimated weight greater than 1,500 g.

- Interval between deliveries—The interval between deliveries for twins is not critical in determining the outcome of twin B. Following the delivery of twin A, the fetal heart rate of twin B should be monitored.

SUPPORT PERSONS IN THE DELIVERY ROOM

Childbirth is a momentous family experience. Obstetric providers should willingly provide opportunities for those accompanying and supporting the woman giving birth to participate in the process. These support persons must be informed about requirements for safety and must be willing to follow the directions of the obstetric staff concerning behavior in the delivery room. They also should understand the normal events and procedures in the labor and delivery area. They must conform to the dress code required of personnel in attendance in a delivery room. Both the obstetrician and the patient should consent to the presence of fathers, partners, or other support persons in the delivery room. Support persons should realize that their major function is to provide psychologic support to the mother during labor and delivery.

The judgment of the obstetric staff, the individual obstetrician, the anesthesiologist, and the pediatric support personnel, as well as the policies of the hospital, determine whether support persons may be present at a cesarean delivery. A written policy developed by all involved hospital staff is recommended.

IMMEDIATE POSTPARTUM MATERNAL CARE

Monitoring of maternal status postpartum is dictated in part by the events of the delivery process, the type of anesthesia or analgesia used, and the complications identified. Postanesthesia pain management should be guided by protocols established by the anesthesiologists and obstetricians, in concert. Blood pressure levels and pulse should be monitored at least every 15 minutes and more frequently if complications are encountered. The woman's temperature should be taken at least every 4 hours.

Nursing staff assigned to the delivery and immediate recovery of a woman should have no other obligations. Discharge from the delivery room, which may involve recovery from an anesthetic, should be at the discretion of the physician or certified nurse–midwife or the anesthesiologist in charge.

When regional or general anesthesia has been used for either vaginal or cesarean delivery, the woman should be observed in an appropriately equipped LDR room or labor–delivery–recovery–postpartum (LDRP) room, or in an appropriately staffed and equipped postanesthesia care unit or equivalent area, until she has recovered from the anesthetic. After cesarean delivery, policies for postanesthesia care should not differ from those applied to nonobstetric surgical patients receiving major anesthesia. Policy should ensure that a physician is available in the facility, or at least is nearby, to manage anesthetic complications and provide cardiopulmonary resuscitation for patients in the postanesthesia care unit. The patient should be discharged from the recovery area only at the discretion of, and after communication between, the attending physician or a certified nurse–midwife, anesthesiologist, or certified registered nurse–anesthetist in charge. Vital signs and additional signs or events should be monitored and recorded as they occur.

Postpartum Tubal Sterilization

In evaluating the feasibility and safety or advisability of immediate postpartum sterilization, consideration must be given to the advent of maternal or neonatal problems and other demands on obstetric and anesthesia staff. If postpartum tubal ligation is planned, the delivery has been uncomplicated, and the anesthetic can be continued safely, there is no contraindication to proceeding directly to the sterilization procedure. Preoperative care and evaluation, therefore, become part of delivery room care, especially if the delivery has taken place in a room designed and equipped for abdominal surgery. The obstetrician and anesthesiologist or certified registered nurse–anesthetist should exercise medical judgment regarding the risks, benefits, and safety of the procedure.

When a woman has had prior or concurrent psychologic difficulties, the risks and benefits of early postpartum sterilization must be carefully considered. In patients who have had medical or obstetric complications during their pregnancy or who have cardiovascular, respiratory, infectious, or metabolic abnormalities during the peripartum period (such as serious anemia, hypovolemia, upper respiratory infections, or hypertension), the procedure should be deferred unless there are overriding medical indications for proceeding. Major physiologic changes occur at delivery in all patients. In particular, cardiovascular stability of the patient should be ensured.

In addition to such maternal considerations, special attention also must be paid to situations in which neonatal outcome is in doubt. Both infant survival and long-term well-being may ultimately influence a decision with respect to desire for a subsequent pregnancy.

Furthermore, consideration of the overall number of patients in relationship to available staffing of the labor-delivery suite also is relevant. An elective procedure, such as tubal ligation, should not be attempted at a time when it might compromise other aspects of patient care. Therefore, the decision to proceed with anesthesia and surgery should not only be a joint one between anesthesiologist and obstetrician, but one that also appropriately involves the patient and nursing and pediatric personnel.

Subsequent Postpartum Care

The medical and nursing staff should cooperatively establish specific postpartum policies and procedures. In the postpartum period, staff should help the woman to learn how to care for the general needs of herself and her neonate and should identify potential problems related to her general health.

The physician should note postpartum orders on the patient's medical record (see "ACOG Discharge/Postpartum Form" in Appendix A). If routine postpartum orders are used, they should be printed or written in the medical record, reviewed and modified as necessary for the particular patient, and signed by the physician before the patient is transferred to the postpartum unit. When an LDR/LDRP room is used, the same guidelines should apply.

Bed Rest, Ambulation, and Diet

It is important for the new mother to sleep, regain her strength, and recover from the effects of any analgesic or anesthetic agents that she may have received during labor. In the absence of complications, she may have a regular diet as soon as she wishes. Because early ambulation has been shown to decrease the incidence of subsequent thrombophlebitis, the mother should be encouraged to walk as soon as she feels able to do so. She should not attempt to get out of bed for the first time without assistance. She may shower as soon as she wishes. It may be necessary to administer fluids intravenously for hydration. If the patient has an intravenous line in place, her fluid and hematologic status should be evaluated before it is removed.

Care of the Vulva

Traditional teaching includes that the patient should be taught to cleanse the vulva from anterior vulva to perineum and anus rather than in the reverse direction. Application of an ice bag to the perineum during the first 24 hours after delivery may help reduce pain and swelling that have resulted from pressure of the neonate's head. Orally administered analgesics often are required and usually are sufficient for relief of discomfort from episiotomy or repaired lacerations. Pain that is not relieved by such medication suggests hematoma formation and mandates a careful examination of the vulva, vagina, and rectum. Beginning 24 hours after delivery, moist heat in the form of a warm sitz bath may reduce local discomfort and promote healing.

Care of the Bladder

Women should be encouraged to void as soon as possible after delivery. Often women have difficulty voiding immediately after delivery, possibly because of trauma to the bladder during labor and delivery, regional anesthesia, or vulvar-perineal pain and swelling. In addition, the diuresis that often follows delivery can distend the bladder before the patient is aware of a sensation of a full bladder. To ensure adequate emptying of the bladder, the patient should be checked frequently during the first 24 hours after delivery, with particular attention to displacement of the uterine fundus and any indication of the presence of a fluid-filled bladder above the symphysis. Although every effort should be made to help the patient void spontaneously, catheterization may be necessary. If the patient continues to find voiding difficult, use of a single indwelling catheter is preferable to repeated catheterization.

Care of the Breasts

The woman's decision about breastfeeding determines the appropriate care of the breasts. Breast care for a woman who chooses to breastfeed is outlined in Chapter 7. The woman who chooses not to breastfeed should be reassured that milk production will abate over the first few days after delivery if she does not breastfeed. During the stage of engorgement, the breasts may become painful and should be supported with a well-fitting brassiere. Ice packs and analgesics can help relieve discomfort during this period. Medications for lactation cessation are discouraged. Women who do not wish to breastfeed should be encouraged to avoid nipple stimulation and should be cautioned against continued manual expression of milk.

Temperature Elevation

The condition of a postpartum patient with an elevated temperature ($\geq38°C$ [$\geq100.4°F$] on two occasions, 6 hours apart) should be evaluated (see "Endometriosis" in Chapter 6). The nursery should be notified if the mother develops a fever at any time during the postpartum period, especially after the first 24 hours. The neonate need not be separated from the woman for infection control.

Postpartum Analgesia

After vaginal delivery, analgesic medication may be necessary to relieve perineal and episiotomy pain and facilitate maternal mobility. This is best addressed by administering the drug on an as needed basis according to postpartum orders. Most mothers experience considerable pain in the first 24 hours after cesarean delivery. Although at one time pain was most often treated by intramuscular injections of narcotics, newer techniques, such as spinal or epidural opiates, patient-controlled analgesia, and potent oral analgesics provide better pain relief and greater patient satisfaction. Regardless of the route of administration, opioids can potentially cause respiratory depression and decrease intestinal motility. Therefore, adequate supervision and monitoring should be ensured for all postpartum patients receiving these drugs.

Immunization—Anti-D Immune Globulin and Rubella

An unsensitized, D-negative woman who delivers a D-positive or D^u-positive neonate should receive 300 μg of anti-D immune globulin postpartum, ideally within 72 hours, even when anti-D immune globulin has been administered in the antepartum period. This dose may be inadequate in circumstances in which there is a potential for greater than average fetal-to-maternal hemorrhage, such as abruptio placentae, placenta previa, intrauterine manipulation, and manual removal of the placenta. In these cases, laboratory analysis should be performed to detect excessive maternal-to-fetal hemorrhage and, therefore, determine the proper dose. If indicated, additional anti-D immune globulin should be given.

A patient who is identified as susceptible to rubella virus infection should receive the rubella vaccine in the postpartum period. The rubella vaccine can be administered before discharge, even if the patient is breastfeeding. Patients should be informed of the possibility of transient arthralgia and low-grade fever after rubella immunization.

Length of Hospital Stay

When no complications are present, the postpartum hospital stay ranges from 48 hours for vaginal delivery to 96 hours for cesarean delivery, excluding the day of delivery. When the physician and the mother want a shortened hospital stay, certain minimal criteria should be met:

- The mother is afebrile, with pulse and respirations of normal rate and quality
- Her blood pressure level is within the normal range
- The amount and color of lochia are appropriate for the duration of recovery
- The uterine fundus is firm
- Urinary output is adequate
- Any surgical repair or wound has minimal edema and no evidence of infection and appears to be healing without complication
- The mother is able to ambulate with ease
- There are no abnormal physical or emotional findings
- The mother is able to eat and drink without difficulty
- Arrangements have been made for postpartum follow-up care
- The mother has been instructed in caring for herself and the neonate at home, is aware of deviations from normal, and is prepared to recognize and respond to danger signs and symptoms

- The mother demonstrates readiness to care for herself and her newborn
- Pertinent laboratory results are available, including a postpartum measurement of hemoglobin or hematocrit
- ABO blood group and Rh D type are known, and, if indicated, the appropriate amount of anti-D immune globulin has been administered
- The mother has received instructions on postpartum activity and exercises and common postpartum discomforts and relief measures
- Family members or other support persons are available to the mother for the first few days following discharge

The medical and nursing staff should be sensitive to potential problems associated with shortened hospital stays and should develop mechanisms to address patient questions that arise after discharge. With a shortened hospital stay, a home visit or follow-up telephone conference by a health care provider, such as a lactation nurse within 48 hours of discharge is encouraged.

When a pregnancy, labor, or delivery is complicated by medical or obstetric disorders, the mother's readiness for discharge may be based on the aforementioned criteria, as modified by the individual judgment of the obstetric care provider. The stability of the woman's medical condition, the need for continued inpatient observation, and treatment and risks of complications should be taken into consideration.

Postpartum Nutritional Guidelines

Postnatal dietary guidelines are similar to those established during pregnancy (see Table 4–2 in Chapter 4). The minimal caloric requirement for adequate milk production in a woman of average size is 1,800 kcal per day. A balanced, nutritious diet will ensure both the quality and the quantity of the milk produced without depletion of maternal stores. Fluid intake by the mother is governed by thirst.

A vitamin-mineral supplement is not needed routinely. Mothers at nutritional risk should be given a multivitamin supplement with particular emphasis on calcium and vitamins B_{12} and D. Iron should be administered only if the mother herself needs it.

Maternal postpartum weight loss can occur at a rate of 2 lb per month without affecting lactation. On average, a woman will retain 2 lb more than her prepregnancy weight at 1 year postpartum. There is no relationship between body mass index or total weight gain and weight retention. Aging, rather than parity, is the major determinant of increases in a woman's weight over time.

Residual postpartum retention of weight gained during pregnancy that results in obesity is a concern. Special attention to lifestyle, including exercise and eating habits, will help these women return to a normal body mass index.

POSTPARTUM CONSIDERATIONS

Before discharge, the mother should receive information about normal postpartum events, including:

- Changes in lochia pattern expected in the first few weeks
- Range of activities that she may reasonably undertake
- Care of the breasts, perineum, and bladder
- Dietary needs, particularly if she is breastfeeding
- Recommended amount of exercise
- Emotional responses
- Signs of complications (eg, temperature elevation, chills, leg pains, episiotomy or wound drainage, increased vaginal bleeding)

The length of convalescence that the patient can expect, based on the type of delivery, also should be discussed. For women who have had cesarean delivery, additional precautions may be appropriate, such as wound care and temporary abstinence from lifting objects heavier than the newborn and from driving motor vehicles. It is helpful to reinforce oral discussions with written information.

The earliest time at which coitus may be resumed safely after childbirth is unknown. Resumption of coitus should be discussed with the couple. Risks of hemorrhage and infection are minimal approximately 2 weeks postpartum. By this time, the uterus has involuted markedly and the endometrium and cervix have begun to reepithelialize.

Thereafter, coitus can be resumed, depending on the patient's desire and comfort and on resolution of contraceptive issues. Sexual difficulties that are common in the early months after childbirth should be discussed. Healing at the episiotomy site can cause the woman some discomfort during intercourse within the first year following delivery. In the lactating woman, the vagina often is atrophic and dry. Lubrication during sexual excitement may be unsatisfactory. Furthermore, the demands of the newborn's care alter the couple's ability to find time for physical intimacy.

Methods of contraception should be fully reviewed and implemented. Nonnursing mothers may begin using a contraceptive soon after delivery if they wish to avoid becoming pregnant. Combined oral contraceptives may be prescribed, or levonorgestrel implants or depot medroxyprogesterone acetate can be initiated before discharge. Nonnursing women may receive depot medroxyprogesterone acetate within 5 days after delivery. Nursing women should delay such an injection until lactation is established.

Nursing mothers may begin using oral contraceptives as soon as their milk supply is established. Progesterone-only contraceptives do not appear to have adverse effects on lactation. An intrauterine device that contains copper also is an option that does not interfere with breast milk. However, intrauterine devices generally are not inserted until 4–6 weeks postpartum. A diaphragm or a cervical cap cannot be fitted adequately during the immediate postpartum period and should be delayed until the 4–6-week examination.

Patients for whom the use of oral contraceptives is contraindicated or who prefer other methods of contraception, such as foam or condoms, should be offered instruction in their use. Spermicides and barrier methods have no effect on breastfeeding. Lubricated condoms may offset vaginal dryness secondary to breastfeeding. Fertility awareness methods, such as the rhythm method, are difficult to practice accurately before the resumption of menses and, therefore, are not recommended.

At the time of discharge, the family should be given the name of the person to contact if questions or problems arise for either the mother or the newborn. Arrangements should be made for a follow-up examination and specific instructions conveyed to the woman, including when contact is advisable.

In general, the following points should be reviewed with the mother or, preferably, with both parents; specific information to be conveyed is discussed within this section.

- Condition of the newborn
- Immediate needs of the newborn (eg, feeding methods and environmental supports)
- Feeding techniques; skin care, including umbilical cord care; temperature assessment and measurement with a thermometer; and assessment of neonatal well-being and recognition of illness
- Roles of the obstetrician, pediatrician, and other members of the health care team concerned with the continuous medical care of the mother and the newborn
- Availability of support systems, including psychosocial support
- Instructions to follow in the event of a complication or emergency
- Importance of maintaining newborn immunization, beginning with an initial dose of hepatitis B virus vaccine

Follow-up Care

The physical and psychosocial status of the mother and the newborn should be subject to ongoing assessment after discharge. The new mother needs personalized care during the postpartum period to hasten the development of a healthy mother–infant relationship and a sense of maternal confidence. Support and reassurance should be provided as the woman masters newborn-care tasks and adapts to her maternal role. Involving the father and encouraging him to participate in the newborn's care not only can provide additional support to the woman but also can enhance the father–infant relationship.

The postpartum period is a time of developmental adjustment for the whole family. Family members now have new roles and relationships, and an effort should be made to assess the progress of the family's adaptation. If a family member—parent or sibling—finds it difficult to assume the new role, the health care team should arrange for sensitive, supportive assistance. This is particularly important for adolescent mothers, for whom it may be necessary to mobilize multiple resources within the community.

Postpartum Visits

Approximately 4–6 weeks after delivery, the mother should visit her physician for a postpartum review and examination (see Appendix H). This interval may be modified according to the needs of the patient with medical, obstetric, or intercurrent complications. A visit within 7–14 days of delivery may be advisable after a cesarean delivery or a complicated gestation.

The review at the first postpartum visit should include obtaining an interval history and performing a physical examination to evaluate the patient's current status and her adaptation to the newborn. Specific inquiries regarding breastfeeding should be made. The examination should include an evaluation of weight, blood pressure levels, breasts, and abdomen, as well as a pelvic examination. Episiotomy repair and uterine involution should be evaluated and a Pap test performed, if needed. Methods of birth control should be reviewed or initiated.

Many women experience some degree of emotional lability in the postpartum period. If this persists or develops into clinically significant depression, intervention may be needed. The emotional status of a woman whose pregnancy had an abnormal outcome also should be reviewed. Counseling should address specific issues regarding her future health and pregnancies. For example, it may be advantageous to discuss VBAC or the implications of diabetes mellitus, intrauterine growth restriction, preterm birth, hypertension, fetal anomalies, or other conditions that may recur in any future pregnancies. Laboratory data should be obtained as indicated. This is a good time to review immunizations, including rubella vaccination for women who are susceptible and did not receive the vaccine immediately postpartum, and to discuss any special problems. The patient should be encouraged to return for subsequent periodic examinations.

The postpartum visit is an excellent time to begin preconceptional counseling for patients who may wish to have future pregnancies (see also "Preconceptional Care" in Chapter 4). This counseling includes risk assessment to facilitate the planning, spacing, and timing of the next pregnancy; health promotion measures; and timely intervention to reduce medical and psychosocial risks. Such intervention may include treatment of infections, counseling regarding behaviors such as those related to sexually transmitted infections, nutrition counseling, supplementation, and appropriate referrals for follow-up care. Although physiologic considerations indicate that a woman can return to a normal work schedule 4–6 weeks after delivery, attention also should be given to maternal–infant bonding.

Bibliography

American Academy of Pediatrics, American College of Obstetricians and Gynecologists. Use and abuse of the Apgar score. ACOG Committee Opinion 174. Elk Grove Village (IL): AAP; Washington, DC: ACOG; 1996.

American Academy of Pediatrics, American Heart Association. Neonatal resuscitation textbook. 4th ed. Elk Grove Village (IL): AAP; Dallas (TX): AHA; 2000.

American College of Obstetricians and Gynecologists. Assessment of fetal lung maturity. ACOG Educational Bulletin 230. Washington, DC: ACOG; 1996.

American College of Obstetricians and Gynecologists. Dystocia and the augmentation of labor. ACOG Technical Bulletin 218. Washington, DC: ACOG; 1995.

American College of Obstetricians and Gynecologists. Fetal heart rate patterns: monitoring, interpretation, and management. ACOG Technical Bulletin 207. Washington, DC: ACOG; 1995.

American College of Obstetricians and Gynecologists. Inappropriate use of the terms fetal distress and birth asphyxia. ACOG Committee Opinion 197. Washington, DC: ACOG; 1998.

American College of Obstetricians and Gynecologists. Induction of labor. ACOG Practice Bulletin 10. Washington, DC: ACOG; 1999.

American College of Obstetricians and Gynecologists. Induction of labor with misoprostol. ACOG Committee Opinion 228. Washington, DC: ACOG; 1999.

American College of Obstetricians and Gynecologists. Operative vaginal delivery. ACOG Practice Bulletin 17. Washington, DC: ACOG; 2000.

American College of Obstetricians and Gynecologists. Response to Searle's drug warning on misoprostol. Committee Opinion 248. Washington, DC: ACOG; 2000.

American College of Obstetricians and Gynecologists. Task Force on Cesarean Delivery Rates. Evaluation of cesarean delivery. Washington, DC: ACOG; 2000.

American College of Obstetricians and Gynecologists. Utility of umbilical cord blood acid-base assessment. ACOG Committee Opinion 138. Washington, DC: ACOG; 1994.

American College of Obstetricians and Gynecologists. Vaginal birth after previous cesarean delivery. ACOG Practice Bulletin 5. Washington, DC: ACOG; 1999.

American College of Obstetricians and Gynecologists, American Society of Anesthesiologists. Optimal goals for anesthesia care in obstetrics. ACOG Committee Opinion 256. Washington, DC: ACOG; Park Ridge (IL): ASA; 2001.

American College of Obstetricians and Gynecologists, American Society of Anesthesiologists. Pain relief during labor. ACOG Committee Opinion 231. Washington, DC: ACOG; Park Ridge (IL): ASA; 2000.

Analgesia and cesarean delivery rates. ACOG Committee Opinion 269. American College of Obstetricians and Gynecologists. Obstet Gynecol 2002;99:369–70.

Induction of labor for vaginal birth after cesarean delivery. ACOG Committee Opinion 271. American College of Obstetricians and Gynecologists. Obstet Gynecol 2002;99:679–80.

Mode of term singleton breech delivery. ACOG Committee Opinion 265. American College of Obstetricians and Gynecologists. Obstet Gynecol 2001; 98:1189–90.

National Institute of Child Health and Human Development. Report of the workshop on acute perinatal asphyxia in term infants. Washington, DC: NICHHD; 1996. NIH publication 96-3823.

Obstetric analgesia and anesthesia. ACOG Practice Bulletin 36. American College of Obstetricians and Gynecologists. Obstet Gynecol 2002;100:177–91.

CHAPTER 6

Obstetric and Medical Complications

Certain complications of pregnancy, labor, or delivery may require more intensive surveillance, monitoring, and special care of the obstetric patient. Often complications can arise without warning. In some cases, early detection and timely intervention can improve outcome. When there is a high risk of complications, it may be advisable to make arrangements for such care in advance. The pediatric and anesthesia service should be made aware of such patients so that appropriate medical care can be planned in advance of the delivery.

Management of Preterm Birth

Preterm birth is defined as delivery before 37 weeks of gestation. It pertains to approximately 11% of all births in the United States and as many as 15% of births from lower socioeconomic populations.

Of all preterm births, 40–50% result from preterm labor, approximately 25–40% from preterm premature rupture of the membranes (PROM), and 20–30% from maternal medical or obstetric complications. Ideally, preterm birth should occur in a hospital setting with personnel and equipment appropriate for the stage of gestation. Very low-birth-weight neonates (weighing < 1,500 g) should be delivered in a subspecialty care facility whenever possible. Although no definitive method of preventing preterm birth has yet been discovered, glucocorticoids are effective in enhancing fetal maturity when a woman is at risk of preterm birth (see "Antenatal Glucocorticoid Administration" in this chapter).

PRETERM LABOR

Strategies for reducing the incidence of preterm birth in the United States have focused on enhanced physician and patient education about the risks for preterm labor, as well as programs to detect uterine activity before term. These approaches are used to ensure that women in preterm labor are evaluated during labor and, when possible, treated at the earliest possible time to prevent preterm birth. Care of the patient who develops preterm labor is directed toward optimizing the outcome for the preterm newborn.

Diagnosis

The timely diagnosis of preterm labor remains problematic. The suggested criteria for diagnosis of preterm labor include:

- Gestation of 20 weeks or greater but less than 37 weeks
- Persistent uterine contractions (four every 20 minutes or eight every 60 minutes)

    and

    — Documented cervical change

    or

    — Cervical effacement of 80% or greater

    or

    — Cervical dilatation of greater than 1 cm

A shortened (less than 2.5 cm in length) cervix as measured by transvaginal cervical ultrasound, fetal fibronectin testing, or a combination of both may be useful in determining women at high risk for preterm labor. However, they are not recommended for routine screening of the general obstetric population. Although a negative fetal fibronectin test result is useful in ruling out imminent preterm labor (ie, within 2 weeks) in symptomatic women, the implications of a positive test result are less clear. There are no current data to support the use of salivary estriol, home uterine activity monitoring, or bacterial vaginitis screening as strategies to identify or prevent preterm birth.

Patients with suspected preterm labor should be examined and observed for 1–2 hours and should have their activity restricted to confirm whether uterine activity is significant and whether the cervix has changed since the most recent examination. After observation, the cervical examination should be repeated, preferably by the same examiner, to help determine whether cervical dilation or effacement is taking place. Because preterm labor often is associated with urinary tract infections, an examination of urine with a microscope and urine culture may be helpful. Based on the test results, antibiotic treatment can be instituted. Ultrasound examination might be considered to confirm gestational age and to assess the presence of any congenital anomalies.

Women diagnosed as having false labor may be discharged once true labor has been excluded. Depending on gestational age and clinical condition, consideration should be given to initiating interventions, such as tocolysis, glucocorticoid therapy, and chemoprophylaxis for group B streptococcal infection, when preterm labor is diagnosed (see "Tocolysis" and "Antenatal Glucocorticoid Administration" in this chapter and "Group B Streptococci" in Chapter 9).

Occult Infection

Because infections have been implicated as both a cause and a consequence of ruptured membranes, the diagnosis of infection is an important component of the evaluation of preterm labor. This diagnosis may be difficult to establish because clinical signs of infection may be absent at the initial evaluation. A variety of organisms, including group B streptococci, *Neisseria gonorrhoeae, Listeria monocytogenes, Mycoplasma* species, *Bacteroides* species, and *Ureaplasma* species have been identified in amniotic fluid. Although the threshold at which colonization is significant enough to result in preterm labor has not yet been defined and the exact proportion of preterm labor that is attributable to infection is unknown, the incidence of infection is highest with ruptured membranes. In the presence of infection, the time from the onset of preterm labor to delivery is shorter and preterm PROM is more likely.

Intraamniotic Infection

Preterm labor may be the first sign of intraamniotic infection in the absence of rupture of the membranes. Organisms may be recovered from the chorioamnion in as many as 60% of women in preterm labor with intact membranes and from the amniotic fluid in 10–15% of women who are not in labor and have intact membranes. Preterm labor at early gestational ages is more likely to be associated with occult intraamniotic infection. Women with poor nutrition or of a low socioeconomic background may be at higher risk for this complication. Intraamniotic infection also may follow amniocentesis or cervical cerclage.

All patients in preterm labor should be evaluated for evidence of chorioamnionitis. Maternal temperature and white blood cell count should be documented and the uterus palpated for tenderness. Maternal or fetal tachycardia could indicate chorioamnionitis. Amniocentesis may be appropriate to detect the presence of occult chorioamnionitis by revealing a low amniotic fluid glucose concentration, the presence of white blood cells, or a positive culture.

When chorioamnionitis is diagnosed during pregnancy, broad-spectrum antibiotic therapy should be initiated and delivery effected. Vaginal delivery should be anticipated, and cesarean delivery should be reserved for standard obstetric indications. The choice of antibiotics should take into consideration the polymicrobial nature of most uterine infections that reflect endogenous vaginal flora. The combination of ampicillin or penicillin, plus an aminoglycoside, provides appropriate coverage of most organisms. If a cesarean delivery is required, anaerobes play a prominent role, and clindamycin or metronidazole should be added to the regimen. Extended spectrum cephalosporins also provide appropriate coverage if a cesarean delivery is needed. Antibiotics should be given intravenously to prevent serious complications of infection in the woman and to prevent or treat transplacental infection of the fetus.

Tocolysis

Although tocolytic agents have been used for the past two decades to prevent or stop labor, it is not readily apparent that their use has decreased the rate of preterm birth or associated perinatal mortality. They do not appear to markedly prolong the length of gestation, but may delay delivery in some patients for at least 48 hours. This delay may provide a window of opportunity for transporting the patient to a regional subspecialty obstetric center and administering antenatal glucocorticoid therapy.

Many clinicians attempt to arrest idiopathic preterm labor by using tocolytic agents at less than 34 weeks of gestation; the use of these agents generally is not recommended after 34 weeks of gestation. Attempts at tocolysis are rarely effective when cervical dilatation has reached 4 cm or more, especially if the cervix is well effaced. The potential risks and benefits of tocolytic therapy must be weighed against the risks of preterm delivery. Conditions that limit the chance of success of tocolysis include incompetent cervix, ruptured membranes, and advanced labor (cervical dilatation ≥4 cm and well effaced).

When preterm labor is suspected, a decision must be made regarding the appropriateness of tocolytic therapy and the choice of agent. Antenatal glucocorticoid therapy should be given to enhance fetal maturation at less than 34 weeks of gestation or whenever fetal lung immaturity has been documented (see "Antenatal Glucocorticoid Administration" in this chapter). The medical history should be reviewed and a physical examination repeated to determine whether there are any contraindications to such therapy. Contraindications to tocolysis that are based on clinical circumstances (particularly gestational age) should take into account the risks of continuing the pregnancy versus those of delivery. General contraindications for tocolytic use include:

- Assessment of fetal status is nonreassuring (except when used for acute intrauterine resuscitation)
- Chorioamnionitis
- Eclampsia or severe preeclampsia
- Fetal demise (singleton)
- Fetal maturity
- Maternal hemodynamic instability

Contraindications for the following specific tocolytic agents include:
- β-mimetic agents
  — Maternal cardiac rhythm disturbance or other cardiac disease
  — Poorly controlled diabetes mellitus, thyrotoxicosis, or hypertension

- Magnesium sulfate
  - Hypocalcemia
  - Myasthenia gravis
  - Renal failure
- Indomethacin
  - Asthma
  - Coronary artery disease
  - Gastrointestinal bleeding (active or past history)
  - Oligohydramnios
  - Renal failure
  - Suspected fetal cardiac or renal anomaly
- Nifedipine—Maternal liver disease

Currently, the two most accepted tocolytic therapies are β-sympathomimetic agents and intravenous magnesium sulfate. Less widely used are calcium channel blockers (such as nifedipine) and prostaglandin synthetase inhibitors (such as indomethacin). Ritodrine hydrochloride remains the only drug approved by the U.S. Food and Drug Administration specifically for the indication of preterm labor. Terbutaline sulfate has actions and side effects similar to those of ritodrine. Although labeled for the treatment of asthma, terbutaline has been used off-label for preterm labor because of its relative advantages in cost, longer half-life, and the convenience of subcutaneous dosing. Magnesium sulfate is similar in efficacy to the β-sympathomimetics and has fewer side effects.

Preterm Premature Rupture of Membranes

Preterm PROM is a major risk factor for obstetric complications because of its association with perinatal infection, preterm delivery, and resultant complications. Preterm PROM is responsible for 25–35% of all preterm deliveries, depending on racial and socioeconomic considerations.

The following factors may be helpful in planning the management of patients with preterm PROM:

- Gestational age
- Presence or absence of chorioamnionitis

- Rectal and vaginal cultures for group B streptococci
- Amniocentesis for Gram stain and culture of amniotic fluid, leukocyte count, glucose concentration, and fetal lung maturity
- Presence or absence of labor
- Possibility of a compromised fetus
- Fetal presentation
- Cervical inducibility

The status of the fetus should be assessed by fetal heart rate monitoring, with particular attention to variable decelerations that are consistent with umbilical cord compression. Determining whether the woman is in labor may be difficult because digital examination of the cervix should be avoided until active labor occurs or until the decision has been made to induce labor.

When preterm PROM occurs, expectant management with close observation usually is attempted. If fetal pulmonary maturity can be confirmed by assessment of amniotic fluid, delivery usually is chosen, especially if the gestational age is known to be greater than or equal to 32 weeks. Many providers will proceed with delivery if preterm PROM has occurred at or beyond 34 weeks of gestation, based on the belief that the risks of complications from infection outweigh the risks of preterm delivery at this point. A hospital's departments of obstetrics and gynecology and pediatrics should develop guidelines for the management of preterm PROM, recognizing the need to individualize patient care. If expectant management is chosen in a woman with preterm PROM, bed rest is indicated. Repeat evaluations should be performed to detect chorioamnionitis and fetal compromise.

The prophylactic use of antibiotics can prolong gestation in women with preterm PROM and may improve perinatal outcome. When used, they should be used according to published protocols. A culture for group B streptococci is not needed if prophylactic antibiotics are used.

The use of glucocorticoids to accelerate fetal pulmonary maturity is recommended for women with preterm PROM at less than 32 weeks of gestation in the absence of clinical chorioamnionitis and may be considered between 32 and 34 weeks of gestation (see "Antenatal Gluco-corticoid Administration" in this chapter). Tocolytic agents may be useful to permit administration of glucocorticoids and antibiotics and to facilitate transfer to a perinatal care center.

When preterm PROM occurs before a viable gestational age, conservative management is unlikely to result in the delivery of a healthy neonate and entails significant risk of maternal morbidity. Such management may produce very preterm neonates, resulting in significant short- and long-term morbidity. Some patients may elect induction of labor with no expectation of neonatal survival or resuscitation. If the woman elects to continue the pregnancy, management at home may be considered. It is strongly suggested that women who have preterm PROM at a previable gestational age be counseled by both an obstetrician and a pediatrician. A woman should participate fully in the decision regarding her pregnancy, and adequate time should be allowed for her to make an informed decision. In the presence of chorioamnionitis, delivery is indicated.

ANTENATAL GLUCOCORTICOID ADMINISTRATION

Following a 1994 consensus conference, the National Institutes of Health concluded that the use of antenatal glucocorticoid therapy to induce fetal maturation is effective in reducing respiratory distress syndrome, intraventricular hemorrhage, and mortality in preterm neonates. These benefits accrue at less than 34 weeks of gestation and are not limited by sex or race. Optimal benefits begin 24 hours after the initiation of therapy and last 7 days, although treatment of less than 24 hours also may improve outcome. Furthermore, antenatal glucocorticoid therapy may complement the benefit of postnatal surfactant therapy.

Following a 2000 consensus conference, the National Institutes of Health reauthorized their 1994 recommendation of giving a single course of glucocorticoids to all pregnant women between 24 and 34 weeks of gestation who are at risk of preterm delivery within 7 days. This panel also recommended that because of insufficient scientific evidence, repeat glucocorticoid courses, including so-called "rescue therapy," should not be routinely used but should be reserved for women enrolled in clinical trials. Treatment should consist of two doses of

12 mg of betamethasone given intramuscularly 24 hours apart or four doses of 6 mg dexamethasone given intramuscularly every 12 hours in patients at risk for preterm delivery between 24 and 34 weeks of gestation with intact membranes or between 24 and 32 weeks of gestation for patients with ruptured membranes.

Data from trials involving the follow-up of children for as long as 12 years indicate that antenatal glucocorticoid therapy does not adversely affect physical growth or psychomotor development. Therefore, with few exceptions, antenatal glucocorticoid therapy is indicated for women with anticipated preterm delivery at less than 34 weeks of gestation. The use of antenatal glucocorticoid therapy after 34 weeks of gestation is not recommended unless there is evidence of fetal pulmonary immaturity. The use of antenatal glucocorticoids for fetal maturation is an example of an intervention technology that yields substantial cost savings in addition to improving health.

BIRTHS AT THE THRESHOLD OF VIABILITY

The anticipated birth of a neonate at the threshold of viability (25 or fewer completed weeks of gestation) presents a variety of complex medical, social, and ethical concerns. It is important to counsel the parents anticipating such a birth about the expectations for outcome of the neonate and the risks and benefits of various approaches to care. Ideally, obstetric and neonatal health care providers will confer before counseling the parents. Each member of the health care team should make every effort to maintain a consistent theme in their discussions with family members regarding the assessment, prognosis, and recommendations for care. If time allows, additional input from other important sources, such as clergy and social workers, can be offered to the parents.

It is recommended that counseling in anticipation of extreme preterm birth include the following information:

- An overview of the potential problems and their treatment and complications
- A range of the most current possible survival rates, allowing for some error in the best estimate of gestational age and estimated fetal weight (see Figs. I–1 and I–2 in the "Introduction")

- The possibility of long-term disabilities, including blindness, cerebral palsy, mental retardation, and requirements for special education
- There are no data to support a benefit of routine cesarean delivery for vertex presentation
- The possibility that expectations for the newborn may change after delivery, based on a more accurate assessment of the gestational age and condition of the newborn
- Care should be taken not to characterize interventions of unproven benefit as "doing everything possible" for the fetus or neonate

In some instances, counseling could result in parents choosing a nonintervention approach, such as remaining in a community hospital or electing vaginal rather than cesarean delivery. Because the benefits of various obstetric management approaches have not yet been established, families should be supported in such decisions. When a decision is made not to resuscitate or to discontinue resuscitation because of nonviability, the family should be treated with dignity and compassion. Support should be provided to the family by physicians, nurses, and other staff beyond the time of the infant's death. Perinatal loss support groups, intermittent contact by telephone, and a later conference with the family to review the medical events surrounding the infant's death and to evaluate the grieving response of the parents often are helpful.

Preeclampsia

Preeclampsia is a disorder of unknown cause that is characterized by hypertension, proteinuria, and edema occurring after 20 weeks of gestation. Preeclampsia complicates approximately 5–8% of pregnancies and is a major cause of maternal and perinatal morbidity and mortality. Efforts to prevent preeclampsia using low-dose aspirin or calcium supplementation have not been successful and are not recommended for routine use in pregnancy.

Treatment of preeclampsia should be directed primarily toward ensuring the safety of the woman, followed closely by the delivery of a healthy, mature neonate. When preeclampsia is diagnosed during the intrapartum period, initial management should include assessing the condition of both the woman and the fetus and administering prophylaxis for maternal seizures. Although the most effective treatment is delivery, other considerations also affect management:

- Severity of preeclampsia
- Gestational age
- Maternal condition
- Fetal condition
- Presence of labor
- Availability of hospital staff and resources
- Capability of hospital staff

Mild preeclampsia before term often can be managed with in-hospital or careful home observation. The disease process is regarded as mild when the following are present:

- Blood pressure levels greater than or equal to 140 mm Hg systolic or greater than or equal to 90 mm Hg diastolic that occurs after 20 weeks of gestation in a woman with previously normal blood pressure levels
- Proteinuria, defined as urinary excretion of greater than or equal to 0.3 g protein in a 24-hour urine specimen

Preeclampsia is considered severe if one or more of the following criteria is present:

- Blood pressure levels of greater than or equal to 160 mm Hg systolic or greater than or equal to 110 mm Hg diastolic on two occasions at least 6 hours apart while the patient is on bedrest
- Proteinuria of greater than or equal to 5 g in a 24-hour urine collection or 3 + or greater on two random urine samples collected at least 4 hours apart
- Oliguria of less than 500 mL in 24 hours

- Cerebral or visual disturbances
- Pulmonary edema or cyanosis
- Epigastric or right upper quadrant pain
- Impaired liver function
- Thrombocytopenia or evidence of hemolysis or both
- Fetal growth restriction

The development of severe preeclampsia usually warrants delivery of the neonate, irrespective of gestational age or fetal maturity. The presence of the HELLP Syndrome, which includes hemolysis, elevated liver enzymes, and low platelet counts, also is an indication for delivery to avoid jeopardizing the health of the woman. There is an increased risk of preeclampsia among women with the antiphospholipid antibody syndrome or one of the heritable thrombophilic disorders. Women with early development of severe preeclampsia should be evaluated for lupus anticoagulant, anticardiolipin antibodies, the factor V Leiden gene mutation, the prothrombin G20210A mutation and deficiencies of antithrombin, protein S and protein C.

Fetuses of women with preeclampsia are at increased risk of a nonreassuring heart rate during labor. Once labor is established, the route of delivery is determined by obstetric factors. Oxytocin augmentation of labor can be used if needed.

SEIZURE PROPHYLAXIS

Magnesium sulfate is the drug of choice for the prevention or treatment of eclamptic convulsions and is superior to phenytoin and diazepam for these purposes. Therapy with magnesium sulfate should be initiated intravenously with a loading dose followed by a continuous infusion of magnesium sulfate. In most situations, clinical assessment of respirations, deep tendon reflexes, and urine output is adequate to monitor for maternal magnesium toxicity without the need to determine the actual maternal serum magnesium levels. If toxic serum levels or side effects are encountered, magnesium sulfate infusion must be discontinued, and calcium gluconate may be administered to reverse these effects.

ANTIHYPERTENSIVE THERAPY

Severe hypertension with a systolic blood pressure level of 160 mm Hg or greater and a diastolic blood pressure level of 110 mm Hg or greater increases the maternal risks of cerebrovascular accidents and congestive heart failure. Reducing the woman's diastolic blood pressure level to 90–100 mm Hg is recommended.

Hydralazine is the most widely used agent for the treatment of acute hypertension in pregnancy, has almost universal efficacy, and is extremely safe. Labetalol is equally effective, although it has a wide range of individual dosing requirements. The calcium antagonist nifedipine, when administered orally (not sublingually) to postpartum patients with severe preeclampsia, offers good blood pressure control and cardiorenal protection. Caution should be used to avoid the possibility of sudden hypotension if a calcium channel blocker (such as nifedipine) is used in conjunction with magnesium sulfate infusion. This effect can be reversed with calcium gluconate.

FLUID BALANCE

Patients with severe preeclampsia are at increased risk of fluid overload and pulmonary edema. Fluid intake and urine output should be assessed hourly before delivery. Total intravenous intake should rarely exceed 100–125 mL per hour. Because intrapartum oliguria is common (especially with oxytocin usage), its presence should not be treated with repetitive "bolus" crystalloid infusions.

Following delivery (especially cesarean delivery), oliguria is most commonly caused by hypovolemia. The initial management of postdelivery oliguria is directed at volume replacement with an infusion of 500 mL of crystalloid over 20 minutes. If oliguria persists after delivery and the woman is anemic, the need for a packed red blood cell transfusion should be considered. Repetitive bolus infusions of crystalloid solution in such patients without red blood cell replacement increase the risk of pulmonary edema and acute renal failure. In rare instances, oliguria that persists despite conservative measures is an indication for invasive hemodynamic monitoring to guide fluid, electrolyte, and blood replacement more accurately.

Deep Vein Thrombosis and Pulmonary Embolism

The risk of venous thromboembolic disease may be increased during pregnancy and is definitely increased during the puerperium in association with increased venous stasis in the lower extremities and increased levels of circulating procoagulants. Risk factors for thromboembolism include cesarean delivery, obesity, trauma, infection, and prolonged bedrest. Women with a personal or family history of venous thromboembolic disease should be evaluated for hereditary and acquired thrombophilic disorders, including:

- Antiphospholipid syndrome (lupus anticoagulant, anticardiolipin antibodies)
- Factor V Leiden gene mutation
- Prothrombin G20210A mutation
- Hyperhomocysteinemia associated with a methylenetetrahydrofolate reductase mutation
- Deficiencies of antithrombin, protein C, protein S

The diagnosis of deep vein thrombosis (DVT) is best made by compression ultrasound examination or impedance plethysmography. Most instances of pulmonary embolism are associated with symptoms such as dyspnea, tachypnea, pleuritic chest pain, and hemoptysis. The diagnosis is most likely in a patient who also has a reduced Pao_2 (<80 mmHg) and an abnormal ventilation or perfusion lung scan. It should be emphasized, however, that a normal arterial blood gas analysis does not rule out a pulmonary embolism.

Anticoagulation is the mainstay of therapy for DVT with or without pulmonary embolism. Acute thromboembolism associated with pregnancy requires an intravenous heparin bolus of 5,000 IU (80 IU/kg) followed by continuous infusion of at least 30,000 IU for 24 hours titrated to achieve full anticoagulation.

Venous thrombosis or pulmonary embolism or both also may be treated effectively with low-molecular-weight heparin. Although laboratory testing appears not to be essential in the nonpregnant patient, the role of monitoring anti-factor Xa levels is not clear in the pregnant patient. The effectiveness of low-molecular-weight heparin is less affected by changes in maternal physiology than is heparin. But there are still changes as the pregnancy progresses. Therefore, it may be warranted to periodically reevaluate anti-factor Xa levels during pregnancy in a woman on adjusted-dose or full anticoagulation. Ideally, dosing should be enough to achieve a peak anti-factor Xa level of 0.5–1.2 U/mL.

Intravenous heparin or low-molecular-weight heparin is continued for 5–7 days or until the symptoms have resolved and there is no evidence of recurrence. Patients should continue anticoagulation with heparin for at least 3 months during and following delivery. Alternatively, warfarin may be used for anticoagulation postpartum and does not contraindicate breastfeeding.

A pregnant woman with a history of DVT or pulmonary embolism, without active disease, may be a candidate for prophylaxis during pregnancy with mini-dose heparin (5,000 U every 12 hours). She should be anticoagulated during the puerperium.

Trauma During Pregnancy

Trauma and other forms of violence are the leading causes of death in women of reproductive age and one of the leading causes of nonobstetric maternal death. Physical trauma is estimated to complicate 1 of every 12 pregnancies. Obstetricians are uniquely qualified to play a vital role in the management of trauma during pregnancy. They understand the effects of altered maternal physiology and anatomy on the management of trauma and its effects on the fetus. The obstetrician's role in ensuring both maternal and fetal well-being is paramount in the management of pregnant trauma victims. Whether acting as a consultant or as a primary physician when seeing a pregnant trauma victim, the obstetrician should provide maternal–fetal care that is timely and systematic to ensure maternal medical stabilization and fetal evaluation.

EVALUATION

Pregnancy should not restrict the use of any of the usual diagnostic, pharmacologic, or resuscitative procedures or maneuvers provided to trauma victims. The more seriously injured the woman, the more important it is to follow a methodic evaluation that ensures her complete assessment and stabilization. Serious or life-threatening maternal injuries could be overlooked if maternal evaluation is not thorough during stabilization. The finding of nonreasurring fetal status by heart rate monitoring or ultrasonography may alert the clinician to more severe maternal injuries than were initially appreciated. To prevent supine hypotension syndrome, deflection of the uterus off the inferior vena cava and abdominal aorta can be obtained by placing the patient in the lateral decubitus position. This position should be maintained throughout evaluation.

Following stabilization, a more detailed secondary survey of the patient, including a thorough ultrasound evaluation of the pregnancy, should be performed. Ultrasonography in this setting can be useful to determine estimated gestational age, placental localization, fetal cardiac function or demise, amniotic fluid volume, and the presence of intraabdominal fluid.

Once the woman's condition has been stabilized, continuous fetal monitoring is recommended when the fetus's gestational age approaches viability. Monitoring and further evaluation are warranted if uterine contractions, a nonreassuring fetal heart rate pattern, vaginal bleeding, significant uterine tenderness or irritability, serious maternal injury, or rupture of the amniotic membranes is present. Monitoring periods of 2–6 hours usually are adequate if there are no uterine contractions, uterine tenderness, or bleeding. Abruptio placentae usually becomes apparent shortly after injury.

Use of open peritoneal lavage to diagnose intraperitoneal hemorrhage has been shown to be safe, sensitive, and specific during pregnancy, particularly in association with abdominal signs and symptoms of intraperitoneal bleeding, altered sensorium, major thoracic injury, unexplained shock, and multiple major orthopedic injuries. This procedure is unnecessary if clinically obvious intraperitoneal bleeding is present or if ultrasound findings are highly suggestive of free blood in the peritoneal cavity.

TREATMENT

In general, aggressive exploratory laparotomy is advocated for gunshot wounds and other penetrating trauma to the abdomen during pregnancy. Laparotomy alone is not an indication to perform cesarean delivery. The fetus usually tolerates surgery and anesthesia well if adequate oxygenation and uterine perfusion are maintained. The uterus should be carefully inspected for injury at the time of laparotomy.

Administration of 300 μg of anti-D immune globulin within 72 hours of injury should protect nearly all (90%) D-negative trauma victims with substantial abdominal trauma and possible D isoimmunization. The Kleihauer–Betke test or a similar quantitative assay of fetal–maternal hemorrhage may be used to detect a fetomaternal transfusion of 30 mL or greater, which may require additional anti-D immune globulin.

Following evaluation and hospital discharge, the patient should be instructed to seek care if she develops vaginal bleeding, leakage of fluid, decreased fetal movement, or severe abdominal pain. Measures to prevent the recurrence of trauma also should be discussed.

Postmortem cesarean delivery more than 10–15 minutes after maternal death is unlikely to result in neonatal survival. If a fetus does survive, there may be a high risk of adverse neurodevelopmental sequelae. After 5 minutes of unsuccessful maternal cardiac resuscitation, perimortem cesarean delivery may facilitate maternal resuscitative efforts and reduce the risks of fetal compromise and death.

Maternal Hemorrhage

Hemorrhage remains one of the leading causes of maternal mortality. Excessive maternal blood loss is the most common cause of hypotension in obstetric patients. Facilities that provide labor and delivery services should be prepared to manage maternal hemorrhage. Written policies should clearly define the steps necessary to treat obstetric hemorrhage, and services should be readily available for use in the labor and delivery area. Proper preparation to manage maternal hemorrhage can be lifesaving. Policies to ensure the need for rapid availability of blood products for transfusion in the event of hemorrhage must be balanced with the need to conserve valuable blood bank reserves.

Hemorrhagic Shock

Obstetric hemorrhage can be of a volume large enough to precipitate a state of generalized circulatory failure, resulting in decreased tissue perfusion that progresses to hypoxia, acidosis, and irreversible tissue damage. The goal of therapy should be timely intervention to identify and remedy the cause of hemorrhage in conjunction with reversing the effects leading to shock. Hemodynamic assessment with a central venous pressure or Swan–Ganz catheter is rarely needed for patients with acute hemorrhagic shock. The central venous pressure and Swan–Ganz catheter may be helpful for managing volume replacement therapy in obstetric patients with sepsis. Policies should be developed to define when to use these catheters in the labor and delivery area and to assign responsibilities for their placement and management, and interpretation of the data from them.

Postpartum Hemorrhage

Factors associated with obstetric hemorrhage include uterine atony (the most common cause of postpartum hemorrhage), uterine inversion, obstetric lacerations, retained placental fragments, placentation abnormalities (such as placenta accreta and succenturiate placental lobe), and maternal coagulopathy. An attempt should be made to identify patients with known risk factors for postpartum hemorrhage. Most postpartum hemorrhage occurs immediately or soon after delivery. Maternal postpartum observation should be tailored to the need for timely identification of signs of excessive blood loss, including hypotension and tachycardia. Maternal vital signs and the amount of vaginal bleeding should be evaluated often. The uterine fundus should be identified and massaged and its size and degree of contraction noted. A dilute solution of oxytocin (20 U/L) routinely administered intravenously after delivery reduces the incidence of postpartum hemorrhage resulting from uterine atony. Labor and delivery areas should have 15-methyl prostaglandin

$F_{2\alpha}$ and ergot alkaloids readily available for further treatment of uterine atony. Any bleeding lacerations of the genital tract should be sutured. If perineal or pelvic pain is present, the patient should be evaluated for a genital tract hematoma.

Appropriate maneuvers, including medical therapy, may fail to control postpartum hemorrhage. The responsible physician and obstetric support staff must be prepared to initiate surgical management when it is deemed necessary. Uterine packing and radiographic embolization of the appropriate pelvic vessels may be appropriate. Because of the rich collateral circulation in the pelvis, surgical ligation of the internal iliac (hypogastric) arteries often fails to control hemorrhage and may result in delay of definitive therapy. Puerperal hysterectomy may be indicated to control hemorrhage in cases of intractable bleeding from uterine atony, uterine rupture, placenta accreta, and leiomyomas. The incidence of placenta accreta has steadily increased, and patients with placenta previa and previous uterine incisions are at increased risk of severe hemorrhage at the time of placental separation. The antenatal use of ultrasonography and magnetic resonance imaging may help to make the diagnosis of placenta accreta before delivery and allow for prudent and appropriate planning and surgical management.

TRANSFUSION

Transfusion therapy is used to prevent or treat hemorrhagic shock and its consequences. Blood loss estimated to be 1,500 mL or greater represents approximately 25% of a pregnant woman's total estimated blood volume (6,000 mL). In some clinical circumstances, a pregnant patient might benefit from transfusion of red blood cells before the blood loss has reached such levels. The circulating blood volume must be maintained in the pregnant patient, and therapy should be directed at the prevention of inadequate cardiac output and resultant decreased tissue perfusion. Component therapy, including fresh-frozen plasma and cryoprecipitate, should be available if needed for temporary correction of clotting factor deficiencies.

Some women have a religious objection to the receipt of any blood product. Written policies to guide the management of these patients during treatment are advisable.

Before Delivery

The goal of red blood cell transfusion therapy is to avoid irreversible tissue damage caused by hypoperfusion from inadequate circulating blood volume. In the obstetric patient, the need for adequate blood volume is made more pressing by the presence of the fetus.

The end point of red blood cell transfusion therapy before delivery varies with the clinical situation. A hematocrit level of 30% or greater has been generally recommended as a goal of therapy in a pregnant patient who is actively bleeding or who is at continued risk for significant obstetric hemorrhage, such as in the presence of placenta previa. In a clinically stable patient who has responded appropriately to therapy, however, the decision to transfuse should be based on individual circumstances. Recombinant human erythropoietin is extremely expensive but may be useful to treat severe but nonacute anemia, particularly in patients who refuse transfusion.

After Delivery

If active bleeding has ceased after delivery, transfusion can be withheld unless there is evidence of symptomatic anemia, hypovolemia, decreased tissue perfusion, or decreased urinary output (less than 30 mL/h). The patient's compensatory mechanisms of increased erythropoiesis and plasma volume expansion, along with iron supplementation, will correct the red blood cell deficit.

When obstetric hemorrhage is diagnosed, packed red blood cells should be typed and cross-matched (prior typed and screened red blood cells are equally safe), and the hospital's blood bank personnel should be notified of the potential for massive transfusion. Until the blood loss is controlled by medical or surgical therapy, it is advisable to ensure the ready availability of packed red blood cell units for use if rapid transfusion is required. Obstetric blood loss of greater than 1,500 mL, or of lesser amounts because of placental causes, may result in inadequate coagulation in otherwise healthy patients.

Endometritis

Postpartum endometritis occurs in 1–3% of vaginal deliveries and in 10–50% of cesarean deliveries. Risk factors for endometritis include cesarean delivery, prolonged rupture of membranes, prolonged labor with multiple vaginal examinations, intrapartum fever, and lower socioeconomic status.

PROPHYLAXIS AGAINST POSTCESAREAN INFECTION

A short course of prophylactic antibiotics significantly lowers the risk of endometritis and abdominal wound infection after nonelective cesarean delivery (ie, cesarean delivery after rupture of membranes or labor of any duration). Intravenous administration of an antibiotic immediately after umbilical cord clamping has been demonstrated to be as effective as administration before the procedure is initiated. For procedures lasting less than 2 hours, a single dose is as effective as a longer course of therapy. If excessive intraoperative blood loss occurs, a second dose may be indicated. A first-generation cephalosporin, such as cefazolin, is as effective as other broad-spectrum agents and is less expensive. Broad-spectrum antibiotics should be reserved for therapy rather than for prophylaxis.

MANAGEMENT

Endometritis usually is diagnosed within a few days after delivery. Infection often is caused by several organisms, including aerobic streptococci (group B β-hemolytic streptococci and the enterococci), gram-negative aerobes (especially *Escherichia coli*), gram-negative anaerobic rods (especially *Bacteroides bivius*), and anaerobic cocci (*Peptococcus* species and *Peptostreptococcus* species). Clinically, endometritis is characterized by fever, uterine tenderness, malaise, tachycardia, abdominal pain, or foul-smelling lochia. Of these, fever is the most characteristic and may be the only sign early in the course of infection.

A woman with postpartum fever should be evaluated by pertinent history, physical examination, blood count, and urine culture. Blood cultures rarely influence therapeutic decisions but could be indicated if septicemia is suspected. Cervical, vaginal, or endometrial cultures need not be routinely performed because these results might not indicate the infecting organism.

Principles for managing postpartum endometritis are as follows:

- Parenteral, broad-spectrum antibiotic treatment should be initiated according to a proven regimen and continued until the patient is afebrile. A combination of clindamycin and gentamicin, with the addition of ampicillin in refractory cases, is recommended for cost-effective therapy.

- Response usually is prompt. If fever persists, a search for alternative etiologies, including pelvic abscess, wound infection, septic pelvic thrombophlebitis, inadequate antibiotic coverage, and retained placental tissue, should be performed.

- Because postpartum endometritis may have neonatal implications, information about the mother's condition should be provided to the neonate's health care providers.

Bibliography

American College of Obstetricians and Gynecologists. Antiphospholipid syndrome. ACOG Educational Bulletin 244. Washington, DC: ACOG; 1998.

American College of Obstetricians and Gynecologists. Premature rupture of membranes. ACOG Practice Bulletin 1. Washington, DC: ACOG; 1998.

American College of Obstetricians and Gynecologists. Prevention of deep vein thrombosis and pulmonary embolism. ACOG Practice Bulletin 21. Washington, DC: ACOG; 2000.

American College of Obstetricians and Gynecologists. Thromboembolism in pregnancy. ACOG Practice Bulletin 19. Washington, DC: ACOG; 2000.

Antenatal corticosteroid therapy for fetal maturation. ACOG Committee Opinion 273. American College of Obstetricians and Gynecologists. Obstet Gynecol 2002;99:871–73.

Antenatal corticosteroids revisited: repeat courses. National Institutes of Health. NIH Consens Statement 2000; Aug. 17-18; 17(2):1–8.

Assessment of risk factors for preterm birth. ACOG Practice Bulletin 31. American College of Obstetricians and Gynecologists. Obstet Gynecol 2001; 98:709–16.

Chronic hypertension in pregnancy. ACOG Practice Bulletin 29. American College of Obstetricians and Gynecologists. Obstet Gynecol 2001;98:177–85.

Diagnosis and management of preeclampsia and eclampsia. ACOG Practice Bulletin 33. American College of Obstetricians and Gynecologists. Obstet Gynecol 2002;99:159–67.

Effect of corticosteroids for fetal maturation on perinatal outcomes. National Institutes of Health. NIH Consensus Statement 1994;12(2):1–24.

Perinatal care at the threshold of viability. ACOG Practice Bulletin 38. The American College of Obstetricians and Gynecologists. Obstet Gynecol 2002; 100:617–24.

Placenta accreta. ACOG Committee Opinion 266. American College of Obstetricians and Gynecologists. Obstet Gynecol 2002;99:169–70.

CHAPTER 7

Care of the Neonate

Delivery Room Care

NEONATAL RESUSCITATION

Both routine assessment and care of the neonate at the delivery and the possible provision of extensive resuscitation should be provided in accordance with the American Heart Association (AHA) and the American Academy of Pediatrics (AAP) Neonatal Resuscitation Program. Although the guidelines for neonatal resuscitation focus on newborns, most of the principles are applicable throughout the neonatal period and early infancy. Hospital medical staff concerned with the care and resuscitation of the newborn, including obstetricians, anesthetists, and pediatricians, should determine the qualifications needed to perform neonatal resuscitation, including completion of AHA and AAP Neonatal Resuscitation Program. At every delivery, there should be at least one person whose primary responsibility is the neonate and who is capable of initiating resuscitation. Either that person or someone else who is immediately available should have the skills required to perform a complete resuscitation, including ventilation with bag and mask, endotracheal intubation, chest compressions, and the use of medications. It is not sufficient to have someone "on call" (either at home or in another area of the hospital) for newborn resuscitations in the delivery room.

Recognition and immediate resuscitation of a distressed neonate requires an organized plan of action and the immediate availability of qualified personnel and equipment as described in the AAP and the AHA *Textbook of Neonatal Resuscitation*. Responsibility for identification and resuscitation of a distressed neonate should be assigned to a qualified individual, who may be a physician, a certified nurse–midwife, advanced practice neonatal nurse, labor and delivery nurse, nurse–anesthetist, nursery nurse, or respiratory therapist. The provision of services and equipment for resuscitation should be planned jointly by the directors of the departments of obstetrics, anesthesia, and pediatrics, with the approval of the medical staff. A physician, usually a pediatrician, should be designated to assume primary responsibility for initiating, supervising, and reviewing the plan for management of depressed neonates in the delivery room. The following issues should be considered in this plan:

- Development of a list of maternal and fetal complications that require the presence in the delivery room of someone specifically qualified in all aspects of newborn resuscitation
- Individuals qualified to perform neonatal resuscitation should demonstrate the following capabilities:
  — Rapid and accurate evaluation of the newborn condition, including Apgar scoring
  — Knowledge of the pathogenesis and causes of a low Apgar score (eg, hypoxia, drugs, hypovolemia, trauma, anomalies, infections, and preterm birth), as well as specific indications for resuscitation
  — Skills in airway management (eg, laryngoscopy, endotracheal intubation, suctioning of the airway), artificial ventilation, cardiac massage, emergency administration of drugs and fluids, and maintenance of thermal stability. Recognition and decompression of a tension pneumothorax by needle aspiration also is a desirable skill.
- Development of procedures to ensure the readiness of equipment and personnel and to provide for periodic review and evaluation of the effectiveness of the system
- Contingency plans for multiple births and other unusual circumstances
- The resuscitation steps should be documented in the medical record along with accurate times
- Development of procedures for transfer of responsibility for care

Apgar Score

Apgar scores are useful for describing the status of the neonate at birth and his or her subsequent adaptation to the extrauterine environment. Apgar scores (Table 7-1) should be obtained at 1 minute and 5 minutes after birth. If the 5 minute Apgar score is less than 7, additional scores should be assigned every 5 minutes for up to 20 minutes.

When necessary, resuscitation should be initiated before the 1-minute Apgar score is obtained. One member of the resuscitation team should assign the Apgar score. Low scores (<3), especially those associated with a delay in the return of tone, are useful in identifying the neonate who is significantly depressed. The change between the 1-minute score and the 5-minute score is useful in assessing the efficacy of resuscitation.

If a low Apgar score is anticipated or assigned, rapid assessment of the neonate's condition is necessary to delineate a plan of care. Umbilical cord blood gas and pH analyses may help to distinguish metabolic acidemia secondary to hypoxia from other causes of low Apgar scores in the depressed neonate.

Maintenance of Body Temperature

Immediately following delivery, the neonate should be put in a warm place and dried completely. Drying the neonate with prewarmed towels

Table 7-1. Criteria for Assigning an Apgar Score

| Sign | Apgar Score | | |
	0	1	2
Heart rate	Absent	<100 beats per minute	≥100 beats per minute
Respirations	Absent	Weak cry; hypoventilation	Good, strong cry
Muscle tone	Limp	Some flexion	Active motion
Reflex irritability	No response	Grimace	Cry or active withdrawal
Color	Blue or pale	Body, pink; extremities, blue	Completely pink

immediately after delivery reduces evaporative heat loss. It is recommended that a radiant warmer with a servocontrolled mechanism be placed in the resuscitation area because such devices allow easy access to the neonate during resuscitation procedures.

Suctioning

The neonate's mouth may be suctioned gently to remove excess mucus or blood. Although clear mucus is suctioned from the mouth routinely in most centers, there is no evidence to support the value of this practice. Vigorous suctioning of the posterior pharynx should be avoided because this may produce significant reflex bradycardia and may damage the oral mucosa, leading to interference with suckling because of pain.

If there is meconium in the amniotic fluid, the mouth and hypopharynx should be thoroughly suctioned with a mechanical device before delivery of the shoulders in a cephalic presentation and immediately after delivery of the head in a breech presentation. If meconium is present and the newborn is depressed, the clinician should intubate the trachea and suction to remove meconium or other aspirated material from beneath the glottis. If the newborn is vigorous, there is no evidence that tracheal suctioning is necessary. Furthermore, injury to the vocal cords is more likely to occur in attempting to intubate a vigorous newborn. When using a mechanical suction apparatus, the suction pressure should be set so that when the suction tubing is occluded the negative pressure does not exceed 100 mm Hg.

Ventilation

The normal neonate breathes within seconds of delivery and usually has established regular respiration within 1 minute after delivery. A neonate who is apneic or gasping or whose heart rate is less than 100 beats per minute requires positive pressure ventilation. For the majority of newborns, bag and mask can provide effective ventilation and serve to initiate spontaneous respirations although it may be difficult to use this method in preterm neonates with noncompliant lungs.

Endotracheal intubation may be performed at various points during a resuscitation. The timing of intubation will be determined by many factors, one of which is the skill of the resuscitator. Individuals not adept at intubation should obtain assistance and focus on providing effective ventilation with bag and mask, rather that waste valuable time trying to intubate. Two conditions require immediate intubation: 1) the presence of a known diaphragmatic hernia, or 2) the presence of meconium in the newborn who has depressed respiratory effort, poor muscle tone, or a heart rate less than 100 beats per minute.

Before applying positive pressure ventilation, it is important to ensure that the airway has been cleared. The head should be placed in a sniffing position, with care to avoid hyperextension of the neck. The mask is held on the face with the thumb and index and/or middle finger encircling much of the rim of the mask, while the ring finger holds the chin in the mask (Fig. 7–1). No fingers (or any part of the mask) should rest on the soft tissues of the neck. Initial lung inflation using 100% oxygen may require 30–40 cm H_2O, while 15–20 cm H_2O often is

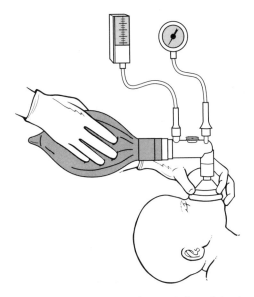

Fig. 7–1. Correctly inflated bag. (Used with permission of the American Academy of Pediatrics. American Academy of Pediatrics, American Heart Association. Neonatal resuscitation textbook. 4th ed. Elk Grove Village [IL]: AAP; Dallas [TX]: AHA; 2000.)

adequate for succeeding breaths, which should be provided at a rate of 40–60 per minute. With rare exceptions, depressed neonates respond promptly to adequate ventilation, and this is the only resuscitation maneuver required.

Symmetric movement of the apices of the chest, equal breath sounds (heard in the axillae), and improvement in heart rate and color indicate satisfactory ventilation. The response of the heart rate is the most useful and readily measurable criterion of adequate ventilation. If the response to ventilation is not prompt, the seal between the face and the mask or the position of the endotracheal tube should be checked. If chest movement and breath sounds appear satisfactory in an intubated neonate, yet the neonate is not responding, a direct laryngoscopy should be performed to insure that the endotracheal tube is in the trachea and inserted to the proper depth.

External Cardiac Massage

If the heart rate does not increase promptly to more than 60 beats per minute after effective ventilation with oxygen, external cardiac massage should be instituted while ventilation is continued. Two techniques are illustrated in Figures 7–2 and 7–3. The thumb technique is preferred although the two-finger method is acceptable. Chest compressions should be carried out at a rate of 90 compressions and 30 ventilations per minute (ratio of 3:1) to a depth of one third of the chest diameter. If there is no response in the heart rate, appropriate drug therapy (and volume expansion, if indicated) should be instituted.

Drugs and Volume Expansion

The use of drugs for resuscitation of the neonate is rarely necessary in the delivery room. When drugs are needed, they should not be administered until ventilation and chest compression have been initiated. The emergency route of administration is the umbilical vein. The infusion of epinephrine into the trachea via an endotracheal tube also may be an effective route of administration. A listing of drugs for resuscitation with their doses should be readily available, preferably in a prominent place in the resuscitation area.

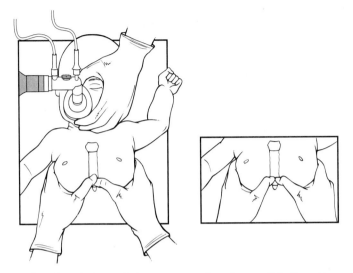

Fig. 7–2. Thumb technique of chest compressions for small (left) and large (right) babies. (Used with permission of the American Academy of Pediatrics. American Academy of Pediatrics, American Heart Association. Neonatal resuscitation textbook. 4th ed. Elk Grove Village [IL]: AAP; Dallas [TX]: AHA; 2000.)

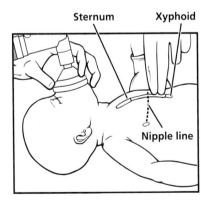

Fig. 7–3. Correct finger position for chest compressions. (Used with permission of the American Academy of Pediatrics. American Academy of Pediatrics, American Heart Association. Neonatal resuscitation textbook. 4th ed. Elk Grove Village [IL]: AAP; Dallas [TX]: AHA; 2000.)

Acidosis. Severely depressed neonates may have combined metabolic and respiratory acidosis. The treatment of acidosis is treatment of the cause. Therefore, respiratory acidosis, which is the result of hypoventilation, is treated by providing positive pressure ventilation. Metabolic acidosis is the result of hypoxemia or hypoperfusion, and the correction of these factors should correct the acidosis.

Significant acidemia is detrimental to myocardial function in the hypoxic heart. Sodium bicarbonate may be useful in a prolonged resuscitation to help correct a documented metabolic acidosis, but its use is discouraged in brief arrests or episodes of bradycardia. In the absence of adequate ventilation, sodium bicarbonate will not improve blood pH significantly. One molar sodium (8.4%) bicarbonate should not be used. One-half molar sodium (4.2%) bicarbonate or lesser concentrations are acceptable.

Bradycardia. For treatment of bradycardia that persists after adequate ventilation and cardiac massage, drugs may be necessary. Epinephrine hydrochloride (1:10,000) may be indicated to treat bradycardia.

Hypovolemia. It is important to recognize that most severely depressed neonates are not hypovolemic and that there may be potential hazards (eg, intracranial hemorrhage) to rapid volume expansion. Conditions associated with hypovolemia include significant hemorrhage from the fetoplacental unit (eg, vasa praevia, fetomaternal bleeding) and compression of the umbilical cord.

If significant hypovolemia is suspected, it should be treated with up to two doses of volume expanders. The neonate's response should be assessed after each infusion. Therapy is stopped when tissue perfusion is adequate.

Narcotic-Induced Respiratory Depression. Respiratory depression as the result of narcotics administered to the mother before delivery is infrequent. If present, prompt and adequate ventilation should be performed until naloxone hydrochloride can be administered and exert its effect. Narcan is contraindicated in a newborn of a narcotic-addicted mother.

Transfer of Responsibility for Resuscitation

Hospital policy should address who will be responsible for assessing and initiating resuscitation of the neonate as required. This policy should indicate circumstances in which a pediatrician (or designated newborn resuscitation personnel) may be called to attend the delivery or to take over resuscitation in an emergency. The process of transfer of responsibility for this care also should be specified.

Neonates are assessed for their individual needs to determine the best facility for care. They may be admitted to the admission and observation area, the intermediate care area, or the intensive care area in the same hospital, or they may be transferred to a hospital that provides specialty or subspecialty care (see "Specialty Care Facility" and "Subspecialty Care Facility" in Chapter 2 and "Transport Procedure" in Chapter 3).

The delivering physician or certified nurse–midwife is responsible for ascertaining that the newborn's adaptations to extrauterine life are proceeding normally and for ensuring immediate postdelivery care of the newborn. Such care may be provided by other health care personnel or transferred to another physician, who will assume responsibility for the ongoing care of the neonate. The care of a newborn with additional needs should be transferred to a physician with appropriate training in neonatal care, as indicated by hospital policy. This policy should delineate the communication that should precede acceptance of this responsibility and the method by which the care of the neonate will be transferred.

Ongoing Care

Resuscitation in the delivery room does not always end with the establishment of normal breathing, heart rate, and color. If the neonate requires ongoing support, a continuing plan for management by personnel who are experienced in the care of such neonates must be established. All neonates who require more than 60 seconds of assisted ventilation or who require epinephrine, volume expanders, or chest compressions should be cared for in an area that can provide careful observation and clinical monitoring to meet the continuing needs of the neonate.

Immediate plans for the neonate should be discussed with the parents (or other support person) before the neonate leaves the delivery room. Whenever possible, the parents should have the opportunity to see and touch the neonate before the neonate is transferred to a nursery. If the neonate is stable and if breastfeeding has been elected by the mother, the neonate should be placed at the breast in the delivery room, within the first hour after delivery. Initial skin-to-skin contact has been associated with a longer duration of breastfeeding.

The physician or other responsible person delivering the neonate also should be advised of the status and plans for the neonate. Communication regarding the potential transfer of care of the neonate must be initiated before the neonate leaves the delivery room, especially when specialized ongoing care is required.

ASSESSMENT OF NEWBORNS IN THE DELIVERY ROOM

An initial evaluation of the neonate's condition should be performed in the delivery room to determine the level of care required. If the neonate's condition is stable, immediate and sustained skin-to-skin contact between the mother and her infant can be provided. Such contact maintains the infant's body temperature and facilitates the opportunity for breastfeeding soon after delivery. Generally, healthy neonates should remain with their mothers.

After appropriate care in the resuscitation area, neonates who are small, sick, or at risk of becoming sick should be transferred to an intermediate or intensive care area in the same hospital or may be transferred to a hospital that provides specialty or subspecialty care.

Because umbilical arterial blood best reflects the fetal condition immediately before delivery, umbilical-artery pH and blood gas measurements may be helpful in ruling out acidemia when a low Apgar score has been assigned. Umbilical venous blood better reflects uteroplacental circulation than it does fetal condition, but if fetal metabolic acidemia is truly present, a venous sample also should indicate its presence. This sample also is helpful when samples of the umbilical artery or chorionic surface artery are unobtainable.

The precise umbilical cord blood pH value that defines chemically significant acidemia is not known; however, umbilical-artery blood pH values of less than 7 (with a metabolic component and a base deficit of >10 mEq/L) realistically represent clinically significant metabolic acidosis.

Neither Apgar score nor pH value alone can define or classify the degree of perinatal asphyxia in a newborn. Many factors other than perinatal asphyxia can result in low 1- and 5-minute Apgar scores.

Therefore, it is recommended that the terms fetal distress and birth asphyxia be discarded as imprecise. If used, the term *asphyxia* should be reserved to describe a neonate with all of the following conditions:

- Profound metabolic or mixed acidemia (pH < 7) on an umbilical-cord artery blood sample, if obtained

- Apgar score of 0–3 for longer than 5 minutes

- Neonatal neurologic manifestations (eg, seizures, coma, or hypotonia)

- Multisystem organ dysfunction (eg, cardiovascular, gastrointestinal, hematologic, pulmonary, or renal system)

Meconium staining of the amniotic fluid, nonreassuring fetal heart rate patterns, low 1-minute Apgar scores, and prolonged labor, in the absence of signs of encephalopathy and seizures, have no predictive value for long-term neurologic injury or cerebral palsy.

IDENTIFICATION AND SECURITY

While the newborn is still in the delivery room, identical bands that indicate the mother's admission number, the neonate's sex, the date and time of birth, and other information specified in hospital policy should be secured to the mother and the newborn. Delivery room and nursery personnel should exercise meticulous care in the preparation and placement of the neonate's identification bands. The nurse in the delivery room should be responsible for preparing and securely fastening these identification bands on the neonate. Footprinting and fingerprinting alone are not adequate methods of patient identification.

The birth records and identification bands should be checked before the neonate leaves the delivery room. When the neonate is taken to the nursery, both the delivery room nurse and the admitting nurse should check the neonate's identification bands and birth records, verify the sex of the neonate, and sign the neonate's medical record. The admitting nurse should fill out the bassinet card and attach it to the bassinet. When the mother is shown her neonate, she should be asked to verify the information on the identification bands and the sex of the neonate. If the condition of the neonate does not allow placement of identification bands (eg, extreme preterm birth), the identification bands should accompany the neonate and should be placed on the incubator or warmer to be attached as soon as is practical.

With multiple births, the umbilical cords should be identified according to hospital policy (eg, use of different number of clamps) so that umbilical cord blood specimens may be correctly labeled. All umbilical cord blood samples must be labeled correctly with an indication that these are samples of the neonate's umbilical cord blood and not that of the mother.

Each institution should develop a newborn security system. This system may include electronic sensor devices as well as instructions to the mother regarding safety precautions designed to avoid abduction when her newborn is rooming in (see "Newborn Security" in Chapter 2).

Routine Neonatal Care

For a healthy neonate born after an uncomplicated pregnancy, an individualized care plan should be established that includes appropriate observation for the stabilization–transition period (the first 6–12 hours) and the remainder of the hospital stay. Health care providers should carefully evaluate and document the neonate's status and care and communicate this information when transferring care to other providers or health care agencies.

PEDIATRIC INFORMATION

Care of the neonate is aided by effective communication of information about the mother and her fetus to the pediatrician or other health care provider. With an uncomplicated pregnancy, labor, and delivery, the information on the medical record accompanying the neonate is sufficient. The obstetric staff should record the following information, which also should be available on a medical record that accompanies the neonate during any transfer of responsibility for care:

- The mother's name, medical record number, blood type, serology result, rubella status, hepatitis B virus test result, and history of substance use or any other socially high-risk circumstances, such as unstable housing, adolescent mother, maternal psychiatric disease, domestic violence, or history of previous child abuse or neglect

- Other maternal test results, if obtained, that are relevant to neonatal care, such as human immunodeficiency virus (HIV) test results and colonization with group B streptococci (in some states, it is necessary to obtain the mother's written authorization before disclosing her HIV status to health care providers, such as her neonate's pediatrician, who are not part of her health care team)

- Intrapartum maternal antibiotic therapy (including type and doses of antibiotics)

- Maternal illness potentially affecting the pregnancy, evidence of chorioamnionitis, and maternal medications (including tocolytics and glucocorticoids)

- Complications of pregnancy associated with abnormal fetal growth, fetal anomalies, or abnormal results from tests of fetal well-being and the corresponding interpretation

- Information regarding the delivery (eg, method and duration of labor), complications of labor (eg, nonreassuring fetal heart rate), duration of rupture of amniotic membranes, and presence or absence of meconium in amniotic fluid or need for resuscitation

- Situations in which lactation may be compromised, such as history of breast surgery, trauma, or previous lactation failure

The obstetric staff should communicate problems before and after delivery in a timely manner to the physician or other health care provider who will be caring for the neonate. For some high-risk pregnancies, a neonatal consultation during the antepartum period may help in obstetric management and assist the parents in understanding what to expect for their neonate. This is of particular importance when fetal abnormalities are significant or a very preterm neonate is expected.

ASSESSMENT OF THE NEWBORN

Intrauterine Growth Status

The neonate's gestational age can be estimated from the mother's menstrual history or the results of an ultrasound examination before 20 weeks of gestation (see "Estimated Date of Delivery" in Chapter 4) and from the physician's assessment of gestational age (Fig. 7–4). The

Neuromuscular maturity

	-1	0	1	2	3	4	5
Posture							
Square Window (wrist)	<90°	90°	60°	45°	30°	0°	
Arm recoil		180°	140–180°	110–140°	90–110°	<90°	
Popliteal angle	180°	160°	140°	120°	100°	90°	<90°
Scarf sign							
Heel to ear							

Physical maturity

Skin	Sticky, friable, transparent	Gelatinous, red, translucent	Smooth, pink, visible veins	Superficial peeling &/or rash, few veins	Cracking, pale areas, rare veins	Parchment, deep cracking, no vessels	Leathery, cracked, wrinkled
Lanugo	None	Sparse	Abundant	Thinning	Bald areas	Mostly bald	
Plantar surface	Heel–toe 40–50 mm:-1 <40 mm:-2	<50 mm, no crease	Faint red marks	Anterior transverse crease only	Creases on ant. 2/3	Creases over entire sole	
Breast	Imperceptible	Barely perceptible	Flat areola– no bud	Stripped areola, 1–2 mm bud	Raised areola, 3–4 mm bud	Full areola, 5–10 mm bud	
Eye/ear	Lids fused loosely (-1), tightly (-2)	Lids open, pinna flat, stays folded	Slightly curved pinna; soft; slow recoil	Well-curved pinna, soft but ready recoil	Formed & firm, instant recoil	Thick cartilage, ear stiff	
Genitals male	Scrotum flat, smooth	Scrotum empty, faint rugae	Testes in upper canal rare rugae	Testes descending, few rugae	Testes down, good rugae	Testes pendulous, deep rugae	
Genitals female	Clitoris prominent, labia flat	Prominent clitoris, small labia minora	Prominent clitoris, enlarging minora	Majora & minora equally prominent	Majora large, minora small	Majora cover clitoris & minora	

Maturity rating

Score	Weeks
-10	20
-5	22
0	24
5	26
10	28
15	30
20	32
25	34
30	36
35	38
40	40
45	42
50	44

Fig. 7-4. The expanded new Ballard Score includes extremely preterm infants and has been refined to improve accuracy in more mature infants. (Ballard JL, Khoury JC, Wedig K, Wang L, Eilers-Walsman BL, Lipp R. New Ballard Score, expanded to include extremely premature infants. J Pediatr 1991;119:417–23.)

gestational age should be assigned by the physician after all data, both pediatric and obstetric, have been assessed. Any marked discrepancy between the presumed duration of pregnancy by obstetric assessment and the physical and neurologic findings in the neonate should be documented on the medical record.

Data from each neonate should be plotted on a birth weight–gestational age chart that is appropriate for the population of neonates in that geographic area. Determination of gestational age and its relationship to weight can be used to identify neonates at risk for postnatal complications. For example, neonates who are either large or small for their gestational ages are at relatively increased risk for hypoglycemia and polycythemia, and appropriate tests (eg, serum glucose screen or hematocrit determination) are indicated.

Risk Assessment

No later than 2 hours after birth, nursery personnel should evaluate the neonate's status and assess risks. Clinical data that are deemed necessary but are initially unavailable should be either obtained or requested at this time. Risks can be assessed through the history and physical examination as documented on the antepartum and intrapartum records. If the neonate's physician (or other health care provider) is not present at the delivery, he or she should be notified of the admission and of the status of the neonate within a time frame established by institutional policy.

Nursery policies should delineate those conditions (eg, low birth weight, small for gestational age) that require specific actions by nurses or immediate notification of a physician. Clinical conditions such as maternal substance use, maternal fever or infection, or low Apgar scores at 5 minutes or more are associated with increased risk for neonatal illness and should prompt immediate notification of the physician. The obstetrician should be notified of the neonate's status in a timely manner, particularly if problems or complications arise.

The neonate's physician or other health care provider, as defined by institutional policy, should examine the apparently normal neonate no later than 24 hours after delivery and within 24 hours before discharge from the hospital. This may be accomplished with one physical examination. The results of the examination should be recorded on the neonate's medical record and discussed with the parents.

IMMEDIATE CARE

Following an initial evaluation of the neonate's condition, a care plan should be established, and the neonate should be carefully observed during the subsequent stabilization–transition period (the first 6–12 hours after birth). If the infant is healthy and stable, the care plan should allow ongoing contact of the mother and the infant during this period. Temperature, heart and respiratory rates, skin color, adequacy of peripheral circulation, type of respiration, level of consciousness, tone, and activity should be monitored and recorded at least once every 30 minutes until the neonate's condition has remained stable for 2 hours. Rooming-in of the mother and her infant is optimal because it allows unrestricted contact and feeding. Hospital staff can easily assess the infant's status in the mother's room until discharge.

The neonate should be observed for any of the following signs of illness:

- Temperature instability
- Change in activity, including refusal of feedings
- Unusual skin color
- Abnormal cardiac or respiratory rate and rhythm
- Delayed or abnormal stools or voiding
- Abdominal distension, bilious vomiting
- Excessive lethargy and sleeping

The normal term neonate passes meconium within the first 24 hours after birth. If a term neonate has not passed meconium by 48 hours after birth, the lower gastrointestinal tract may be obstructed. Urine is normally passed within the first 12 hours after birth. Failure to void within the first 24 hours may indicate genitourinary obstruction or abnormality.

Eye Care

Prophylaxis against gonococcal ophthalmia neonatorum is mandatory for all neonates, including those born by cesarean delivery. A variety of topical agents appear to be equally efficacious. Acceptable prophylactic regimens are application of a 1–2-cm ribbon of sterile ophthalmic ointment containing tetracycline (1%) or erythromycin (0.5%) in single-use tubes or an ophthalmic solution of povidone-iodine (2.5%). Care should be taken to ensure that the agent reaches all parts of the conjunctival sac. The eyes should not be irrigated with saline or distilled water after application of any of these agents; however, after 1 minute, excess solution or ointment can be wiped away with sterile cotton. Application may be delayed up to 1 hour after birth, and often can be delayed until after the first breastfeeding.

Vitamin K

To prevent vitamin K-dependent hemorrhagic disease of the newborn, every neonate should receive a single parenteral dose of natural vitamin K1 oxide (phytonadione) within 1 hour of birth. Oral administration of vitamin K has not been shown to be as efficacious as parenteral administration. Furthermore, no commercial oral vitamin K preparation is approved for use in the United States.

Weighing

Each neonate should be weighed shortly after birth, or after the first breastfeeding, and daily thereafter. The neonate must be kept warm during weighing. The scale pan should be covered with clean paper before each neonate is weighed. The accuracy of the nursery scales should be checked once per month.

Clothing

Most neonates require only a cotton shirt or gown without buttons in addition to a soft diaper. They may be clothed only in a diaper during hot weather if the nursery is not air-conditioned. A supply of soft, clean, cotton clothing, bed pads, sheets, and blankets should be kept at the bedside. Nontoxic dyes should be used to mark clothing, blankets, or other items used in the care of newborns.

Skin Care

Skin care, including bathing, may be important for the health and appearance of the individual neonate and for infection control within the nursery. The first bath should be postponed until the neonate's thermal stability is ensured. The medical and nursing services of each hospital should develop guidelines regarding the time of the first bath, circumstances and method of skin cleansing, and the roles of personnel and parents.

The effects on the neonate's skin should be considered in selecting skin care techniques. Some agents are absorbed and may be toxic; others change skin flora and may increase the risk of infection. Whole-body bathing of the neonate may not be necessary. Localized skin care or techniques that minimize exposure to water may reduce the neonate's heat loss. Sterile cotton sponges (not gauze) soaked with warm water may be used to remove blood and meconium from the neonate's face, head, and body. Alternatively, the neonate can be cleansed with a mild, nonmedicated soap and then rinsed with water. Careful drying of the neonate's skin and removal of blood after delivery may minimize the risk of infection with potentially contaminating microorganisms, such as hepatitis B virus, herpes simplex virus, and HIV. If the neonate's skin is not grossly soiled, it may not require much cleansing.

For the remainder of the neonate's stay in the hospital nursery, the buttocks and perianal regions should be cleansed with fresh water and cotton, or with a mild soap and water, at diaper changes. Ideally, agents used on the newborn's skin should be dispensed in single-use containers, or each neonate should have a personal dispenser.

Various antiseptic compounds for skin care have been studied to determine their safety and effectiveness in preventing colonization and infection in neonates. Hexachlorophene, although relatively effective against gram-positive bacteria, particularly *Staphylococcus aureus*, should not be used routinely for bathing neonates because of its potential for neurotoxic effects in neonates. Although iodophors are good antiseptics, they have not been proved to be both safe and effective for routine skin care. Chlorhexidine gluconate, a compound that is poorly absorbed through intact skin, is useful for bathing or for localized skin care.

No single method of umbilical cord care has proved to be superior in preventing colonization and disease. Current methods include the local application of antimicrobial agents, such as bacitracin, or triple-dye. The skin absorption and toxicity of triple-dye in newborns have not been carefully studied. Alcohol used alone is not effective in preventing umbilical cord colonization and omphalitis.

Circumcision

Existing scientific evidence demonstrates potential medical benefits of newborn male circumcision; however, these data are not sufficient to recommend routine neonatal circumcision. The exact incidence of complications after circumcision is not known, but data indicate that the rate is low and that the most common complications are local infection and bleeding. Given this understanding, parents should make the determination in the interest of the neonate. To make an informed choice, the parents of all male neonates should be given accurate and unbiased information on circumcision and be given an opportunity to discuss this decision. If circumcision is performed, analgesia should be provided. Swaddling, sucrose by mouth, and acetaminophen administration may reduce the stress response but are not sufficient for the operative pain and cannot be recommended as the sole method of analgesia. Although local anesthesia and EMLA cream provides some anesthesia benefit, both ring blocks and dorsal penile blocks have proved more effective.

The uncircumcised penis is easy to keep clean. The foreskin usually does not fully retract for several years and should not be forced. Gentle washing of the genital area while bathing is sufficient for normal hygiene. Later, when the foreskin is fully retractable, boys should be taught the importance of washing underneath the foreskin on a regular basis.

Preventive Care

Hepatitis Immunization

Immunization against hepatitis B virus often is initiated in the nursery. Each hospital should establish procedures to assess the neonate's status regarding hepatitis exposure and timely, appropriate intervention and immunization (see "Hepatitis B Virus" in Chapter 9).

Universal Neonatal Screening

Newborn screening is a preventive public health procedure that should be available to all neonates. The diseases or abnormalities that are subjected to universal screening should be determined and implemented by the local and state health authority or agency. Although all states have newborn screening programs, some neonates with disorders included in the newborn screening battery will be missed, even when properly screened. This may be because of individual or biologic variations, very early discharge, or administrative or laboratory error.

An adequate neonatal screening program involves laboratory tests, education, administration, follow-up, management, and evaluation components. Systematic follow-up and management should be part of the comprehensive newborn screening program. A comprehensive screening program includes the following components:

- Education of parents and practitioners about newborn screening and about their participation in the activity
- Reliable acquisition and transportation of adequate specimens
- Reliable and prompt performance of screening tests
- Prompt retrieval and follow-up of individuals with abnormal test results
- Accurate diagnosis of individuals with confirmed positive test results
- Education, genetic counseling, and psychosocial support for families with affected neonates
- Appropriate intervention and treatment of affected individuals

Every hospital should establish routines to provide total participation of all newborns in the screening program in accordance with state law. Preterm neonates, neonates receiving parenteral feeding, or neonates being treated for illness should have a specimen of blood serum obtained for screening at or near age 7 days if a specimen has not been obtained before that time, regardless of feeding status. An adequate specimen should be provided to the laboratory for analysis. Umbilical cord blood is not adequate for detection of phenylketonuria or other disorders in which metabolite accumulation occurs after birth and after the initiation of feeding. If a neonate requires transfusion or dialysis before the routine time for acquisition of the newborn screening specimen, appropriate modifications should be made in the screening procedure to allow accurate diagnosis. If the initial specimen is obtained from the neonate before 12–24 hours after delivery (timing depends on type of laboratory method used), then a second specimen should be obtained at age 1–2 weeks to decrease the probability that phenylketonuria and other disorders with metabolite accumulation will be missed as a consequence of testing on the first day of life. Repeat testing also should be performed if clinically indicated regardless of the initial screening results.

The responsibility for transmitting the screening test results to the physician or other health care provider should rest with the authority or agency that performed the test. Screening status should be entered into the patient's medical record. The pediatrician and other health care providers should recognize the need for careful documentation of newborn screening test results on each neonate entering the practice for the purpose of comprehensive care.

In the absence of risk factors and symptoms, screening for hypertension or hypotension by blood pressure measurements, for hyperglycemia or hypoglycemia by blood glucose screening, and for polycythemia or anemia by hematocrit determination are not warranted. Screening for blood glucose and hematocrit abnormalities is appropriate for high-risk neonates, such as those born to mothers who have diabetes mellitus and in cases of intrauterine growth restriction and twin-to-twin transfusion.

Hearing Screening

The prevalence of newborn hearing loss is approximately 1–2 per 1,000 live births, with an incidence of 1 per 1,000 in the normal newborn nursery population and 20–40 per 1,000 in the newborn intensive care unit population. In accordance with the recommendations of the AAP Task Force on Newborn and Infant Hearing and the Joint Committee on Infant Hearing, every hospital with obstetric service should develop and implement a universal newborn hearing screening program to ensure appropriate screening, tracking and follow-up, identification and intervention, and evaluation. A protocol for screening should be developed at each hospital, defining how each step in the program will be carried out. Screening should be performed with a physiologic measure, either automated auditory brainstem response or otoacoustic emission, or a combination of the two. Every effort should be made to complete screening before discharge from the hospital. Many programs use a two-step screening protocol, where all infants will have an initial screen with either automated auditory brainstem response or otoacoustic emission. If they pass the screen, then no further testing is done; if they fail the first screen, a repeat screening test is performed before discharge, usually with automated auditory brainstem response. The fail rate of newborn hearing screening (ie, the referral rate for diagnostic hearing testing after completion of screening) should be less than 4%.

Until universal newborn hearing screening is fully implemented, neonates should be evaluated if they have the following risk factors (which will only identify 50% of all newborns with significant hearing loss):

- Family history of hereditary childhood sensorineural hearing loss
- In utero infection, such as cytomegalovirus (CMV), rubella, syphilis, herpes, or toxoplasmosis
- Craniofacial anomalies, including neonates with morphologic abnormalities of the pinnae and ear canals
- Birth weight less than 1,500 g
- Hyperbilirubinemia at a serum level requiring exchange transfusion
- Ototoxic medications, including, but not limited to, aminoglycosides used in multiple courses or in combination with loop diuretics

- Bacterial meningitis
- Apgar score of 0–4 at 1 minute or 0–6 at 5 minutes after birth
- Mechanical ventilation lasting 5 days or longer
- Stigmata or other findings associated with a syndrome known to include a sensorineural or conductive hearing loss

All infants who pass the newborn hearing screening test, and particularly those with any risk factor, should be reevaluated periodically throughout childhood with objective measures of hearing (see the AAP periodicity table). A significant number of children may develop progressive or late-onset hearing loss, and continued surveillance is essential to identify these children in a timely manner.

All infants who fail the newborn screen should receive complete diagnostic testing by qualified pediatric specialists by age 3 months, with intervention provided by age 6 months. Tracking and close follow-up are essential to ensure that children receive the appropriate and necessary evaluation and intervention. Ongoing evaluation of the screening program also is essential for quality assessment.

Visiting Policies

The father, or supporting person, should be encouraged to remain with the mother throughout the intrapartum and postpartum periods. Whenever possible, parents of neonates in continuing care, intermediate care, or intensive care areas should be allowed unrestricted visits. Provisions should be made for feeding (particularly breastfeeding), handling, and holding these neonates. Flexible and liberal visiting policies for families are encouraged.

Some institutions offer sibling classes to prepare other children in a family for the event of childbirth. Contact with the mother and newborn in the hospital helps prepare siblings for the new family member and is reassuring for younger children. The presence of siblings may be appropriate in labor, at delivery, or in the postpartum period, as local policy permits. The children must be accompanied by an adult to help them understand what is occurring and to remove them if circumstances demand.

Physical contact of siblings with neonates is a topic of current concern because of the possible transmission of viral infectious diseases. If siblings are allowed to have direct contact with the newborn, the visit may take place in the mother's private room or, if the mother is not in a private room, in a special sibling visitation area. Thorough hand-washing should be required. Parents should share the responsibility of preventing the exposure of their newborn to a sibling with a contagious illness. Contact of the newborn with children other than siblings should be avoided.

An institution that allows sibling visitation should have clearly defined, written policies and procedures that are based on currently available information. Basic guidelines for sibling visits, which may serve as the basis for policy formulation, are listed as follows:

- Sibling visits should be encouraged for both healthy and ill newborns.
- Before the visit, a nurse or physician should interview the parents at a site outside the unit to assess the current health of each sibling visitor. No child with fever or symptoms of an acute illness, such as upper respiratory infection or gastroenteritis, should be allowed to visit. Siblings who have been recently exposed to a known communicable disease (eg, chickenpox) should not be allowed to visit.
- Children should be prepared in advance for their visit.
- All visitors should be adequately observed and monitored by the medical and nursing staff.
- Visiting siblings should visit only their sibling.
- Children should carefully wash their hands before patient contact.
- Throughout the visit, sibling activity should be supervised by parents or a responsible adult.

Because available data on the risks and benefits of sibling visitation are limited, continued evaluation and reporting are needed. Evaluation should include both psychologic and infectious-disease factors. Institutions that have not introduced sibling visitation should consider the opportunity to use controlled trials to study the effects of these programs. Institutions offering controlled sibling visitation in neonatal intensive care units have noted no adverse effects, but more study is needed before a general recommendation can be made.

Discharge

The hospital stay of the mother and the neonate should be long enough to allow identification of problems and to ensure that the mother is sufficiently recovered and prepared to care for herself and her neonate at home. Many neonatal cardiopulmonary problems that are related to the transition from the intrauterine to the extrauterine environment usually become apparent during the first 12 hours after birth. Other neonatal problems, such as jaundice, ductal-dependent cardiac lesions, and gastrointestinal obstruction, may require a longer period of observation by skilled and experienced personnel. Likewise, significant maternal complications, such as endometritis, may not become apparent during the first day after delivery. The length of stay should therefore be based on the unique characteristics of each mother–newborn dyad, including the health of the mother, the health and stability of the neonate, the ability and confidence of the mother to care for herself and her neonate, the adequacy of support systems at home, and access to appropriate follow-up care. All efforts should be made to keep mothers and neonates together and to ensure simultaneous discharge.

The timing of discharge from the hospital should be the decision of the physicians caring for the mother and the neonate. The decision of when to discharge should be made in consultation with the family and should not be based on arbitrary policies established by third-party payers.

A shortened hospital stay (< 48 hours after delivery) for healthy term newborns can be accomplished but is not appropriate for every mother and neonate. Each mother–neonate dyad should be evaluated individually to determine the optimal time of discharge. Institutions should develop guidelines through their professional staff in collaboration with appropriate community agencies, including third-party payers, to establish hospital stay programs for mothers and their healthy term newborns. State and local public health agencies also should be involved in the oversight of existing hospital stay programs for quality assurance and monitoring.

Neonatal Considerations

The following minimum criteria should be met before a newborn is discharged from the hospital after an uncomplicated pregnancy, labor, and delivery. It is unlikely that the fulfillment of these criteria and conditions can be met in less than 48 hours after birth:

- The antepartum, intrapartum, and postpartum courses for both the mother and the neonate are uncomplicated.

- Delivery was vaginal.

- The neonate is a single birth at 38–42 weeks of gestation, and birth weight is appropriate for gestational age according to appropriate intrauterine growth curves.

- The neonate's vital signs are documented to be normal and stable for the 12 hours before discharge, including a respiratory rate of fewer than 60 breaths per minute, a heart rate of 100–160 beats per minute, and an axillary temperature of 36.1–37°C (97–98.6°F) in an open crib with appropriate clothing.

- The neonate has urinated and has passed at least one stool.

- The neonate has completed at least two successful feedings, and documentation has been made that the neonate is able to coordinate sucking, swallowing, and breathing while feeding. If breastfeeding, an actual feeding should be observed by a caregiver knowledgeable in breastfeeding and documentation of latch, milk transfer, maternal pain, maternal comments, and infant satiety made in the medical record.

- Physical examination reveals no abnormalities that require continued hospitalization.

- There is no evidence of excessive bleeding at the circumcision site for at least 2 hours.

- There is no evidence of significant jaundice in the first 24 hours of life (noninvasive means of detecting jaundice may be useful).

- The mother's (or, preferably, both parents') knowledge, ability, and confidence to provide adequate care for the neonate are documented by the fact that the following training and information has been received:

— Condition of the neonate

— The breastfeeding mother–neonate dyad should be assessed by trained staff regarding nursing position, latch-on, adequacy of swallowing, and woman's knowledge of urine and stool frequency.

— Umbilical cord, skin, and newborn genital care as well as temperature assessment and measurement with a thermometer should be reviewed.

— The mother should be able to recognize signs of illness and common newborn problems, particularly jaundice.

— Instruction in proper newborn safety (eg, proper use of a car seat and positioning for sleeping) should be provided.

• Family members or other support persons, including health care providers such as the family pediatrician or his or her designees, who are familiar with newborn care and are knowledgeable about lactation and the recognition of jaundice and dehydration are available to the mother and the neonate for the first few days after discharge

• Instructions to follow in the event of a complication or emergency

• Laboratory data are available and have been reviewed, including:

— Maternal syphilis, hepatitis B virus surface antigen (HbsAg), and HIV status

— Umbilical cord or newborn blood type and direct Coombs' test result, as clinically indicated

• Screening tests have been performed in accordance with state requirements. If a test was performed before 24 hours of milk feeding, a system for repeating the test during the follow-up visit must be in place in accordance with local or state policy

• Initial hepatitis B vaccine has been administered or an appointment scheduled for its administration and the importance of maintaining newborn immunizations stressed

- A physician-directed source of continuing medical care for both the mother and the neonate has been identified. For newborns discharged before 48 hours after delivery, an appointment has been made for the neonate to be examined within 48 hours of discharge. The follow-up visit can take place in a home or clinic setting, as long as the personnel examining the neonate are competent in newborn assessment and the results of the follow-up visit are reported to the neonate's physician or designees on the day of the visit
- Family, environmental, and social risk factors have been assessed. When risk factors are present, the discharge should be delayed until they are resolved or a plan to safeguard the newborn is in place. Such factors may include, but are not limited to:
  — Untreated parental substance use or positive urine toxicology test results in the mother or the newborn
  — History of child abuse or neglect
  — Mental illness in a parent who is in the home
  — Lack of social support, particularly for single, first-time mothers
  — No fixed home
  — History of untreated domestic violence, particularly during this pregnancy
  — Adolescent mother, particularly if other risk factors are present

All newborns having a shortened hospital stay should be examined by experienced health care providers within 48 hours of discharge. This follow-up visit should be considered an independent service to be reimbursed as a separate package and not as part of a global fee for labor, delivery, and routine nursery services. If it cannot be assured that this examination will take place, discharge should be deferred until a mechanism for follow-up evaluation is identified. The follow-up visit is designed to fulfill the following functions:

- Assess the newborn's general health, hydration, and degree of jaundice and identify any new problems
- Review feeding pattern and technique, including observation of breastfeeding for adequacy of position, latch-on, and swallowing
- Assess historical evidence of adequate stool and urine patterns

- Assess quality of mother–neonate interaction and details of newborn behavior
- Reinforce maternal or family education in neonatal care, particularly regarding feeding and sleep position
- Review results of laboratory tests performed at discharge
- Perform screening tests in accordance with state regulations and other tests that are clinically indicated
- Identify a plan for health care maintenance, including a method for obtaining emergency services, preventive care and immunizations, periodic evaluations and physical examinations, and necessary screening

HIGH-RISK NEONATES

Discharge planning for high-risk neonates should begin shortly after admission. This is to ensure a smooth transition from the hospital to the home (see "Hospital Discharge of the High-Risk Neonate" in Chapter 8).

Education and Psychosocial Factors

The reduction in the average length of a patient's hospital stay has compromised the opportunity for parent education. Hospital resources that have traditionally been extended to parents can no longer be accommodated within the shortened hospital stay. Physicians should be willing to accept, understand, and respond to parent inquiries that arise throughout the perinatal period and should make every effort to ensure that the educational aspects of care are provided before and after hospitalization.

Videotapes that have been previewed and approved by the obstetric and pediatric staff, printed materials, and counseling by hospital personnel (eg, postpartum and nursery nurses, registered dietitians and nutritionists, lactation specialists, and physical therapists) have been helpful to parents. Other beneficial activities are group or individual educational sessions held regularly during the postpartum period to teach and discuss patient self-care, including exercises and self-examination of the breasts; parent–neonate relationships; care of the neonate, including bathing and feeding; and child growth and development. Family-planning techniques appropriate to the patient's needs and desires also should be explained in detail (see "Postpartum Considerations" in Chapter 5).

The newborn undergoes rapid changes in physiology that should be explained to the parents. The neonate's cardiovascular, pulmonary, renal, and neurologic maturation should be observed by the parents with the guidance of qualified personnel. Parents should be familiar with normal and abnormal changes in wake–sleep patterns, temperature, respiration, voiding, stooling, and the appearance of the skin, including jaundice. They also should observe and become familiar with the behavior, temperament, and neurologic capabilities of the newborn. Awareness of newborn cardiopulmonary resuscitation techniques also may be helpful.

During the postpartum hospital stay, health care personnel can provide the mother with professional assistance when she is most likely to be uncomfortable and can help her to anticipate how she may feel once she is home. The mother may be unsure of the normal physical changes that occur after delivery and of her ability to care for the newborn. The mother should be evaluated when she is with her neonate to identify any problems she is having so that appropriate instructions can be provided before and after discharge. Prenatal instructions given to prepare the family for the neonate's care at home also should be reinforced.

Both in-hospital and community agencies often are available to assist the family. Information on public and private groups that provide services to families with newborns, and the circumstances under which these organizations may be asked for such assistance, should be available in the hospital. Information sources may include:

- The in-hospital social service department, as an integral part of the interdisciplinary effort to coordinate hospital and discharge activities, to obtain public or private assistance, and to render psychosocial support

- Members of the home care services, for home visits to assess the parents' child-rearing skills, the home environment, the mother's emotional stability, and the neonate's status and development (under the physician's direction, these nurses may administer drugs or provide other types of therapy)

- Groups that lend support and provide education on special activities (eg, breastfeeding)

Sleep Position and Sudden Infant Death Syndrome

Sudden infant death syndrome (SIDS) is a leading cause of newborn mortality after 1 month and before age 1 year in the United States. Recent investigations on the hazards of prone sleeping and reviews of the epidemiology of SIDS with attention to sleep position have resulted in the recommendation that healthy neonates not be placed in the prone position for sleeping. Supine positioning (lying wholly on the back) carries the lowest risk of SIDS and is preferred; however, the side position is still significantly safer than the prone position. Additionally, parents should be instructed to avoid excessively loose or soft bedding materials by which the neonate's airway may become occluded. For neonates with gastroesophageal reflux disease, obstructive sleep apnea, or certain congenital malformations, the physician should recommend specific sleep positioning. Preterm infants in the newborn intensive care unit should be placed supine as determined by physician judgment as far in advance of discharge as possible.

Decreases in deaths caused by SIDS have been documented in countries where parents have changed from placing neonates in prone positions to back positions for sleeping. No serious adverse effects to the newborn because of supine positioning have been reported. Home monitoring has not been shown to reduce the incidence of SIDS in any population studied.

FOLLOW-UP CARE

The physical and psychosocial status of the mother and the neonate should be subject to ongoing assessment after discharge. The mother needs personalized care during the postpartum period to hasten the development of a healthy mother–newborn relationship and a sense of maternal confidence. Support and reassurance should be provided as the mother masters neonatal-care tasks and adapts to her maternal role. Involving the father or other close support person and encouraging participation in the neonate's care not only can provide additional support to the mother but also can enhance the relationship between the newborn and the family.

The postpartum period is a time of developmental adjustment for the whole family. Family members now have new roles and relationships, and an effort should be made to assess the progress of the family's adaptation. If a family member finds it difficult to assume the new role, the health care team should arrange for sensitive, supportive assistance. This is particularly important for adolescent mothers, for whom it may be necessary to mobilize multiple resources within the community.

Neonatal Considerations

The frequency of follow-up visits for normal neonates varies with patient, locale, and community practices. The interval should be consistent with the AAP's guidelines on preventive health care. Regular follow-up visits and good records of development should be maintained.

The intervals of follow-up visits required by high-risk neonates should be determined by the needs of the individual infant and family. It may be necessary to examine some of these infants weekly or bimonthly at first. Neurologic, developmental, behavioral, and sensory status should be assessed more than once during the first year in high-risk infants to ensure early identification of problems and referral for remedial care. A perinatal follow-up program with an appropriate staff of multidisciplinary personnel is useful in providing these assessments.

Physicians and other professionals who provide follow-up care to women and infants should be aware of and look for the following physical, social, and psychologic factors associated with child abuse:

- Preterm birth
- Neonatal illness with long periods of hospitalization, especially in neonatal intensive care units
- Single parenthood
- Adolescent motherhood
- Closely spaced pregnancies
- Infrequent family visits to hospitalized infants
- Substance use

Children born preterm have been shown to have a greater incidence of irritability, hyperkinesis, and increased dependency. Prolonged hospitalization inevitably disrupts family relationships, particularly the parent–child relationship. Infants and parents with such a history or with other factors associated with child abuse require closer follow-up than does the average family. The interaction of the parents, especially the mother, with the infant should be evaluated periodically. The infant or child who fails to thrive may be a victim of neglect, if not outright abuse, and a causal relationship between neglect and failure to thrive should always be suspected. In every state, providers of health care to children are legally obligated to report suspected child abuse.

Adoption

Health care for neonates who are to be adopted should focus on the needs of the child, the adoptive family, and the birth parents. These neonates may have acute and long-term medical, psychologic, and developmental problems because of their genetic, emotional, cultural, psychosocial, or medical backgrounds. The pediatrician should perform a careful medical assessment of the child and should counsel the adopting family appropriately. Just as a birth family cannot be certain that its biologic child will be healthy, an adoptive family cannot be guaranteed that a child will not have future health problems. Most adopted children, even those from high-risk backgrounds, are healthy. Those with certain disorders and special problems, however, also can be successfully adopted. The risks should be defined and carefully explained to the family so that problems can be anticipated and addressed expediently.

The pediatrician's role is not to judge the advisability of a proposed adoption, but to apprise the prospective parents and any involved agency clearly and honestly of any special health needs detected at examination or anticipated in the future. Pediatricians evaluating a newborn for adoption should obtain an extensive history from the birth parents and enter these data into the formal medical record. There may never again be a comparable opportunity to obtain this information. If the pediatrician is unable to interview the parents personally, an adoption agency social worker who is trained to do a skilled genetic and medical interview should obtain a complete prenatal and postpartum history. The prenatal history should include information on the birth parents' lifestyle that may affect the fetus at birth or later in development. Physicians and adoption agency social workers should be trained to obtain lifestyle information in a manner that is sensitive to psychologic and cultural issues. Such information includes parental use of alcohol or other drugs and history of sexual practices that increase the risk of sexually transmitted diseases in both birth parents. The increased risk of genetically inherited disorders by neonates of incestuous mating may require special consultations. After reviewing whatever history is available, the pediatrician should examine the adopted child carefully and perform metabolic, genetic, and other assessments as indicated.

Physicians must be careful with semantics when dealing with the adoptive family. This is an "adoptive family," not only an "adopted child." The term *parents* applies to the parents in the adoptive family; the *birth parents* are those who conceived the child. *Real* or *natural parent(s)* are confusing terms that should be eliminated because they may reflect negatively on adoptive families and imply a temporary or less-than-genuine relationship between adoptive families and their children.

The physician should be aware of state laws on adoption procedures. Hospital nurseries should have policies regarding the handling of adoptions in accordance with these laws. Policies should reflect sensitivity toward both the adoptive family as well as the birth parents. Although adoption is generally an elective decision initiated by the birth parents, they often need support adjusting to the separation from their neonate.

Neonatal Nutrition

BREASTFEEDING

At birth, the neonate's intestinal-tract host defense mechanism against bacterial and viral agents is not completely developed. Colostrum and mature human milk contain a number of factors that promote immunologic development of the gastrointestinal tract and help to protect the newborn from infection.

There are diverse and important advantages to infants, mothers, families, and society for breastfeeding and the use of human milk for infant feeding. These include health, nutritional, immunologic, developmental, psychologic, social, economic, and environmental benefits. Human milk supports optimal growth and development of the infant while decreasing the risk of a variety of acute and chronic diseases.

Prenatal counseling and education regarding methods of newborn feeding may allow correction of misperceptions about feeding methods. Virtually all mothers who are hesitant to breastfeed can do so successfully with appropriate counseling, education, and knowledgeable support. If, after these interventions, the mother chooses not to breastfeed, she should be supported in her decision.

Initiation of Breastfeeding

The successful management of breastfeeding begins during pregnancy. Prenatal care should include discussion of prior breastfeeding experience, feeding plans, and breast care. Ascertainment of history of breast surgery, trauma, or prior lactation failure is important as these situations may present special challenges to successful breastfeeding. The breasts should be examined to determine whether the nipples are inverted or flat; special help after delivery may be necessary. The areolar glands provide adequate lubrication during pregnancy and breastfeeding, and the use of special soaps or ointments should be discouraged. During prenatal visits to the pediatrician, the decision to breastfeed should be reinforced. The integration of breastfeeding into the total care of the newborn in the first months of life should be discussed.

The mother should be offered the opportunity and be encouraged to breastfeed her newborn as soon as possible after delivery. Breastfeeding may be initiated in the first hour of life, unless medically contraindicated. The mother should be guided so that she can help the newborn latch on to the breast properly. Enough of the areola (at least 1/2 in.) should be in the neonate's mouth to permit the tongue to stroke the areola over the collecting ductals against the hard palate in the act of sucking.

From the time of delivery to discharge from the hospital, the mother and her newborn should be together as much as possible. Newborns should be nursed whenever they show signs of hunger, such as increased alertness or activity, mouthing, or rooting. Crying is a late indicator of hunger.

When awake, the newborn should be encouraged to feed frequently (8–12 times per day until satiety (usually 10–15 minutes on each breast) to help stimulate milk production. In the early weeks after birth, nondemanding neonates may need to be aroused to feed if 4 hours have elapsed since the last nursing. Usually, it is wise to alternate the breast used to initiate the feeding and to equalize the time spent at each breast over the day. When satisfied, the newborn will fall asleep or unlatch.

Intermittent bottle-feeding of a breastfed newborn may lessen the success of breastfeeding. If the newborn's appetite is partially satisfied by water or formula supplements, the newborn will take less from the breast, and milk production will be diminished. Therefore, bottle-feeding a healthy breastfed neonate should be discouraged. It is uncommon for breastfeeding newborns to need any supplementation during the first week of life. Routine water and milk supplementation is contraindicated for healthy, term newborns and most large preterm newborns.

Monitoring the Breastfed Newborn

Although breastfed infants have widely varying patterns of wakefulness, sleep, feeding, and elimination, especially during the first week after birth, an adequately nourished newborn usually is considered to be one who takes at least eight feedings per day and sleeps well between feedings. It also is important to ensure that the neonate urinates at least six times per day, stools at least three times per day in the first week of life, and gains weight over time. After lactogenesis (onset of copious milk production, normally by the end of the first week after delivery), the healthy neonate commonly feeds 8–12 times per day and produces a small, moist stool with many of the feedings. A physician, nurse or other health care provider should examine the neonate during the first 2 weeks of life, regardless of the newborn's age on discharge. If discharge occurs at younger than 48 hours, the neonate should be reexamined within 48 hours of discharge for breastfeeding behavior, weight gain or loss, evidence of significant jaundice, and hydration status. The neonate, the mother, and the breastfeeding process should be further evaluated with an outpatient visit if any of the following occur:

- Significant maternal breast pain
- Infant feeds less than eight times per day
- Urination is fewer than six times per day
- Bowel movements are fewer than three per day

Infants of primiparous women or mothers breastfeeding for the first time should be evaluated by age 1 week, and all infants should be examined at age 2 weeks, regardless of previous progress or problems. Weight loss beyond age 3 days, weight loss more than 7% of birth weight, or failure to regain birth weight by age 2 weeks in the term neonate requires a careful evaluation of the feeding techniques being used and the adequacy of breastfeeding. Exclusive breastfeeding is ideal nutrition and sufficient to support optimal growth and development for the healthy term infant for approximately the first 6 months after delivery. In families with a strong history of allergy, breastfeeding is likely to be especially beneficial. Newborns weaned before age 12 months should not receive cow's milk feedings but should receive iron-fortified newborn formula.

Contraindications to Breastfeeding

Contraindications to breastfeeding include certain maternal infectious diseases and maternal medications. Endometritis or mastitis being treated with antibiotics is not a contraindication to breastfeeding. Mothers with active herpes simplex virus infection may breastfeed their neonates if they have no vesicular lesions in the breast area, as long as the woman observes careful handwashing techniques (see "Handwashing" in Chapter 10).

Despite the demonstrated benefits of breastfeeding, there are some situations in which breastfeeding is not in the best interest of the newborn. These include the newborn with galactosemia, the newborn whose mother uses illegal drugs, the newborn whose mother has untreated active tuberculosis, and the newborn whose mother is HIV-infected. Mothers with active tuberculosis may breastfeed their neonates only after they have received adequate therapy and are considered noninfectious. The neonate should be examined for infection and provided with appropriate treatment, if necessary. Newborns born to CMV-seronegative women who seroconvert during lactation and preterm newborns with low concentration of transplacentally acquired antibodies to CMV can develop symptomatic disease with sequelae from acquiring CMV though breastfeeding. Decisions regarding breastfeeding of preterm newborns by mothers known to be CMV-seropositive should consider both the potential benefits of human milk and the risk of CMV transmission.

Pasteurization of milk appears to inactivate CMV; freezing milk at –20°C (–4°F) will decrease viral titers but does not reliably eliminate CMV. Mothers who test positive for HBsAg may breastfeed, but their newborns must receive hepatitis B virus immune globulin and vaccine.

Evidence exists suggesting the presence of hepatitis C virus in the breastmilk of infected mothers. However, to date there has been no report in the literature documenting the transmission of hepatitis C infection to neonates from breastmilk. Currently, maternal hepatitis C infection is not considered a contraindication to breastfeeding. Women should be advised of the available information regarding risks to the neonate so that they can make an informed decision (see "Cytomegalovirus" in Chapter 9).

Human immunodeficiency virus has been found in the milk of HIV-infected women. The relative risk of infection of newborns from this source is unknown. In the United States and other developed countries where formula is safe and readily available, women infected with HIV should be counseled against breastfeeding their neonates. They also should not serve as milk donors.

The effects on the newborn of medications taken by a nursing mother have been closely studied. The AAP Committee on Drugs reviewed the current data on the transfer of drugs and other chemicals into human milk (Tables 7–2 to 7–7). There are only a few drugs that, taken by the

Table 7–2. Cytotoxic Drugs That May Interfere With Cellular Metabolism of the Nursing Infant

Drug	Reason for Concern, Reported Sign or Symptom in Infant, or Effect on Lactation
Cyclophosphamide	Possible immune suppression, unknown effect on growth or association with carcinogenesis, neutropenia
Cyclosporine	Possible immune suppression, unknown effect on growth or association with carcinogenesis
Doxorubicin*	Possible immune suppression, unknown effect on growth or association with carcinogenesis
Methotrexate	Possible immune suppression, unknown effect on growth or association with carcinogenesis, neutropenia

*Drug is concentrated in human milk.

Used with permission of the American Academy of Pediatrics. Transfer of drugs and other chemicals into human milk. Pediatrics 2001;108:776–89.

Table 7–3. Drugs of Abuse for Which Adverse Effects on the Infant During Breastfeeding Have Been Reported*

Drug	Reported Effect or Reasons for Concern
Amphetamine[†]	Irritability, poor sleeping pattern
Cocaine	Cocaine intoxication—irritability, vomiting, diarrhea, tremulousness, seizures
Heroin	Tremors, restlessness, vomiting, poor feeding
Marijuana	Only one report in literature, no effect mentioned, very long half-life for some components
Phencyclidine	Potent hallucinogen

*The Committee on Drugs strongly believes that nursing mothers should not ingest drugs of abuse, because they are hazardous to the nursing infant and to the health of the mother.

[†]Drug is concentrated in human milk.

Used with permission of the American Academy of Pediatrics. Transfer of drugs and other chemicals into human milk. Pediatrics 2001;108:776–89.

Table 7–4. Radioactive Compounds That Require Temporary Cessation of Breastfeeding*

Compound	Recommended Time for Cessation of Breastfeeding
Copper 64 (^{64}Cu)	Radioactivity in milk present at 50 h
Gallium 67 (^{67}Ga)	Radioactivity in milk present for 2 wk
Indium 111 (^{111}In)	Very small amount present at 20 h
Iodine 123 (^{123}I)	Radioactivity in milk present up to 36 h
Iodine 125 (^{125}I)	Radioactivity in milk present for 12 d
Iodine 131 (^{131}I)	Radioactivity in milk present 2–14 d, depending on study
Iodine[131]	If used for treatment of thyroid cancer, high radioactivity may prolong exposure to infant
Radioactive sodium	Radioactivity in milk present 96 h
Technetium 99m (^{99m}Tc), ^{99m}Tc macro-aggregates, ^{99m}Tc O$_4$	Radioactivity in milk present 15 h to 3 d

*Consult nuclear medicine physician before performing diagnostic study so that radionuclide that has the shortest excretion time in breast milk can be used. Before study, the mother should pump her breast and store enough milk in the freezer for feeding the infant; after study, the mother should pump her breast to maintain milk production but discard all milk pumped for the required time that radioactivity is present in milk. Milk samples can be screened by radiology departments for radioactivity before resumption of nursing.

Used with permission of the American Academy of Pediatrics. Transfer of drugs and other chemicals into human milk. Pediatrics 2001;108:776–89.

Table 7–5. Drugs for Which the Effect on Nursing Infants Is Unknown but May Be of Concern*

Drug	Reported or Possible Effect
Antianxiety	
Alprazolam	None
Diazepam	None
Lorazepam	None
Midazolam	—
Perphenazine	None
Prazepam[†]	None
Quazepam	None
Temazepam	—
Antidepressants	
Amitriptyline	None
Amoxapine	None
Bupropion	None
Clomipramine	None
Desipramine	None
Dothiepin	None
Doxepin	None
Fluoxetine	Colic, irritability, feeding and sleep disorders, slow weight gain
Fluvoxamine	—
Imipramine	None
Nortriptyline	None
Paroxetine	None
Sertraline[†]	None
Trazodone	None
Antipsychotic	
Chlorpromazine	Galactorrhea in mother, drowsiness and lethargy in infant, decline in developmental scores
Chlorprothixene	None
Clozapine[†]	None
Haloperidol	Decline in developmental scores
Mesoridazine	None
Trifluoperazine	None

(continued)

Table 7–5. Drugs for Which the Effect on Nursing Infants Is Unknown but May Be of Concern* *(continued)*

Drug	Reported or Possible Effect
Others	
Amiodarone	Possible hypothyroidism
Chloramphenicol	Possible idiosyncratic bone marrow suppression
Clofazimine	Potential for transfer of high percentage of maternal dose, possible increase in skin pigmentation
Lamotrigine	Potential therapeutic serum concentrations in infant
Metoclopramide†	None described, dopaminergic blocking agent
Metronidazole	In vitro mutagen, may discontinue breastfeeding for 12–24 h to allow excretion of dose when single-dose therapy given to mother
Tinidazole	See metronidazole

*Psychotropic drugs, the compounds listed under anti-anxiety, antidepressant, and antipsychotic categories, are of special concern when given to nursing mothers for long periods. Although there are very few case reports of adverse effects in breastfeeding infants, these drugs do appear in human milk and, thus, could conceivably alter short-term and long-term central nervous system function. See discussion in text of psychotropic drugs.

†Drug is concentrated in human milk relative to simultaneous maternal plasma concentrations.

Used with permission of the American Academy of Pediatrics. Transfer of drugs and other chemicals into human milk. Pediatrics 2001;108:776–89.

Table 7–6. Drugs That Have Been Associated With Significant Effects on Some Nursing Infants and Should Be Given to Nursing Mothers With Caution*

Drug	Reported Effect
Acebutolol	Hypotension, bradycardia, tachypnea
5-Aminosalicylic acid	Diarrhea (one case)
Atenolol	Cyanosis, bradycardia
Bromocriptine	Suppresses lactation, may be hazardous to the mother
Aspirin (salicylates)	Metabolic acidosis (one case)
Clemastine	Drowsiness, irritability, refusal to feed, high-pitched cry, neck stiffness (one case)
Ergotamine	Vomiting, diarrhea, convulsions (doses used in migraine medications)
Lithium	One-third to one-half therapeutic blood concentration in infants
Phenindione	Anticoagulant—increased prothrombin and partial thromboplastin time in one infant; not used in United States

(continued)

Table 7–6. Drugs That Have Been Associated With Significant Effects on Some Nursing Infants and Should Be Given to Nursing Mothers With Caution* (*continued*)

Drug	Reported Effect
Phenobarbital	Sedation; infantile spasms after weaning from milk containing phenobarbital, methemoglobinemia (one case)
Primidone	Sedation, feeding problems
Sulfasalazine (salicylazosulfapyridine)	Bloody diarrhea (one case)

*Blood concentration in the infant may be of clinical importance.

Used with permission of the American Academy of Pediatrics. Transfer of drugs and other chemicals into human milk. Pediatrics 2001;108:776–89.

Table 7–7. Food and Environmental Agents: Effects on Breastfeeding

Agent	Reported Sign or Symptom in Infant or Effect on Lactation
Aflatoxin	None
Aspartame	Caution if mother or infant has phenylketonuria
Bromide (photographic laboratory)	Potential absorption and bromide transfer into milk
Cadmium	None reported
Chlordane	None reported
Chocolate (theobromine)	Irritability or increased bowel activity if excess amounts (≥16 oz/d) consumed by mother
Chlorophenothane, benzene hexachlorides, dieldrin, aldrin, hepatachlorepoxide	None
Fava beans	Hemolysis in patient with G-6-PD deficiency
Fluorides	None
Hexachlorobenzene	Skin rash, diarrhea, vomiting, dark urine, neurotoxicity, death
Hexachlorophene	None; possible contamination of milk from nipple washing
Lead	Possible neurotoxicity
Mercury, methylmercury	May affect neurodevelopment

(continued)

Table 7–7. Food and Environmental Agents: Effects on Breastfeeding (*continued*)

Agent	Reported Sign or Symptom in Infant or Effect on Lactation
Methylmethacrylate	None
Monosodium glutamate	None
Polychlorinated biphenyls and polybrominated biphenyls	Lack of endurance, hypotonia, sullen, expressionless facies
Silicone	Esophageal dysmotility
Tetrachloroethylene cleaning fluid (perchloroethylene)	Obstructive jaundice, dark urine
Vegetarian diet	Signs of B_{12} deficiency

Used with permission of the American Academy of Pediatrics. Transfer of drugs and other chemicals into human milk. Pediatrics 2001;108:776–89.

mother, are absolute contraindications to breastfeeding. Physicians are encouraged to review available data and recommendations from reputable sources before advising against breastfeeding when mothers are taking medications. The mother should discuss the use of these medications with her obstetrician and child's physician if she wishes to continue breastfeeding. They must determine whether the drug therapy is really necessary, whether safer drugs are available, and whether the neonate's drug exposure may be minimized by having the woman take the medication after feedings. If the drug presents a risk to the neonate, the neonate should be carefully monitored to detect any adverse effects, and consideration should be given to measuring blood concentrations. Oral contraceptives may be used by breastfeeding mothers once lactation has been established.

HUMAN MILK COLLECTION AND STORAGE

There are many situations where a mother might be separated from her infant, necessitating her to express and store her breast milk. A healthy infant whose mother is occupied outside of home (eg, work, school) can maintain exclusive breast-milk feeding by providing expressed milk to be given in her absence. Furthermore, hospitalized infants may benefit significantly from receipt of their mother's breast milk. Therefore, it is important to encourage and support mothers in providing their infants expressed milk, and to inform them about proper methods of expressing and storing their breast milk.

The use of donor breast milk generally is discouraged. Concern over transmission of infectious diseases has led to heat treatment of all banked human milk, reducing its beneficial aspects. In addition, the composition of donor human milk depends on the donor's diet, environmental exposure, and lifestyle and may pose unknown risks to the newborn. There is general agreement that the use of pooled donor human milk is the least satisfactory regimen for feeding newborns or infants and is discouraged. Consequently, human milk banks have declined in number in the United States and have avoided the use of pooled milk. Careful monitoring of donors and laboratory evaluation of donated milk is required by the Human Milk Banking Association of North America.

Women who donate breast milk for other newborns should be interviewed carefully regarding past and current infectious diseases, use of drugs and medicines, and other factors that may impair the quality or safety of the breast milk that they provide. Before they are accepted as milk donors, they should be tested for HIV, HBsAg, hepatitis C, and tuberculosis. Because seroconversion may occur, ideally the breast milk should be stored and the donor retested at 4–6 months for HIV infection before the milk is consumed. Women with positive test results should not be accepted as donors. These tests should be repeated periodically for donors who continue to provide milk or who seek reinstatement as a donor. The potential risks should be explained to mothers whose newborns are to receive donated milk. Decisions regarding the use of CMV-seropositive donor milk to preterm newborns should consider both the potential benefits of human milk and the risk of CMV transmission.

Mothers who have tested positive for the HIV antibody or HBsAg should not provide stored breast milk for their neonates while in the nursery because of the risk to other newborns. Although mothers who are HBsAg positive may breastfeed their neonates after the neonates have received hepatitis B immune globulin and vaccine, it is preferable not to store breast milk that is potentially contaminated with hepatitis B virus in the nursery.

All mothers who provide breast milk for their newborns should be instructed in the proper techniques of milk collection to prevent bacterial contamination. Careful handwashing is critical, and the nipples should be wiped with cotton and plain water before the breast milk is expressed. Although manual expression, when performed correctly, yields relatively clean milk, many women prefer to use a breast pump. All parts of the pump that are in contact with the milk should be washed carefully with hot, soapy water after each use.

Expressed breast milk can be refrigerated in sterile glass or plastic containers for 48 hours without an increase in bacterial contamination. If it must be stored for longer periods, it can be frozen in the freezing compartments of refrigerators for 2–3 weeks, or in a deep freeze at $-20°C \pm 2°C$ ($-4°F \pm 3.6°F$) for several months.

Frozen expressed breast milk should be thawed quickly under running water, using precautions to avoid contamination from the water, or thawed gradually in the refrigerator at $4°C$ ($39.2°F$). It should not be left at room temperatures for long periods, nor should it be subjected to extremely hot water or to microwave ovens. The very high temperatures that may be reached with the latter methods can destroy valuable components of the breast milk and result in thermal injury to the neonate. Once the breast milk has been thawed, it may be refrigerated for up to 24 hours.

There is no consensus on standards of the microbiologic quality of expressed breast milk. In general, each milliliter of expressed human milk contains 10^3–10^4 colony-forming units of normal skin bacteria, such as *Staphylococcus epidermidis* and diphtheroids; this breast milk can be fed to newborns with no ill effects. The presence of gram-negative rods in the breast milk may indicate a problem in the collection technique. Feeding intolerance has been reported with breast milk containing more than 10^2 colony-forming units of gram-negative bacteria per milliliter, and higher levels have been associated with suspected sepsis. Bacteria levels in breast milk can be controlled by heat treatment, which entails heating the breast milk to $62.5°C$ for 30 minutes. Heat treatment also inactivates HIV. Heat treatment leads to a 15% loss of secretory immunoglobulin A, a 25% loss of lactoferrin and folate, a 75% loss of phosphatase, and total elimination of beneficial cellular elements.

Routine screening of expressed milk samples for bacterial count is rarely indicated. Further, when expressed milk is to be given by continuous infusion at room temperature, thereby creating a risk of bacterial proliferation in the container and tubing, the syringe and tubing should be changed every 4–6 hours.

Formula Preparation

Formula selection and control should be directed by the physician. New formulas should be reviewed by the appropriate hospital committees and the director of the nursery before use. For mothers who intend to breastfeed their newborns, distribution of formula packages on discharge should be discouraged. For mothers who intend to feed their newborns with formula, the distribution of formula packages on discharge should be consistent with the physician's written orders. The physician should write orders for the formula to be used and the amount to be given at each feeding.

Most hospitals now use prepared formula units with separate nipples that are readily attached to the bottles just before use. These units need not be refrigerated and may be stored in a convenient, clean, cool area. The sterile cap should be kept on the nipple until the neonate is ready to be fed.

If there is a special area where nipples are uncapped and placed on the bottle, it should be kept very clean and should be used only for formula preparation. Alternatively, nipples may be uncapped and attached to bottles at the mother's bedside just before feeding. The formula and nipple unit should be used as soon as possible, certainly within 4 hours after the bottle is uncapped, and then discarded.

Vitamin and Mineral Supplementation

The vitamin D content of human milk is low (22 IU/L), and rickets can occur in deeply pigmented breastfed neonates or in those with inadequate exposure to sunlight. As adequate exposure to sunlight is difficult to guarantee and because supplementation at the recommended dose is safe, vitamin D supplementation at 400 IU per day should be considered for breastfed neonates.

Recent recommendations by the American Dental Association and the AAP indicate that fluoride supplementation for both breastfed and bottlefed newborns can begin at age 6 months.

Although the iron content of human milk is low, the bioavailability is high—50% of the iron is absorbed by newborns who are exclusively breastfed. Breastfed newborns should be given supplemental elemental iron (2–3 mg/kg per day) or iron-containing complementary foods when they reach age 6 months. Iron-containing formulas with up to 12 mg of elemental iron per liter of formula should be used for all formula-fed newborns. Further iron supplementation is not necessary. Newborns consuming commercial newborn formulas do not need vitamin and mineral supplementation for the first 6 months of life.

Bibliography

American Academy of Pediatrics. Committee on Nutrition. Soy protein-based formulas: recommendations for use in infant feeding. Pediatrics 1998;101: 148–53.

American Academy of Pediatrics, American College of Obstetricians and Gynecologists. Use and abuse of the Apgar score. ACOG Committee Opinion 174. Elk Grove Village (IL): AAP; Washington, DC: ACOG; 1996.

American Academy of Pediatrics, American Heart Association. Neonatal resuscitation textbook 4th ed. Elk Grove Village (IL): AAP Dallas (TX); Dallas (TX): AHA; 2000.

American Academy of Pediatrics Committee on Accident and Poison Prevention. Safe transportation of newborns discharged from the hospital. Pediatrics 1990;86:486–7.

American Academy of Pediatrics Committee on Drugs: The transfer of drugs and other chemicals into human milk. Pediatrics 1994;93:137–50.

American Academy of Pediatrics Committee on Early Childhood, Adoption & Dependent Care. Initial medical evaluation of an adopted child. Pediatrics 1991;88:642–4.

American Academy of Pediatrics, Committee on Nutrition. Pediatric nutrition handbook. 4th ed. Elk Grove (IL): AAP; 1998.

American Academy of Pediatrics Vitamin K Ad Hoc Task Force. Controversies concerning vitamin K and the newborn. Pediatrics 1993;91:1001-3.

American College of Obstetricians and Gynecologists. Inappropriate use of the terms fetal distress and birth asphyxia. ACOG Committee Opinion 197. Washington, DC: ACOG; 1998.

American College of Obstetricians and Gynecologists. Utility of umbilical cord blood acid-base assessment. ACOG Committee Opinion 138. Washington, DC: ACOG; 1994.

Ballard JL, Khoury JC, Wedig K, Wang L, Eilers-Walsman BL, Lipp R. New Ballard Score, expanded to include extremely premature infants. J Pediatr 1991;119:417-23.

Breastfeeding and the use of human milk. American Academy of Pediatrics. Work Group on Breastfeeding. Pediatrics 1997;100:1035-39.

Circumcision. ACOG Committee Opinion 260. American College of Obstetricians and Gynecologists. Obstet Gynecol 2001;98:707-8.

Circumcision policy statement. American Academy of Pediatrics. Task Force on Circumcision. Pediatrics 1999;103:686-93.

Does bed sharing affect the risk of SIDS? American Academy of Pediatrics. Task Force on Infant Positioning and SIDS. Pediatrics 1997;100:272.

Erenberg A, Lemons J, Sia C, Trunkel D, Ziring P. American Academy of Pediatrics, Task Force on Newborn and Infant Hearing, 1998-1999. Pediatrics 1999;103:527-30.

Guidelines for home care of infants, children, and adolescents with chronic disease. American Academy of Pediatrics Committee on Children with Disabilities. Pediatrics 1995;96:61-4.

Hepatitis C virus infection. Committee on Infectious Diseases. American Academy of Pediatrics. Pediatrics 1998;101:481-5.

Hospital discharge of the high-risk neonate-proposed guidelines. American Academy of Pediatrics Committee on Fetus and Newborn. Pediatrics 1998; 102:411-7.

Hospital stay for healthy term newborns. American Academy of Pediatrics Committee on Fetus and Newborn. Pediatrics 1995;96:788-90.

Human milk, breastfeeding, and transmission of human immunodeficiency virus in the United States. American Academy of Pediatrics Committee on Pediatric AIDS. Pediatrics 1995;96: 977-79.

The initiation or withdrawal of treatment for high-risk newborns. American Academy of Pediatrics Committee on Fetus and Newborn. Pediatrics 1995; 96:362-3.

Iron fortification of infant formulas. American Academy of Pediatrics. Committee on Nutrition. Pediatrics 1999;104:119–23.

Joint Committee on Infant Hearing year 2000 position statement: principles and guidelines for early hearing detection and intervention programs. Logan (UT): National Center for Hearing Assessment & Management; 2000. Available at http://www.infanthearing.org/jcih/index.html. Retrieved June 17, 2002.

Kattwinkel J, Niermeyer S, Nadkarni V, Tibballs J, Phillips B, Zideman D, et al. An advisory statement from the Pediatric Working Group of the International Liaison Committee on Resuscitation. Pediatrics 1999;103:e56.

National Institute of Child Health and Human Development. Report of the workshop on acute perinatal asphyxia in term infants. Washington, DC: NICHD; 1996. NIH publication 96-3823.

Newborn screening fact sheets. American Academy of Pediatrics. Committee on Genetics. Pediatrics 1996;98:473–501.

Positioning and sudden infant death syndrome (SIDS): update. American Academy of Pediatrics. Task Force on Infant Positioning and SIDS. Pediatrics 1996;98:1216–18.

Recommended childhood immunization schedule–United States, January–December 1999. American Academy of Pediatrics. Committee on Infectious Diseases. Pediatrics 1999;103:182–5.

The role of the primary care pediatrician in the management of high-risk newborn infants. American Academy of Pediatrics. Committee on Practice and Ambulatory Medicine and Committee on Fetus and Newborn. Pediatrics 1996;98:786–88.

Safe transportation of premature and low birth weight infants. American Academy of Pediatrics. Committee on Injury and Poison Prevention and Committee on Fetus and Newborn. Pediatrics 1996;97:758–60.

Update on timing of hepatitis B vaccination for premature infants and for children with lapsed immunization. American Academy of Pediatrics Committee on Infection Diseases. Pediatrics 1994;94:403–4.

CHAPTER 8

Neonatal Complications

Because of advances in knowledge and controversies surrounding certain issues, some neonatal conditions and treatments require particular attention. Whenever possible, therapies should be based on the best evidence available, preferably from well-designed, randomized, controlled trials.

Hyperbilirubinemia

Although bilirubin may be toxic to the central nervous system and may cause neurologic impairment, the factors that determine the toxicity of bilirubin to the brain cells of neonates are many, complex, and incompletely understood. Factors include those that affect serum albumin concentration and the binding of bilirubin to albumin, the penetration of bilirubin into the brain, and the vulnerability of brain cells to the toxic effects of bilirubin. In addition, the interrelationships between serum bilirubin concentrations and kernicterus (a condition characterized by a definitive neurologic syndrome, staining, and neuronal injury within specific brainstem nuclei) and residual bilirubin encephalopathy (brain damage caused by bilirubin) are not clear. Whether hyperbilirubinemia causes mild neurologic impairment less severe than frank bilirubin encephalopathy is not known, nor is it known at what bilirubin concentration or under what circumstances the risk of brain damage exceeds that of treatment. In addition to uncertainty about the cause and effect of the disorder, differences in patient populations, geographic locations, and practice settings contribute to variations in the management of hyperbilirubinemia.

BILIRUBIN TOXICITY

A direct association between severe, unconjugated hyperbilirubinemia, kernicterus, and bilirubin encephalopathy has been demonstrated in neonates with erythroblastosis fetalis. In the past, survivors often manifested serious sequelae, particularly the athetoid form of cerebral palsy, hearing loss, paralysis of upward gaze, and dentoalveolar dysplasia. In most studies of otherwise healthy term neonates without hemolysis, total serum bilirubin concentrations of less than 25 mg/dL (428 μmol/L) have not been associated with either cognitive or serious neurologic abnormalities.

Studies of preterm neonates have failed to identify a specific serum bilirubin concentration as a risk factor for kernicterus. Autopsy findings of yellow-stained cerebral tissues in preterm neonates whose bilirubin concentrations never exceeded 10 mg/dL (171 μmol/L) have been reported. Some published guidelines for the management of jaundice in such neonates have suggested early phototherapy and exchange transfusion at bilirubin concentrations of as low as 10 mg/dL (171 μmol/L). Several studies of preterm neonates, however, have failed to confirm a relationship between serum bilirubin concentrations and later neurodevelopmental handicap, particularly if serum bilirubin concentrations did not exceed 20 mg/dL (342 μmol/L). In the studies reporting kernicterus in preterm neonates at low bilirubin concentrations, noteworthy clinical findings were a lack of the classic encephalopathic syndrome and the concurrent presence of other disorders which had the potential to result in a central nervous system insult—respiratory failure with hypoxia and hypercarbia, sepsis, and intraventricular hemorrhage. Therefore, the management decision for exchange transfusion for prevention of kernicterus in the preterm neonate should include consideration of other coexisting pathophysiologic processes.

DETECTION AND MANAGEMENT OF JAUNDICE

Data from numerous studies of bilirubin toxicity are so complex that it is difficult to derive a single rational approach to treat neonates with jaundice. One principle is well accepted—if the neonate's clinical course suggests that the jaundice is not physiologic, the cause should be investigated. The most important step in evaluating a newborn with jaundice is to determine if hemolysis is the contributing process. In general, jaundice presenting within the first 24 hours following birth is hemolytic in origin and requires investigation. Jaundice that persists beyond 2 weeks requires further investigation, including measurement of both total and direct serum bilirubin concentrations. Elevation of the direct serum bilirubin always requires further investigation and possible intervention.

Term Neonates with Hemolytic Disease

Clinical observation of term neonates with hemolytic disease has confirmed that the occurrence of clinical kernicterus is highly unlikely if serum unconjugated bilirubin concentrations are less than 20 mg/dL (342 µmol/L). The physician may elect to perform an exchange transfusion before the serum bilirubin concentration reaches 20 mg/dL (342 µmol/L) if several determinations of bilirubin levels indicate that the concentration is likely to reach that level in spite of all other appropriate medical management including phototherapy.

Term Neonates Without Hemolytic Disease

There are no properly designed studies, or even observational data, on preterm or term neonates without hemolytic disease on which to base clinical guidelines for the treatment of neonates with serum bilirubin concentrations of less than 20 mg/dL (342 µmol/L). Follow-up data for apparently healthy term neonates whose serum bilirubin concentrations were as high as 25 mg/dL (428 µmol/L) showed no apparent ill effects from these concentrations. On the basis of these observations, the American Academy of Pediatrics (AAP) developed guidelines for managing healthy term neonates (defined as those born at ≥37 weeks of gestation) who have hyperbilirubinemia but no signs of illness or apparent hemolytic disease (Table 8–1).

Preterm Neonates

In the past, some physicians have recommended, as a result of the aforementioned autopsy studies, initiating phototherapy early and performing exchange transfusions in selected preterm neonates who have serum bilirubin concentrations of as low as 10 mg/dL (171 µmol/L). However,

Table 8–1. Management of Hyperbilirubinemia in the Healthy Term Newborn

	Total Serum Bilirubin Levels (mg/dL)			
Age (hours)	Consider Phototherapy*	Phototherapy	Exchange Transfusion if Intensive Phototherapy Fails	Exchange Transfusion and Intensive Phototherapy
<24	Term neonates who are clinically jaundiced at <24 hours are not considered "healthy" and require evaluation			
25–48	≥12	≥15	≥20	≥25
49–72	≥15	≥18	≥25	≥30
≥73	≥17	≥20	≥25	≥30

*Phototherapy at these levels is a clinical option; that is, the intervention is available and may be used on the basis of individual clinical judgment.

Used and modified with permission of the American Academy of Pediatrics. Practice parameter: management of hyperbilirubinemia in the healthy term newborn. American Academy of Pediatrics. Provisional Committee for Quality Improvement and Subcommittee on Hyperbilirubinemia. Pediatrics 1994;94:558–65.

this approach cannot guarantee the prevention of kernicterus. As the risks of exchange transfusion are significant and the benefit in this population unproved, most neonatologists allow serum bilirubin concentrations to reach 15–20 mg/dL (257–342 µmol/L) before considering exchange transfusion.

Relationship Between Breastfeeding and Jaundice

Breastfeeding has a significant effect on the level as well as the duration of unconjugated hyperbilirubinemia, as compared with formula fed infants. This relationship is seen in two ways. The first is known as breast milk jaundice, characterized as an extension of physiologic jaundice beyond the first week of age. Although formula fed infants generally have serum bilirubin levels less than 1.5 mg/dL by age 10–14 days, breastfed infants commonly have levels greater than 5 mg/dL for several weeks after delivery. This increased unconjugated hyperbilirubinemia is caused by an as yet unidentified factor in human milk that promotes an increase in intestinal absorption of bilirubin. Jaundice persisting beyond the first week of life should be monitored to ensure that it is unconjugated hyperbilirubinemia, that levels of bilirubin are not increasing, and that other pathologic causes for the jaundice are not present.

A second way in which breastfeeding is related to hyperbilirubinemia is a pathologic one, which is a result of an inadequate intake of human milk in breastfed infants. This breastfeeding failure, or "breast-non-feeding jaundice," most often occurs in association with a primiparous or first-time breastfeeding mother with a near-term infant. Early hospital discharge is an additional risk factor. Because of inadequate milk production, which is unrecognized by the woman and health care providers, the infant may lose up to 30% of its birth weight over 7–14 days following hospital discharge associated with marked hyperbilirubinemia. There have been reports of mortality and kernicterus associated with this type of lactation failure. Proper education and support of the mother and the infant, along with early and continued follow-up after hospital discharge to evaluate the feeding process and the health of the neonate are essential in preventing such problems. If failure of milk production is confirmed, infants should be promptly provided necessary medical evaluation and support (including appropriate rehydration) and changed to newborn formula, because establishing lactogenesis at that point is unlikely to be successful.

Some evidence indicates that frequent breastfeeding (8–10 times per 24 hours) may reduce the incidence of hyperbilirubinemia. Supplementing nursing with water or dextrose-water will not decrease serum bilirubin concentrations in jaundiced, healthy, breastfeeding neonates. When an indirect serum bilirubin concentration is elevated by some pathologic cause, there is no reason to discontinue breastfeeding. However, if the serum unconjugated bilirubin level in a breastfed, term, healthy infant is increasing and is higher than 20 mg/dL, the physician has several options to reduce the level. Breastfeeding may be continued and the infant treated with phototherapy, while infant and mother undergo thorough evaluation and assistance with the feeding process. Alternatively, breastfeeding may continue and the infant supplemented with newborn formula. Finally, complete substitution of breast milk with infant formula for 24–48 hours will almost always result in a rapid decrease in serum bilirubin concentrations. This can be combined with phototherapy. Women who must temporarily cease nursing should be given positive and enthusiastic support. They should be encouraged to maintain lactation by using a breast pump or manual expression during the period of interrupted nursing. They also should be reassured that the nutritional value of their milk is not compromised by the use of these methods.

HYDRATION

There is no evidence that excess fluid administered to the neonate decreases the serum bilirubin concentration. Some neonates who are admitted to the hospital with high bilirubin concentrations also may be mildly dehydrated and may need supplemental fluid intake to correct dehydration. In the absence of dehydration, routine supplementation (with dextrose-water) of neonates receiving phototherapy is not indicated. However, in sick very low-birth-weight (LBW) neonates receiving phototherapy, excess evaporative water loss is known to occur and frequently necessitates increased fluid intake or environmental humidity or both for replacement or prevention of ongoing losses.

PHOTOTHERAPY

Phototherapy is effective in reducing serum bilirubin concentrations in neonates with nonhemolytic jaundice. Phototherapy is less effective in neonates with ABO and CDE (Rh) hemolytic disease, reducing, but not eliminating, the need for exchange transfusions in these neonates. Exchange transfusion is the treatment of choice when the bilirubin concentration appears to pose an imminent threat to the health of the neonate.

There is no standardized method for delivering phototherapy. However, detailed recommendations on phototherapy can be found in the hyperbilirubinemia practice parameters of AAP. Commonly used phototherapy units contain daylight, cool white, blue, or "special blue" fluorescent tubes. Other units use tungsten-halogen lamps in different configurations, either freestanding or as part of a radiant-warming device. Fiber optic systems have been developed that deliver high-intensity light to a fiber optic blanket.

The efficacy of phototherapy is influenced by the energy output (irradiance), in the blue spectrum (measured in $\mu W/cm^2$), the spectrum of light source, and the surface area of the neonate exposed to the light source. The irradiance of a unit should be monitored and bulbs changed as needed to maintain maximum energy output. It is acceptable to interrupt phototherapy during feeding or brief parental visits. Intensive phototherapy can be achieved by use of blue lights, decreasing the distance of the source from the neonate, and increasing the surface area exposed to the lights. The neonate's temperature should be monitored frequently while phototherapy is being applied.

Although phototherapy has many biologic effects, it has no known lasting toxic effects in the human neonate. Because experiments in animals have documented retinal damage from phototherapy, the neonate's eyes should be covered with opaque patches during exposure to phototherapy light. Known potential complications from improper monitoring of eye patch placement include malposition and obstruction of the nares, inadequate securing allowing lid opening and resultant corneal abrasion, and conjunctivitis from use without intermittent removal to assess the condition of the covered tissues.

With the introduction of early discharge of term and near-term neonates, the determination of a neonate's suitability for early discharge has required heightened awareness of normal course of physiologic hyperbilirubinemia. Recent data suggest that there is some predictability to the progressive rise in serum bilirubin concentrations from nonpathologic sources. It is suggested that for neonates who are otherwise candidates for early discharge, a predischarge serum bilirubin determination can be helpful in predicting risk for a subsequent increase to more concerning concentrations. A neonate with early onset jaundice (within the first 24 hours) should have hemolysis excluded as a cause before being considered for early discharge.

Some neonates with uncomplicated nonhemolytic jaundice may be treated with phototherapy at home. Guidelines should be developed by each institution to define criteria for neonates who are eligible for home phototherapy. Home care requires appropriate follow-up and supervision by a health care professional with access to serum bilirubin determinations as clinically indicated. With proper instruction of the parents or guardians, phototherapy can be provided by using a freestanding device or a fiber optic blanket. If serum bilirubin concentrations do not decrease in response to conventional phototherapy, admission to the hospital may be indicated for more intensive phototherapy or exchange transfusion and for evaluation of the underlying cause.

Clinical Considerations in the Use of Oxygen

The hazards associated with the nonindicated administration of supplemental oxygen to preterm neonates have been recognized for many years. Studies conducted in the 1950s indicated that prolonged oxygen therapy without clinical indication was associated with increased rates of retinopathy of prematurity, formerly called retrolental fibroplasia. The ensuing blanket restriction of ambient oxygen therapy resulted in a marked decrease in retinopathy of prematurity at the cost of a marked increase in morbidity and mortality. Current practice includes the prudent use of supplemental oxygen as needed, based on an objective determination of oxygen requirements.

When supplemental oxygen therapy is considered, the potential risks, in terms of both hypoxia and hyperoxia, should be weighed. Clinical judgment of physical signs alone as a guide to the amount of supplemental oxygen needed is acceptable for short periods, emergencies, or abrupt clinical changes. However, the ease of noninvasive determinations of oxygen saturation should preclude the continued use of supplemental oxygen without an objective assessment.

Administration and Monitoring

In an emergency, high concentrations of supplemental oxygen may be administered by a face mask or endotracheal tube. When a neonate requires oxygen therapy beyond the emergency period, the oxygen should be warmed and humidified, and the concentration or flow should be carefully regulated and monitored. Oxygen can be delivered via an endotracheal tube, oxygen hood, nasal prong, or incubator. Oxygen analyzers should be calibrated in accordance with manufacturers' recommendations. Orders for oxygen therapy should be written in terms of desired ambient concentration or flow and should indicate the intervals at which the concentration (or flow rate, when nasal prongs are used) should be routinely checked. Alternatively, orders should be written to adjust FIO_2 or flow within a stated range to maintain oxygen saturation within specific limits. There should be an institutional policy for ordering, delivering, and documenting oxygen therapy and monitoring.

An important development in the care of neonates who require oxygen therapy has been the ability to monitor oxygenation continuously with noninvasive techniques. The transcutaneous oxygen analyzer provides an indirect measurement of Pao_2, and the pulse oximeter measures oxyhemoglobin saturation. Because neither technique measures Pao_2 directly, they should be used as adjuncts to, rather than substitutes for, arterial blood gas sampling, especially in neonates with moderate to severe respiratory distress.

Periodic measurement of Pao_2 in samples from an umbilical or peripheral artery catheter is the most reliable method of assessing the effectiveness of oxygen therapy. If an indwelling arterial catheter is not in place, peripheral artery puncture can be used, but repeated sampling from these sites is not always possible. When arterial blood sampling is not possible, arterialized capillary sampling is an acceptable alternative. This measurement produces fairly reliable estimates of arterial pH and arterial carbon dioxide ($Paco_2$) but usually underestimates true Pao_2.

In neonates whose condition is unstable, noninvasive measurements should be correlated with Pao_2 at least every 8–12 hours. More frequent analyses of arterial blood gas may be indicated for the assessment of pH and Pao_2. In neonates whose condition is stable, correlation with arterial blood gas samples may be performed less frequently.

The use of either transcutaneous oxygen measurement or pulse oximetry may shorten the time required to determine optimum inspired oxygen concentration and ventilator settings in the acute care setting. Both measurements are particularly useful in monitoring oxygen therapy in neonates who are recovering from respiratory distress or who require long-term supplemental oxygen. Because transcutaneous oxygen measurements underestimate oxygenation in older neonates with bronchopulmonary dysplasia (BPD), pulse oximetry may be a more suitable method for monitoring oxygen therapy in these neonates.

In consideration of the current, but incomplete, understanding of the effects of oxygen administration, the following recommendations are offered:

- Supplemental oxygen should not be used without a specific indication, such as cyanosis, low Pao_2, or low oxygen saturation.

- The use of supplemental oxygen other than for resuscitation should be monitored by regular assessments of Pao_2 and oxygen saturation.

- The duration of time that oxygen therapy may be administered in nurseries lacking the capability of appropriate Pao_2 or oxygen saturation monitoring before consideration of transfer to a higher level unit is contingent on the gestational age of the neonate and the severity of the oxygenation deficit. In general, neonates delivered at less than 36 weeks of gestation or those requiring more than 40% ambient oxygen should be stabilized and transferred promptly.

- For neonates who require oxygen therapy for acute care, measurements of blood pressure levels, blood pH, and $Paco_2$ should accompany measurements of Pao_2. In addition, a record of blood gas measurements, details of the oxygen delivery system (eg, ventilator, settings, continuous positive airway pressure), and ambient oxygen concentrations (or liter of flow per minute, if nasal prongs are used) should be maintained.

- When supplemental oxygen is administered to a preterm neonate, attempts should be made to maintain Pao_2 at 50–80 mm Hg. Oxygen tensions in this range should be adequate for tissue needs, given normal hemoglobin concentrations and blood flow. Even with careful monitoring, however, Pao_2 may fluctuate outside this range, particularly in neonates with cardiopulmonary disease.

- It is prudent when oxygen therapy is needed for a preterm neonate to discuss the reasons for using supplemental oxygen and the associated risks and benefits with parents.

- Hourly measurement and recording of the concentration of oxygen delivered to the neonate is recommended

- Except for an emergency situation, air-oxygen mixtures should be warmed and humidified before being administered to newborns.

RETINOPATHY OF PREMATURITY

Myriad factors other than hyperoxia may contribute to the pathogenesis of retinopathy of prematurity. Prolonged ventilatory support (especially when accompanied by episodes of hypoxia and hypercapnia) and clinical conditions, including acidosis, shock, sepsis, apnea, anemia, patent ductus arteriosus, and vitamin E deficiency also have been associated with retinopathy of prematurity.

To date, a safe level of Pao_2 in relation to retinopathy of prematurity has not been established. Retinopathy of prematurity has occurred in preterm neonates who have never received supplemental oxygen therapy and in neonates with cyanotic congenital heart disease in whom Pao_2 levels never exceeded 50 mm Hg. Conversely, retinopathy of prematurity has not developed in some preterm neonates after prolonged periods of hyperoxia. Recent data have demonstrated no additional progression of active prethreshold retinopathy of prematurity when supplemental oxygen was administered at pulse oximetry saturations between 96% and 99%. Further, continuous close monitoring of transcutaneous oxygen tension has not resulted in a decrease in the incidence of retinopathy of prematurity.

On the basis of published data, the following statements regarding retinopathy of prematurity and oxygen use are warranted:

- Retinopathy of prematurity is not preventable in some neonates, especially extremely LBW neonates.
- Many factors other than hyperoxia are important in the pathogenesis of retinopathy of prematurity.
- Transient hyperoxia alone cannot be considered sufficient to cause retinopathy of prematurity.
- Strict adherence to existing standard of care for supplemental oxygen therapy will not completely prevent complications or side effects.
- An ophthalmologist with experience in retinopathy of prematurity and indirect ophthalmoscopy should examine the retinas of all preterm neonates (ie, those delivered at ≤28 weeks of gestation or weighing ≤1,500 g at birth). The examination should be performed at 4–6 weeks of chronologic age or at 31–33 weeks post-

menstrual age (gestational age at birth plus chronologic age), as determined by the neonate's attending pediatrician or neonatologist.

- Scheduling of follow-up examinations is best determined from the findings of the first examination, using the International Classification of Retinopathy of Prematurity. Neonates with threshold disease should be considered candidates for peripheral retinal ablative therapy of at least one eye within 72 hours of diagnosis.

- If a neonate at risk for retinopathy of prematurity is transferred to another hospital during the period of susceptibility for development or progression of the disease, the status of monitoring examinations must be communicated to the physician assuming responsibility for the neonate's subsequent care.

- A written hospital policy designating responsibility for tracking and scheduling ophthalmologic examinations of preterm neonates at risk for retinopathy of prematurity is useful and strongly encouraged.

Drug Exposure

Neonatal Implications

The use of illicit substances by women of childbearing age has led to increased numbers of neonates having had in utero exposure and subsequent risk of adverse effects from a variety of drugs. Both licit substances, alcohol and tobacco, and illicit "street drugs" have the potential of adversely affecting fetal growth and development and postnatal adaptation. Fetal drug exposure often is unrecognized because of the lack of overt symptomatology or structural abnormality following birth. In such circumstances neonates may be discharged to homes where they are at increased risk for a complex of medical and social problems, including abuse and neglect. Frequently the lifestyle choices of the woman using illicit substance(s) includes exposure to sexually transmitted diseases—human immunodeficiency virus (HIV) and acquired immunodeficiency syndrome (AIDS), herpes, hepatitis, and syphilis, in particular—with significant consequences to her fetus if she becomes infected. In addition, there may have been little or no prenatal care, further increasing risks for the fetus.

Illicit drugs may reach the fetus via placental transfer, or may reach the newborn through breast milk. The specific effect on the fetus and newborn varies with the respective substances. An opiate exposed fetus may experience withdrawal in utero when the woman undergoes withdrawal, either voluntary or under supervision, and after birth when the delivery of the drug by way of the placenta ceases. Although the incidence of breastfeeding by substance-using women is low in general, nursing women should be counseled about the adverse effects of substance use.

Universal screening of women and newborns for substance use is not recommended. However, because of both immediate as well as potential long-term adverse effects from in utero drug exposure on the neonate, it is imperative that a thorough maternal substance use history be obtained. Toxicology screening of maternal blood or urine or neonatal urine or meconium samples may be useful when there are clinical indications of drug effect. Screening of meconium provides a more comprehensive and accurate indication of exposure over a longer gestational period than does screening of neonatal urine. Physicians and nursery staff should be competent in the recognition of signs of neonatal withdrawal. There are a number of useful systematic scoring schemata for assessing severity and each nursery unit should have a written policy for implementation of a scoring system for neonatal withdrawal.

Documentation of in utero illicit substance exposure should preclude early discharge following birth. Appropriate planning for discharge and subsequent follow-up care requires social work assessment and may include referral for child protective services if there is a concern about the future well-being of the neonate.

PEDIATRIC IMPLICATIONS

Long-term effects on learning and school performance, behavioral problems, and emotional instability of children exposed to illicit drugs in utero remain major concerns. There is evidence that all drugs of abuse have an impact on the endogenous neurotransmitter systems of the brain. Exposure during development may alter the development and functions of these systems, which may have a long-lasting impact on behavioral and cognitive outcomes. Environmental factors also place drug-exposed children at high risk for physical, sexual and emotional abuse, neglect, and developmental delay. Long-term follow-up is indicated from medical, developmental, and social aspects. Pediatricians should, therefore, work with state social service agencies and state legislatures to extend the assistance now available through child protective services. Until this is accomplished, pediatricians should consider recruiting the assistance of the local child protective services agency to provide multidisciplinary treatment and support for the affected woman, child, and family. In general, a coordinated multidisciplinary approach in the development of a plan without criminal sanctions has the best chance of helping children and families.

Respiratory Distress Syndrome

Respiratory distress syndrome (RDS) is associated with preterm birth-related surfactant deficiency. Multiple randomized, controlled clinical trials indicate the benefits of surfactant replacement therapy, including reduction in the severity of RDS, improvement in survival rate, and fewer pulmonary complications. However, coexistent morbidity, such as necrotizing enterocolitis, nosocomial infections, patent ductus arteriosus, intraventricular hemorrhage, and BPD appear primarily unaffected. Long-term outcome of treated neonates has shown neither beneficial nor adverse effects on growth and neurodevelopment.

SURFACTANT REPLACEMENT THERAPY

Universal availability of surfactant replacement therapy raises concerns about its potential misuse. A major concern is that very LBW neonates with multisystem disorders may be treated with surfactant and stay in nurseries where their other diseases and morbidities cannot be addressed adequately. Caring for these neonates in nurseries that do not have the full range of required capabilities may affect overall outcome adversely. Therefore, the availability of surfactant therapy should not alter the referral criteria for high-risk maternal and neonatal transfers, specifically early-gestational-age and very LBW neonates.

As systems of neonatal health care adapt to modified patterns of disease in LBW neonates, the following recommendations should be incorporated:

- Surfactant therapy should be used only in institutions in which facilities and personnel are available for the management of multisystem disorders in LBW neonates.

- An institutionally approved protocol for administering surfactant therapy should be a component of a quality-assessment program.

- Surfactant replacement therapy should be directed by physicians who are trained in the respiratory management of LBW neonates and have knowledge and experience in mechanical ventilation.

- Nursing and respiratory therapy personnel who are experienced in the management of LBW neonates, including the use of mechanical ventilation, should be available when surfactant therapy is administered.

- The equipment necessary for managing and monitoring the condition of LBW neonates, including that needed for mechanical ventilation, should be available when surfactant therapy is administered.

- Radiology and laboratory support to manage a broad range of needs of very LBW neonates should be immediately available.

- At institutions that do not meet these requirements to offer surfactant therapy, and when timely transfer of a high-risk newborn to an appropriate institution cannot be achieved, surfactant therapy may be given, but only by a physician who is skilled in endotracheal intubation. Neonates should be transferred if appropriate from such institutions, as soon as feasible, to a center with appropriate facilities and trained staff to care for multisystem morbidity in LBW neonates.

Hemorrhagic and Periventricular White Matter Brain Injury

CLINICAL CONSIDERATIONS

Neonates born at 32 weeks of gestation or less or at birth weights of 1.5 kg or less are those at highest risk for hemorrhagic and other injury to the brain. Both the incidence and severity increase with decreasing gestational age. Their vulnerability arises from the vascular and cellular immaturity of the developing brain and may be compounded by inadequate protective cerebral autoregulation of blood flow during the frequent periods of physiologic instability characteristic of this group of newborns. Periventricular, intraventricular hemorrhage, which is the most frequent hemorrhagic lesion, ranges from a small germinal matrix bleed to varying amounts of intraventricular blood to massive intraparenchymal hemorrhage or hemorrhagic infarction. Most periventricular, intraventricular hemorrhage occurs in the first 72 hours after birth. Post hemorrhagic hydrocephalus secondary to periventricular, intraventricular hemorrhage is apparent within 2–4 weeks after delivery. Periventricular leukomalacia is the most frequent white matter lesion identified. Residual lesions following brain injury include minimal to extensive cystic lesions in the periventricular white matter and ventriculomegaly secondary to diffuse cerebral atrophy. Porencephaly may develop following severe localized ischemic or hemorrhagic cortical infarction. These lesions evolve over the course of several weeks after the precipitating insult. Both hemorrhagic and other brain injury can occur in the same neonate, although the pathophysiologic processes are different.

SURVEILLANCE

Portable bedside cranial ultrasonography is the most frequent imaging modality used to diagnose and follow the evolution of both hemorrhagic and ischemic lesions. There can be great variability in the interpretation. The quality of the images is affected by the choice of equipment and the expertise of the sonographer in obtaining consistent positioning of the sensor.

It is recommended that each center establish a protocol for screening cranial ultrasound examinations in at-risk neonates. In the absence of the need to make a diagnosis for clinical reasons, the initial study can be performed between 3 and 14 postnatal days. Follow-up studies to monitor for the evolution of severity or emergence of a complication may be timed based on the clinical course and the known progression of such. Current experience suggests that the best correlation with subsequent risk for neurodevelopmental sequelae is found from the results of studies performed at approximately 40 weeks postmenstrual age. This potentially identifies those neonates who are most in need of comprehensive follow-up.

Prevention

As yet, no single intervention has been found to consistently prevent either periventricular, intraventricular hemorrhage or other lesions although many approaches have been tried. A coordinated perinatal approach to reduce the severity and impact of episodes of hemodynamic instability is important. Currently, there is good evidence that glucocorticoids given to women in preterm labor for acceleration of fetal lung maturation also decrease the incidence and severity of periventricular, intraventricular hemorrhage in susceptible fetuses.

Hypoxic Cardiorespiratory Failure

Hypoxic cardiorespiratory failure in neonates born at or near term may be caused by such conditions as primary persistent pulmonary hypertension, RDS, aspiration of meconium, pneumonia or sepsis, and congenital diaphragmatic hernia. Conventional therapies, which have not been validated by randomized controlled trials, include administration of high oxygen concentrations, hyperventilation, high frequency ventilation, the induction of alkalosis, neuromuscular blockade, and sedation. Despite aggressive conventional therapy, neonatal cardiorespiratory failure has been associated with a high mortality rate and with persistent respiratory dysfunction necessitating chronic medical management in many survivors. Two major modalities of alternative rescue treatments have been developed in the past two decades that have been shown to increase survival—extracorporeal membrane oxygenation (ECMO) and inhaled nitric oxide.

EXTRACORPOREAL MEMBRANE OXYGENATION

The technique for providing lung rest by use of a mechanical membrane oxygenator has been incorporated into the management of neonates who, having failed to respond to conventional therapy, are at extreme risk for death from hypoxic cardiorespiratory failure. Although the numbers of newborns receiving ECMO therapy have been declining in the past 5 years, all studies indicate that there is a core group of patients who will benefit from this therapy.

Because of the high resource use, the need for concentrated experience for optimal outcomes, and the decreasing numbers of neonates who require ECMO treatment, the following guidelines for the development of ECMO centers have been promulgated:

- Demonstrated regional need for the establishment of an ECMO center
- Demonstrated management of a regional neonatal or perinatal care program in a tertiary (subspecialty) perinatal care center
- Availability of skilled personnel
- Organized and functioning neonatal transport system
- Institutional guidelines for initiating ECMO therapy
- Established program for neurodevelopmental follow-up of neonatal intensive care unit graduates

Questions remain about the long-term safety of ECMO therapy although recent reports of outcomes have been encouraging with a large majority of survivors being found to be normal. Both the primary disease process that precipitated the hypoxic respiratory failure and the severity of the clinical condition before the initiation of ECMO strongly affect the outcome.

Inhaled Nitric Oxide

Inhaled nitric oxide is a selective pulmonary vasodilator. Several prospective randomized clinical trials have shown that inhaled nitric oxide improves oxygenation and reduces the risk for ECMO therapy in neonates with hypoxic cardiorespiratory failure. Inhaled nitric oxide has been approved by the U.S. Food and Drug Administration for treatment of hypoxic cardiorespiratory failure in term and near-term neonates. Although approved for use, the efficacy of inhaled nitric oxide and an optimal dosing strategy remains to be established. Its use should be limited to neonates meeting the clinical criteria of published clinical trials. Preterm neonates may experience more toxicity than term and near-term neonates.

It is critical that neonates with hypoxic cardiorespiratory failure receive care in institutions that have personnel—including physicians, nurses, and respiratory therapists who are qualified to use multiple modes of ventilation—and readily accessible radiologic and laboratory support. Neonates who are failing conventional therapies should be transferred in a timely manner to centers capable of providing alternative treatments. Institution-specific guidelines for transfers should be developed.

Management of Anemia in Preterm Neonates

Anemia of prematurity results from multiple factors and varies with the degree of immaturity, the postnatal age, the nutritional status and intake, and the nature and severity of neonatal illness. Appropriate management requires accurate assessment of the role of the various etiologies with therapeutic interventions determined by that assessment. At times, the need for adequate oxygen carrying capacity necessitates packed red blood cell transfusion on an acute basis while awaiting response to other interventions to correct the anemia producing process. However, transfusion poses risks of transmission of pathogens, particularly with exposure to multiple donors.

Current evidence indicates that anemia occurring in the first 2–3 weeks after delivery can be accounted for by the volume of blood sampling obtained for clinical management. Once growth begins, adequate protein intake becomes important. The balance of oxidative substrate (polyunsaturated free fatty acids), antioxidant (vitamin E), and oxidant (iron) in the diet during growth also may play a role in red blood cell survival. As growth accelerates with advancing postnatal age, depletion of iron stores begins to impact erythropoiesis. Underlying all of these factors is the very LBW neonate's limited capacity to increase erythropoietin production in response to anemia. This further decreases red blood cell production and increases the likelihood of dilutional anemia from an expanding blood volume.

Recent controlled clinical trials have shown that adherence to protocols with strict indications for transfusion reduced both the volume of blood transfused and donor exposure without adverse clinical consequences. Prophylactic use of recombinant human erythropoietin in clinical trials, both administered early in the neonatal course and initiated after several weeks, has demonstrated a limited reduction in the number of transfusions and the volume of transfused blood; the impact of reduced donor exposure has not been studied in most trials. In none of these studies was the need for transfusion eliminated altogether.

It would seem prudent from the available evidence to recommend that a multiprong approach to limiting transfusion be used, particularly in very LBW neonates. Both the causation as well as the correction of anemia of prematurity must be addressed. This would include judicial use of blood sampling (using noninvasive oxygen monitoring extensively), maintenance of optimal nutritional intake whenever possible, adherence to a protocol with strict indications for transfusion of packed red blood cells, and establishment of a system of blood banking that limits donor exposure to the maximum possible extent. Routine use of human recombinant erythropoietin for all preterm neonates is not recommended at this time. There may be specific groups of very LBW neonates (eg, Jehovah's Witnesses) in whom its use would be beneficial.

Bronchopulmonary Dysplasia

Historical Perspective

The introduction of mechanical ventilatory support for the treatment of RDS in the early 1960s was followed by the emergence of a syndrome of chronic respiratory failure, which was described initially in 1968 and named BPD or chronic lung disease of newborns. It was recognized to follow prolonged exposure to high oxygen concentrations and positive pressure mechanical ventilation. By the late 1980s a decrease in the incidence of BPD was observed. Subsequent to the universal application of surfactant replacement therapy in the early 1990s, a shift in birth-weight-specific survival to hospital discharge occurred with larger numbers of very LBW neonates surviving, particularly extremely LBW neonates—weighing less than 1 kg at delivery. A new spectrum of BPD is now recognized among extremely LBW survivors.

Therapeutic Approaches—Prevention

Multiple strategies and pharmacologic interventions have been proposed to decrease the induction of inflammation in the lungs of very LBW neonates. Few have been adequately supported by controlled clinical trials of appropriate size and rigorous design to support recommendation for universal implementation. The prevention of RDS and the requirement for mechanical ventilation by the antenatal administration of glucocorticoids to women at risk of preterm delivery decreases the at-risk population. Vitamin A supplementation has been shown to be safe and to result in a modest decrease in the risk of BPD in ventilated extremely LBW neonates. Assisted ventilation strategies to avoid deleterious hyperinflation are desirable but strong supportive evidence for most specific individual strategies are lacking. Permissive hypercapnia (ie, accepting higher Pco_2 levels than previously was customary) has been suggested but controlled studies in neonates to demonstrate its safety and efficacy have not been reported. High-frequency ventilation using various modalities and strategies has not been found to be consistently efficacious. The use of synchronized ventilation, if achievable, would seem prudent to avoid volutrauma. High volumes of fluid intake in the first week have been shown to contribute to the persistence of a patent ductus arteriosus and perhaps to the development of BPD. However, no single fluid regimen has been shown to be safer and more efficacious; fluid restriction often means caloric restriction as well. Other modalities directed at specific antecedents of inflammatory injury have included antioxidants (vitamin E and superoxide dismutase), erythromycin (prophylaxis or treatment for Ureaplasma), and early postnatal steroids. None of these can be recommended at this time either because of safety issues (early postnatal steroids) or unconfirmed efficacy (vitamin E is not beneficial); erythromycin and superoxide dismutase have not been adequately studied.

THERAPEUTIC APPROACHES—TREATMENT

Once BPD is established, current evidence and clinical experience support that diuretics and inhaled bronchodilator agents improve pulmonary function and, therefore, may facilitate reduction in ventilatory support and extubation. Oxygen supplementation is a consistent component of care but the most efficacious therapeutic range of oxygen saturation has not been established. Episodes of spontaneous desaturation are a frequent occurrence in neonates with BPD. Oxygen supplementation has been shown to improve growth and decrease the likelihood of progression to pulmonary hypertension. Both inhaled and systemic glucocorticoid therapy have facilitated reduction in ventilatory support and hastened extubation. However, neonates treated with systemic glucocorticoids are at risk of experiencing a number of adverse effects, including an arrest or decrease in growth rate, possibly an increase in neurodevelopmental abnormalities, as well as an increased incidence of gastrointestinal hemorrhage, intestinal perforation, nosocomial sepsis, hyperglycemia, hypertension, and adrenal suppression. Growth failure without steroid exposure is well recognized to accompany severe BPD; energy expenditure has been shown to be significantly higher in neonates with BPD. Lung healing is impaired by inadequate nutritional intake. Therefore, although not supported by controlled trials, provision of calories, minerals and protein to sustain a growth rate comparable with non-BPD gestational age peers seems a logical approach. Immunoprophylaxis for viral respiratory illnesses, RSV, and influenza has reduced the post hospitalization morbidity of neonates with BPD.

NUTRITIONAL NEEDS OF PRETERM NEONATES

Optimal nutrition is critical in the management of small preterm neonates. There is no standard for the precise nutritional needs of preterm neonates comparable with the human milk standard for term neonates. Present recommendations are designed to provide nutrients to approximate the rate of growth and composition of weight gain for a normal fetus of the same postmenstrual age and to maintain normal concentrations of blood and tissue nutrients. However, the presence of acute neonatal illness and the immaturity of a variety of organ systems may make provision of optimal nutrition, without inducing additional morbidity, especially difficult. This is particularly true for the sickest and most immature neonates during the initial days and weeks of life.

Parenteral Nutrition

Parenteral administration of amino acids, glucose and fat is an important aspect of the nutritional care of preterm neonates, particularly those who weigh less than 1,500 g. The high incidence of respiratory and other morbidities, combined with intestinal immaturity, dictates the need for slow advancement of the volume of enteral feedings. Parenteral nutrition can supplement the gradually increasing enteral feedings so that total intake by both routes meets the neonate's nutritional needs.

Positive nitrogen balance, indicating an anabolic state, is achieved with amino acid intakes of 2–3 g/kg per day, and with parenteral lipid and glucose energy intakes of 50–60 kcal/kg per day. With nonprotein energy intakes of 80–85 kcal/kg per day and amino acid intakes of 3–4 g/kg per day, nitrogen retention may occur at the fetal rate. Growth generally requires a minimum parenteral nonprotein energy intake of approximately 70 kcal/kg per day. Current evidence indicates that parenteral administration of amino acid and glucose may be safely initiated within 24 hours of birth. Provision of amino acids at 1.5 g/kg per day, with at least 35 kcal/kg per day of nonprotein energy, will prevent negative nitrogen balance and is well-tolerated, even in the most immature neonates (whose normal fetal amino acid supply is approximately 3.8 g/kg/d). As nonprotein energy and amino acid intake is increased, a balanced supply of glucose and intravenous lipid generally is recommended to prevent some of the metabolic complications of parenteral nutrition.

Enteral Nutrition

The method of enteral feeding chosen for each neonate should be based on gestational age, birth weight, and clinical condition. Often enteral feedings are delayed in the small preterm neonate because of extreme immaturity, perceived increased risk of necrotizing enterocolitis, or significant respiratory or other morbidity. However, evidence indicates that early introduction of "trophic" or "priming" feedings are safe, well-tolerated, and associated with significant benefits. The actual route of enteral feeding (nasogastric, orogastric, gastrostomy, transpyloric, nipple) is again determined on the basis of gestational age, clinical condition, and oromotor integrity (ability to coordinate sucking, swallowing, and breathing).

Human milk from the preterm neonate's mother has a number of special features that make its use desirable in feeding preterm neonates. Fresh or properly stored refrigerated human milk contains immunologic and antimicrobial factors that are protective against infection. Fat digestion is facilitated by the lipase present and the structure of triglycerides found in human milk. However, human milk does not provide adequate protein, calcium, phosphorus, sodium, trace metals, and some vitamins to meet the tissue and bone growth needs of the very LBW neonate. Dry and liquid human milk fortifiers that are nutritionally balanced to correct these deficiencies when added to human milk are commercially available.

Preterm neonates who weigh more than 2,000 g at birth generally achieve adequate growth when fed their mother's milk or a regular 67-kcal/dL term neonate formula. However, calcium and phosphorus retention rates are slower than fetal accretion rates. They may require vitamin supplementation during the period when the volume of formula or human milk ingested does not provide the recommended daily vitamin intake, particularly of vitamin D (Table 8–2).

Table 8–2. Comparison of Enteral Intake Recommendations for Growing Preterm Neonates in Stable Clinical Condition

Nutrients per 100 kcal*	Consensus Recommendations		AAPCON[†]	ESPGAN-CON[†]
	<1,000 g	>1,000 g		
Water, mL	125–167	125–167	—	115–154
Energy, kcal	100	100	100	100
Protein, g	3–3.16	2.5–3	2.9–3.3	2.25–3.1
Carbohydrate, g	—	—	9–13	7–14
Lactose, g	3.16–9.5	3.16–9.8	—	—
Oligomers, g	0–7	0–7	—	—
Fat, g	—	—	4.5–6	3.6–7
Linoleic acid, g	0.44–1.7	0.44–1.7	0.4+	0.5–1.4
Linolenic acid, g	0.11–0.44	0.11–0.44	—	>0.055
$C_{18:2}/C_{18:3}$	>5	>5	—	5–15
Vitamin A, IU	583–1,250	583–1,250	75–225	270–450
With lung disease	2,250–2,333	2,250–2,333	—	—
Vitamin D, IU	125–333	125–333	270	800–1,600/d
Vitamin E, IU	5–10	5–10	>1.1	0.6–10
Supplement, human milk	2.9	2.9	—	—
Vitamin K, µg	6.66–8.33	6.66–8.33	4	4–15
Ascorbate, mg	15–20	15–20	35	7–40
Thiamine, µg	150–200	150–200	>40	20–250
Riboflavin, µg	200–300	200–300	>60	60–600
Pyridoxine, µg	125–175	125–175	>35	35–250
Niacin, mg	3–4	3–4	>0.25	0.8–5
Pantothenate, mg	1–1.5	1–1.5	>0.3	>0.3
Biotin, µg	3–5	3–5	>1.5	>1.5
Folate, µg	21–42	21–42	33	>60
Vitamin B$_{12}$, µg	0.25	0.25	>0.15	>0.15
Sodium, mg	38–58	38–58	48–67	23–53
Potassium, mg	65–100	65–100	66–98	90–152
Chloride, mg	59–89	59–89	—	57–89
Calcium, mg	100–192	100–192	175	70–140
Phosphorus, mg	50–117	50–117	91.5	50–87
Magnesium, mg	6.6–12.5	6.6–12.5	—	6–12
Iron, mg	1.67	1.67	1.7–2.5	1.5
Zinc, µg	833	833	>500	550–1,100

(continued)

Table 8–2. Comparison of Enteral Intake Recommendations for Growing Preterm Neonates in Stable Clinical Condition *(continued)*

Nutrients per 100 kcal*	Consensus Recommendations			
	<1,000 g	>1,000 g	AAPCON[†]	ESPGAN-CON[†]
Copper, μg	100–125	100–125	90	90–120
Selenium, μg	1.08–2.5	1.08–2.5	—	—
Chromium, μg	0.083–0.42	0.083–0.42	—	—
Manganese, μg	6.3	6.3	>5	1.5–7.5
Molybdenum, μg	0.25	0.25	—	—
Iodine, μg	25–50	25–50	5	10–45
Taurine, mg	3.75–7.5	3.75–7.5	—	—
Carnitine, mg	2.4	2.4	—	>1.2
Inositol, mg	27–67.5	27–67.5	—	—
Chlorine, mg	12–23.4	12–23.4	—	—

*Based on a need for 120 mg/kg per day
[†]AAPCON indicates American Academy of Pediatrics, Committee on Nutrition; ESPGAN-CON, European Society of Paediatric Gastroenterology and Nutrition, Committee on Nutrition of the Preterm Infant
Used and modified with permission of the American Academy of Pediatric. Pediatric nutrition handbook, 4th ed, Copyright of the American Academy of Pediatrics, 1998.

Special formulas for very LBW neonates contain additional protein, easily absorbed carbohydrates (glucose polymers and lactose), and easily digested and absorbed lipids (15–50% medium-chain triglycerides). The calcium and phosphorus contents are increased to achieve a bone mineralization rate equivalent to the fetal rate. The sodium content also is increased. Trace metals and vitamins have been added to meet the increased needs of the very LBW neonate. Weight gain and bone mineralization closer to that of the reference fetus and improved long-term growth and development have been shown following the use of formulas for preterm neonates as compared with that of formulas for term neonates.

Traditionally, very LBW preterm formula-fed neonates were changed to a standard term neonate formula in preparation for hospital discharge. However, this practice has been reevaluated. Formulas that provide increased protein, energy, and mineral intake to meet the continuing growth needs of the small preterm neonate have been developed. These are now available in the community at a cost slightly higher than that of standard formulas. Their use has been shown to result in greater linear growth, weight gain, and bone mineralization when compared with the use of term neonate formula. Small preterm neonates and neonates with other morbidities (eg, BPD) may benefit from the use of such formulas for several months after hospital discharge.

Surgical Procedures in the Neonatal Intensive Care Unit

Neonates in the neonatal intensive care unit often require surgical procedures during hospitalization. These procedures range from establishing venous access to laparotomy for necrotizing enterocolitis or thoracotomy for ligation of a patent ductus arteriosus. The transport of an acutely ill neonate to the operating room may be associated with a number of risks, including hypothermia, changes in blood pressure levels, and dislodging of an intravenous catheter or endotracheal tube. For this reason, in many centers, selected surgical procedures are performed within the neonatal intensive care unit. Studies of central venous catheter insertion, extracorporeal membrane oxygenation cannulation or decannulation, patent ductus arteriosus ligation, laparotomy, and other procedures have suggested that this approach can be safe and effective and may result in improved outcome. In addition, both cryo and argon laser ablation of the retina has been performed in neonatal intensive care units. There are unique personnel and environmental safety precautions required when lasers are used.

With the exception of relatively minor procedures, surgery must be performed in an area of the neonatal intensive care unit that is separate from other neonates, is equipped with adequate lighting and working space, and permits ongoing monitoring and anesthetic management. Personnel should wear appropriate operating room attire, and strict sterile techniques must be used.

Hospital policies governing all surgical procedures performed within the neonatal intensive care unit, including management of anesthesia, should be developed in conjunction with the institutional operating room committee to ensure that appropriate guidelines are met.

Analgesia

Pain consists of the perception of painful stimuli (nociception) and the psychologic response to painful stimuli (anxiety). Recent studies measuring a variety of physiologic factors, including oxygen saturation, beta-endorphin, glucose, cortisol, and epinephrine concentrations, confirm that neonates of all gestational ages have a nociceptive response to pain stimuli. Observations of neonate behavior suggest that anxiety also is a component of the infantile pain response, but its character, intensity, and duration remain undetermined. Therefore, the true significance of anxiety in the newborn remains unknown. Measures for assessing pain in the newborn have been developed and validated. However, despite these advances in understanding and assessment, prevention of unnecessary pain from planned invasive procedures and noxious stimuli remains limited.

Pain is most effectively managed by limiting or avoiding noxious stimuli and providing analgesia. Any unnecessary noxious stimuli (acoustic, visual, tactile, vestibular) of neonates should be avoided, if possible. Simple comfort measures such as swaddling, nonnutritive sucking, and positioning (if not contraindicated because of medical or surgical concerns) should be used whenever possible for minor procedures. Oral administration of sucrose reduces pain associated with painful procedures. The risks and benefits of pain management techniques must be considered on an individualized basis. Pharmacologic analgesia should be chosen carefully.

Intraoperative and Postoperative Pain Management

For major surgical procedures, general anesthesia by inhalation of anesthetic gases, intravenous administration of narcotic agents, or regional techniques can be safe and effective. The use of paralytic agents without analgesia during surgery cannot be condoned. Anesthesia for surgical procedures for all newborns should be administered by specially trained physicians and the choice of technique and agent carefully based on a comprehensive assessment of the neonate, efficacy and safety of the drug, and the technical requirements of the procedure.

The use of analgesic agents is important in the immediate postoperative period and should be continued as required. Both continuous infusions of opioids and continuous caudal or epidural blockade can be used to provide a steady course of pain relief but both require careful management and continuous monitoring of cardiorespiratory and hemodynamic status.

Pain Management for Minor Surgical and Other Invasive Procedures

Analgesia for minor invasive procedures, such as chest tube insertion or incisional placement of central venous lines, usually can be provided with superficial infiltration of local anesthetic agents. For circumcision, either a regional nerve block (ring block or dorsal penile nerve block) or topical anesthetic cream is recommended.

Sedation for Prolonged Endotracheal Intubation

Use of analgesic and anxiolytic agents in newborns for amelioration of the discomfort associated with prolonged endotracheal intubation should be undertaken only after careful consideration of the observed response to pain and anxiety, as demonstrated by the individual neonate, and the side effects of the commonly used agents.

Certain concepts that must be remembered include:

- Sedatives and anxiolytics do not provide analgesia.
- Chronic use of many sedatives or hypnotics may lead to tolerance, dependency, and withdrawal.
- Neurodevelopmental outcome from chronic sedation of neonates is unknown.
- Sedatives or hypnotics may cause respiratory and cardiovascular depression.
- Combined treatment with a sedative or hypnotic and an opioid requires a decreased dosage of each.
- Agitation in the chronically ventilated neonate may indicate the need for adjustment in ventilatory settings or reduction in noxious environmental stimuli.

Recommendations

The following recommendations about the use of analgesia in neonates can be made:

- Validated pain assessment tools must be used in a consistent manner.

- Environmental and nonpharmacologic interventions should be provided as baseline measures to prevent, reduce, or eliminate stress and pain.

- Pharmacokinetic and pharmacodynamic properties and efficacy in neonates should be known for pharmacologic agents administered to newborns.

- Agents known to compromise cardiorespiratory function should be administered only by individuals experienced in airway management and in settings with the capacity for continuous cardiorespiratory monitoring.

- Each institution should develop, implement, and regularly update patient care policies to assess, prevent, and manage pain in newborns.

Immunization

GENERAL POLICY

A policy for immunization of neonates, both preterm and term neonates requiring prolonged hospital stays, should be implemented in each neonatal intensive care unit. Preterm neonates should begin the immunization series at the usual chronological age of 2 months, unless otherwise indicated for a specific vaccine or disease process. Some very LBW neonates have been found to have a reduced level of immune response when the usual timing of immunizations is followed. Additional studies are needed to define the optimal schedule for this group of infants. Vaccine doses should never be reduced either for very LBW or preterm infants. Term neonates who remain in the hospital at age 2 months likewise should receive vaccines according to the recommended schedule. Thiomersal-free vaccines should always be used.

Acellular pertussis and inactivated polio vaccines should be used for the initial immunization series as recommended by the AAP *Red Book.*

VACCINE-SPECIFIC ISSUES

The optimal time to initiate hepatitis B vaccination for preterm neonates with birth weights of less than 2 kg whose mothers are HBsAg negative has not been determined. Extremely preterm (<28 weeks of gestation), very LBW and more mature preterm infants all demonstrate consistently high rates of seroconversion following the first dose of hepatitis B vaccine comparable with term neonates. However, subsequent antibody levels in these neonates after the recommended three-dose hepatitis B vaccine series have been reported to be less than that found in term infants 9 to 12 months after initiation of the series. Therefore, initiation of hepatitis B immunization in preterm infants with a birth weight less than 2 kg whose mothers are HbsAg negative should be delayed until just before hospital discharge or until age 2 months when other vaccines are given. If the maternal HBsAg is positive, all neonates with birth weights of less than 2 kg should receive both hepatitis B immune globulin and hepatitis B vaccine at different sites within 12 hours of birth. When born to women with an unknown HbsAg status, this same group of at-risk infants should receive the hepatitis B vaccine, and if the mother's HbsAg status cannot be determined within the first 12 hours after delivery, hepatitis B immune globulin should be given as well. The initial dose of hepatitis B vaccine given to preterm infants born to HbsAg-positive women should not be counted as part of the required three-dose hepatitis B immunization series.

Neonates with BPD or severe congenital heart disease should be immunized against influenza beginning at age 6 months. Immunization of family members and other caretakers against influenza is recommended as well. In addition, staff of neonatal intensive care units should receive influenza vaccine annually before the onset of the influenza virus season.

The addition of pneumococcal conjugate vaccine to the routine immunization schedule for infants will require specific recommendations for use in preterm neonates. These recommendations will be based on ongoing studies to assess vaccine safety and efficacy in this select pediatric population. Centers are encouraged to explore the availability of a Vaccine for Children funding source for assistance in the provision of immunizations to high-risk neonates.

PASSIVE IMMUNIZATION

Palivizumab or respiratory syncytial virus intravenous immune globulin prophylaxis should be administered before hospital discharge to preterm neonates with BPD if the discharge will occur during the respiratory syncytial virus season and continue on a monthly basis until the season ends locally. There may be an advantage to the use of respiratory syncytial virus intravenous immune globulin in decreasing the incidence of serious nonrespiratory syncytial virus respiratory infections in neonates younger than age 6 months and, therefore, ineligible to receive the influenza vaccine. Preterm neonates delivered at less than 32 weeks of gestation and who are judged to be at increased risk either because of immaturity, increased environmental exposure, or age at the onset of the local respiratory syncytial virus season also are candidates for respiratory syncytial virus prophylaxis.

The Neonate with Anticipated Early Death

Hospice care for neonates may be chosen by families whose neonate has an irreversible, fatal disease. The site for such care may vary with local community resources and family wishes. Although less well-studied than for older children, the components of neonatal hospice care are not unlike those established for pediatric hospice care. These components include:

- Involvement of skilled professionals
- Control of distressing symptoms and provision of physical comfort
- Coordinated, multidisciplinary service delivery
- Social support of the family
- Follow-up and bereavement care

Enhancing the quality of the remaining life for the neonate and family is more important than the site of care delivery.

Death of a Neonate

Loss of a pregnancy or death of a neonate touches many aspects of a family's life. The intense emotions of grieving can be confusing and overwhelming. Every effort should be made to determine the cause of the loss and to understand the family's grief response and facilitate healthy coping and adjustment. Efforts to obtain organs for donation are strongly encouraged.

In-Hospital Support and Counseling

Bereavement counseling support has an important impact on family members' ability to adjust to their loss and to continue with their lives. Counseling should be tailored to the specific circumstances surrounding the death; should be sensitive to specific ethical, cultural, religious, and family considerations; and should be provided by specific staff within the hospital. The period after a neonatal death always has an element of confusion because of the continuing grief, the tasks of informing relatives and friends, and the need to make final arrangements.

The time in the hospital before and after the neonate has died is the parents' only opportunity to create a memory of the neonate and experience being the neonate's parent. Therefore, involvement of the parents in as much of the bedside care of even critically ill neonates as is commensurate with safety and their needs is of major importance. When a neonatal death is anticipated or after an unexpected death, specific management procedures can be useful in facilitating parental adjustment to the loss:

- Offer the parents and extended family, if desired, an opportunity to see, hold, and spend time with the neonate both before and immediately after the death.
- Facilitate involvement with the clergy, priest, or spiritual adviser of the family's choice in preparing the family for the death and supporting them afterwards.

- Encourage the family to name the neonate, if they have not done so previously, for it is easier to connect memories to a neonate if parents can refer to the neonate by name.

- Obtain pictures and remembrances (eg, identification tags, footprints, a lock of hair, birth and death certificates, height and weight records, a receiving blanket for the neonate). Even if the parents say initially that they do not want these mementos, they frequently ask for them days, weeks, or months later.

- Provide information about options for burial, cremation, funerals, or memorial services. Encourage both parents to take an active part in making these arrangements.

- Visit the parents daily while the mother is in the hospital; listen to them sympathetically, and give them information as it becomes available.

- Provide reliable preliminary information from the appropriate medical professionals concerning the cause and circumstances of death.

- Physicians should be aware that the staff's potential reactions—a sense of guilt, failure, and uncertainty—may cause them to avoid the parents thereby impeding discussion of the deceased neonate with the family.

- Ensure that the parents have access to support from their families and friends. Anticipate with parents the difficulties they may have in sharing information about the loss with other children, family, and friends. Provide information and suggestions on how they might handle difficult situations or times.

- Explain the grieving process so that the parents understand the usual reactions. Parents frequently demonstrate reactions of acute grief, such as somatic disturbances, a preoccupation with the newborn's appearance or probable future appearance, guilt, hostility, and loss of ability to function. Mourning should be allowed and encouraged to proceed.

- Encourage the parents to communicate their thoughts and feelings openly with one another. Help them understand and accept the differences in how each of them grieves.

- Provide written materials for the parents to read in the hospital and after discharge. Although there can be no substitute for a multidisciplinary group of professionals carefully organized to provide support, written materials can provide concrete information about specific procedures, such as autopsy and funeral arrangements, as well as guidance on long-term issues, such as grief, marriage, explanations for young children, and consideration of another pregnancy. These materials can be designed by the individual hospital or obtained through various associations.

Finally, because families may come from a distance and may not be well acquainted with the attending physicians, it is especially important that specialty and subspecialty referral centers designate a member of the team to be an advocate for the family during the hospital stay and after discharge.

The designated individual also should be responsible for documenting the management and follow-up of each death. Too often families are lost to follow-up, as physicians, nurses, and families avoid sharing the sadness of bereavement.

ASSESSMENT

When a neonatal death occurs, a special effort should be made to determine the cause of death. This process is helpful for several reasons:

- It helps the family to understand the medical reasons for the death.
- It provides a basis for counseling the family about future pregnancies, including family planning, genetic counseling, and obstetric and neonatal management.
- It provides correct diagnoses for statistical reporting and analysis of perinatal care outcomes.

Requesting an autopsy after the death of a neonate must be handled with sensitivity and gentleness. Selecting the right time to introduce the idea is critical. It can be helpful when it is apparent that a neonate is dying, particularly when the underlying cause is uncertain, to introduce the idea of a postmortem examination to the parents. Its value, as a means of gaining information that will be helpful in answering their questions in the future, often is perceived as a compelling reason for consent. Involvement of the primary care physician and the mother's obstetrician in the request for autopsy consent also may facilitate the family's acceptance of the idea. If there is reluctance for consent for a complete examination of the body, consideration should be given to a limited one, to obtaining specimens of body fluids for microbial culture or other analyses as indicated, and to obtaining postmortem imaging studies if such could further elucidate the cause of death. In all neonatal deaths, every effort should be made to obtain histopathologic examination of the placenta, membranes, and umbilical cord. When an underlying genetic disorder is suspected and premortem testing is incomplete, advance planning for appropriate specimen retrieval with or without a full autopsy should occur. In every instance the family should initially receive the final results of the autopsy and other examinations in person, if possible, and in a written report in conjunction with a verbal explanation of the findings.

Each unit should have a formal process for periodic review of all neonatal deaths. In addition, when there has been an unexpected clinical deterioration leading to a death, a contemporaneous review of the specific clinical events and decisions with all the involved staff participating can be helpful to resolve interpersonal conflicts, relieve feelings of guilt or failure, and improve both understanding and team interaction. Such sessions usually are best led by the attending neonatologist although, on occasion, employment of an uninvolved facilitator can be useful.

Post-Loss Follow-up

The responsibility for ongoing bereavement counseling depends on the specific circumstances of the death and on the family's relationship to the physician. Usually a multidisciplinary approach is best. In the case of neonatal death, it is coordinated by the neonatologist. In general, such counseling should include:

- An initial session 4–6 weeks after the death
- Assessment of the grieving process
- Additional genetic services if indicated
- Review of preliminary autopsy data
- Answers for parents' specific questions

- Education and reassurance regarding the normal grieving process
- Follow-up visits as indicated by the individual family needs
- Referral of family members to bereavement support groups or bereavement counselors

Persisting Apnea of Prematurity

CLINICAL CONSIDERATIONS

The persistence of symptomatic apnea of prematurity beyond the postmenstrual age of 36 weeks may occur in very LBW neonates. This may be the only remaining issue to be resolved for neonate readiness for discharge from the hospital. Neonates with extremely LBW (<1 kg) and BPD are those most prone to delay in maturation of respiratory control. Although preterm neonates have been found to have a higher incidence of sudden infant death syndrome, no correlation between apnea of prematurity and sudden infant death syndrome has been established. Within the survivors of preterm birth, neonates with BPD have a higher incidence of sudden, unexplained death than those without.

USE OF HOME CARDIORESPIRATORY MONITORS

The use of home cardiorespiratory monitors for neonates with delayed maturation of respiratory control may facilitate early hospital discharge without undue family stress. Studies of the predictability of cardiopulmonary polygraphic studies (polysomnography) have not found a strong correlation between documented apnea or bradycardia episodes and subsequent serious alarm events. In the absence of objective measurements that clearly identify neonates at risk for significant cardiorespiratory instability, clinicians have used an empiric approach of requiring an event-free interval of some days before discharge. The precise number of days without apnea or bradycardia episodes that defines full maturation and diminished risk after discharge has not been determined. Therefore, the definition of cardiorespiratory stability and the decision to use home monitoring to facilitate transition to home care remain a matter of individual clinical judgment, taking into consideration the neonate's clinical course and unresolved medical problems.

Hospital Discharge of the High-Risk Neonate

DISCHARGE PLANNING

The care of each high-risk neonate after discharge must be carefully coordinated to provide ongoing multidisciplinary support of the family. The discharge planning team should include parents, the primary care physician, the neonatologist, neonatal nurses, and the social worker. Other professionals (eg, nutritionist, physical therapist) may be included as needed. The initiation of discharge planning should begin when it is evident that recovery is certain, although the exact date of discharge may not be predictable. The goal of the discharge plan is to ensure successful transition to home care. The essential elements are a physiologically stable neonate, a family who can provide the necessary care without undue strain and with appropriate support services in place within the community, and a primary care physician who is prepared to assume the responsibility with appropriate backup from specialist physicians and other professionals as needed.

It is prudent that each institution establish guidelines for discharge of high-risk neonates. These should allow for individual physician judgment and flexibility. The determination of readiness for care at home of a neonate after neonatal intensive care is complex. Careful balancing of neonate safety and well-being with family needs and capabilities is required. Consideration of the availability and adequacy of community resources and support services is essential. The final decision for timing of hospital discharge, which is the responsibility of the attending physician, must be tailored for the unique constellation of issues posed by each situation.

TECHNOLOGY-DEPENDENT NEONATES

With the increased survival rates of LBW neonates and the development of specialized home care services, many neonates with unresolved medical problems are being discharged from hospitals with continuing requirements for monitoring or respiratory support or alternative feeding methods. These neonates include those with BPD with requirement for oxygen supplementation, persistent apnea of prematurity, feeding disorders, or postoperative short bowel syndrome problems. The appropriate management of these neonates will require coordination of care between the center-based subspecialty team, the primary care physician, the home health care agency, and equipment providers.

SPECIAL CONSIDERATIONS

Discharge planning for neonates who have been transported back to community hospitals for convalescent care should follow the same principles as that for neonates being discharged from a subspecialty center unit. Appropriate follow-up during the most critical periods for neonates at risk for adverse sensorineural outcomes (ie, the very LBW neonate for progression of retinopathy of prematurity and hearing screening for all high-risk neonates) needs to be coordinated between the two units before transfer of the neonate.

Coordination of follow-up care after discharge between local resources and center-based ones is encouraged to improve efficiency and decrease time demands on the family. When the need for services from multiple disciplines is identified before discharge, a multidisciplinary center-based clinic may be the least cumbersome option.

It is important in choosing home care service providers for surveillance, ancillary treatment services, and parent support to ascertain that the staff are qualified to evaluate and treat neonates. It is essential that previous performance and existing quality control programs be considered when choosing a home health care agency to provide personnel for in-home care of the technology-dependent neonate.

READINESS FOR HOSPITAL DISCHARGE

The following recommendations are offered as a framework for consideration as each individual neonate and care giving situation is evaluated and the discharge decision made.

Neonate Readiness for Hospital Discharge

The responsible physician should assess the following factors when determining a neonate's readiness to be discharged from the hospital:

- A sustained pattern of weight gain of sufficient duration
- Adequate maintenance of normal body temperature with the neonate fully clothed in an open bed with normal ambient temperature (24–25°C)
- Competent suckle feeding, breast or bottle, without cardiorespiratory compromise
- Physiologically mature and stable cardiorespiratory function of sufficient duration
- Appropriate immunizations have been administered
- Appropriate metabolic screening has been performed
- Hematologic status has been assessed and indicated therapy instituted
- Nutritional risks have been assessed and indicated therapy and dietary modification instituted
- Sensorineural assessments, hearing and funduscopy, have been completed as indicated
- Review of hospital course has been completed, unresolved medical problems identified, and plans for treatment instituted as indicated

Home Care Plan Readiness

An individualized home care plan has been developed with input from all of the appropriate disciplines. Specific and detailed plans for neonates with complex multiple system problems, particularly for those requiring technological assistance, are necessary. For neonates at psychosocial risk, arranging for appropriate psychosocial surveillance and family support is essential.

Family and Home Environmental Readiness

In evaluating family and home environmental readiness, assessments of the family care giving capabilities, resource requirements, and home physical facilities have been completed, including:

- Identification of at least two family members, one of whom is an adult, and assessment of their ability, availability, and commitment

- Psychosocial assessment for parenting risks
- A home environmental assessment that may include an on-site evaluation; for home care of the technology-dependent neonate, documentation by an on-site assessment of the availability of 24-hour telephone access, electricity, in-house water supply, and heating are required and necessary modification of home facilities confirmed
- Review of available financial resources and identification of adequate financial support; home care of the technology-dependent neonate cannot be achieved without this

Parents and other family members have demonstrated the necessary capabilities to provide all components of care including:

- Feeding, whether breast, bottle, or an alternative technique, including formula preparation and vitamin and mineral supplementation as required
- Basic neonate care including bathing; skin, umbilical cord, and genital care; temperature measurement; dressing; and comforting
- Neonate cardiopulmonary resuscitation and emergency intervention as indicated
- Assessment of clinical status, including understanding and detecting the general early signs and symptoms of illness, as well as the signs and symptoms specific to the individual neonate's condition
- Neonate safety precautions including proper neonate positioning during sleep and use of car seats
- Special safety precautions for airway maintenance, alternative feeding methods, and other mechanical and prosthetic devices as indicated
- Administration of medications (dosage, timing, storage) and recognition of signs and symptoms of toxicity
- Equipment operation, maintenance, and problem-solving for each mechanical support device as indicated
- Appropriate technique for each required special care procedure (eg, ostomy care, artificial airway, neonate stimulation, reflux precautions)

Community and Health Care System Readiness

Follow-up care needs and resources have been identified including:

- Primary care physician identified, and responsibility for care of neonate accepted
- Pediatric medical and surgical subspecialty physicians and other providers (eg, nurse specialists, nutritionists, physical therapists) identified and appropriate arrangements made
- Neurodevelopmental follow-up arranged
- Home nursing visits arranged as indicated
- Appropriate communication has been exchanged with and hospital discharge summaries and home care plans provided to all involved
- Emergency intervention and transportation plans have been developed and emergency service providers identified and notified as indicated.

Follow-up of High-Risk Neonates

General Considerations

The designation of high-risk encompasses a broad range of potential adverse outcomes and neonate groups but without distinguishing between types of risk or vulnerable populations. The organization of follow-up care is influenced by the group being followed and the specific goals which may include:

- Primary care—monitoring growth and preventive care and guidance
- Management of unresolved medical problems
- Early detection of abnormality or delayed developmental progress
- Early intervention and habilitation
- Neonate safety
- Parent education
- Evaluation of treatment

- Documentation of outcomes
- Neurosensory follow-up
- Environmental and psychosocial concerns
- Referral to other community resources

Beyond the outcomes of healthy growth and avoidance of disease common to primary care of all newborns, two categories of outcome—neurodevelopmental and psychosocial—will be addressed specifically, as well as the care of neonates with unresolved medical problems at hospital discharge.

Involvement of the Primary Care Physician

The neonate's primary care physician should share in the responsibility for providing continuity of care with the subspecialty or specialty care center. Frequently, the more detailed developmental and psychologic evaluations and the initial management of complex, unresolved medical problems are primarily the responsibility of the care center. As the recovery progresses, medical care is shifted more to the primary care physician. With recent changes in the structure of health care financing, the primary care physician may be delegated the responsibility for referral to subspecialty consultation and care. Within any format of shared patient care delivery, it is imperative that all professionals communicate information in a timely manner and share in the planning and execution of the long-term care for neonates with multidisciplinary service needs.

Surveillance and Assessment

The intervals of follow-up visits required by high-risk neonates should be determined by the needs of the individual neonate and family. It may be necessary to examine some of these neonates weekly or semimonthly at first. Neurologic, developmental, behavioral, and sensory status should be assessed more than once during the first year in high-risk neonates to ensure early identification of problems and referral for remedial care. A perinatal follow-up program with an appropriate staff of multidisciplinary personnel is useful in providing these assessments.

Physicians and other professionals who provide follow-up care to women and neonates should be aware of and look for the physical, social, and psychologic factors associated with child abuse, including:

- Preterm birth
- Neonatal illness with long periods of hospitalization, especially in neonatal intensive care units
- Single parenthood
- Adolescent motherhood
- Closely spaced pregnancies
- Infrequent family visits to hospitalized neonates
- Substance use

Children born preterm have been shown to have a greater incidence of irritability, hyperkinesis, and increased dependency. Prolonged hospitalization inevitably disrupts family relationships, particularly the parent–child relationship. Neonates and parents with such a history or with other factors associated with child abuse require closer follow-up than the family and newborn without risk factors. The interaction of the parents, especially the mother, with the neonate should be evaluated periodically. The neonate or child who fails to thrive may be a victim of neglect, if not outright abuse, and a causal relationship between neglect and failure to thrive should always be suspected. In every state, providers of health care to children are legally obligated to report suspected child abuse.

Growth parameters of the neonate should be assessed, including continued monitoring of the adequacy of weight gain, linear growth, and head growth. Growth should be plotted on standardized birth-weight-appropriate growth curves with the appropriate age correction for gestational age at birth. Review of nutritional intake and calculation of caloric intake are essential in case management.

Physical examination should assess neuromotor, cardiac, pulmonary, gastrointestinal and nutritional status as well as any hernias, anomalies, or orthopedic deformities. Residual scars from invasive procedures during the neonatal course should be monitored for satisfactory healing. On occasion, referral for reconstructive procedures may be necessary.

Medication dosage should be reevaluated, doses increased with weight gain and age, and blood concentrations monitored as indicated. Immunization status should be reviewed and age appropriate administration maintained. Follow-up audiologic and visual assessments should be obtained when indicated.

Neurologic assessment should include an appraisal of muscle tone, development, protective and deep tendon reflexes, and visual and auditory responses. In addition, developmental progress should be monitored both by parental report of milestone acquisition and by assessment using a standard developmental screening tool, such as the Denver II Developmental Screening Test. When neurologic findings are suspect or developmental delays are suspected, neonates should be referred for more in-depth assessment, either to a neonatal follow-up program or to equivalent facilities or programs capable of providing detailed neurodevelopmental assessments. Neonates at greatest risk for adverse neurodevelopmental outcome (eg, ≤1,500 g birth weight, posthypoxic ischemic encephalopathy or neonatal seizures, hypoxic cardiorespiratory failure, complex multiple congenital anomalies) should have as a minimum, formal neurodevelopmental testing with a battery of standardized tests at 1 and 2 years corrected age. This will allow for recognition of aberrant development in all domains (gross motor; fine motor and adaptive; visual perceptive and problem solving; hearing, language, and speech; socialization). Primary care physicians should ensure that such testing is completed irrespective of the results of developmental screening. Universal standardized testing of these populations will greatly enhance the evaluation of prenatal and neonatal interventions. The results will be useful in forming intervention strategies for those children who are identified as having functional deficits.

EARLY INTERVENTION

Intervention programs for high-risk neonates have been established under federal legislation to provide early detection of developmental delay and other disabilities. Intervention services may be provided to age 3 years for individual neonates with confirmed neurodevelopmental delay or other disability. Programs also offer therapeutic guidelines for families, parent support groups, and respite care programs. Although no definitive data confirm the beneficial effects of infant stimulation programs, indications are that early intervention may improve the social adaptation, limit the residual functional disability, and provide valuable family support.

Bibliography

American Academy of Pediatrics. Committee on Fetus and Newborn. Use of inhaled nitric oxide. Pediatrics 2000;106:344–5.

American Academy of Pediatrics. Pickering LK, editor. 2000 Red book: report of the Committee on Infectious Diseases. 25th ed. Elk Grove Village (IL): AAP; 2000.

American Academy of Pediatrics. Task Force on Prolonged Infantile Apnea. Prolonged infantile apnea: 1985. Pediatrics 1985;76:129–31.

American Academy of Pediatrics Committee on Fetus and Newborn: Recommendations on extracorporeal membrane oxygenation. Pediatrics 1990;85: 618–9.

American Academy of Pediatrics, Committee on Nutrition. Pediatric nutrition handbook. 4th ed. Elk Grove Village (IL): AAP; 1998.

American Association of Blood Banks. Standards for blood banks and transfusion services. 20th ed. Bethesda (MD): AABB; 2000.

American College of Obstetricians and Gynecologists. Fetal and infant mortality review manual: a guide for committees. Washington, DC: ACOG; 1998.

Antenatal corticosteroid therapy for fetal maturation. ACOG Committee Opinion 273. American College of Obstetricians and Gynecologists. Obstet Gynecol 2002;99:871–3.

Drug-exposed infants. American Academy of Pediatrics. Committee on Substance Abuse. Pediatrics 1995;96:364–7.

Guidelines for home care of infants, children, and adolescents with chronic disease. American Academy of Pediatrics Committee on Children with Disabilities. Pediatrics 1995;96:161–4.

Hospital discharge of the high-risk neonate—proposed guidelines. American Academy of Pediatrics. Pediatrics 1998;102:411–7.

Practice parameter: management of hyperbilirubinemia in the healthy term newborn. American Academy of Pediatrics. Provisional Committee for Quality Improvement and Subcommittee on Hyperbilirubinemia. Pediatrics 1994; 94:558–65.

Prevention and management of pain and stress in the neonate. American Academy of Pediatrics. Committee on Fetus and Newborn. Committee on Drugs. Section on Anesthesiology. Section on Surgery. Canadian Paediatric Society. Fetus and Newborn Committee. Pediatrics 2000;105:454–61.

Screening examination of premature infants for retinopathy of prematurity. A joint statement of the American Academy of Pediatrics, the American Association for Pediatric Ophthalmology and Strabismus, and the American Academy of Ophthalmology. Pediatrics 1997;100:273.

Supplemental Therapeutic Oxygen for Prethreshold Retinopathy of Prematurity (STOP-ROP), a randomized, controlled trial. I: primary outcomes. Pediatrics 2000;105:295–310.

Surfactant replacement therapy for respiratory distress syndrome. American Academy of Pediatrics. Committee on Fetus and Newborn. Pediatrics 1999; 103:684–5.

CHAPTER 9

Perinatal Infections

Certain infections that occur in the antepartum or intrapartum period may have a significant effect on the fetus and newborn. Care of the mother antepartum and intrapartum and of the newborn soon after birth can reduce the frequency of or ameliorate many serious problems, and it can minimize the risk of subsequent transmission of infection in the nursery. Communication and cooperation among all perinatal care personnel are essential to obtain the best results. The infections discussed in this chapter have been selected on the basis of new and evolving information that affects management.

Viral Infections

CYTOMEGALOVIRUS

Approximately 1% of all newborns are infected with cytomegalovirus (CMV) in utero and excrete CMV after birth. Although the majority of congenital CMV infections are asymptomatic, approximately 5% of infected neonates are symptomatic at birth.

Transmission occurs via transplacental passage of the virus, contact of the fetus with infectious secretions at the time of birth, through ingestion of infected breastmilk, or via transfusion of blood from seropositive donors. Transmission via transfusion has been virtually eliminated by the use of blood from CMV-negative donors, the use of frozen deglycerolized red blood cells, or by filtration to remove white blood cells. Newborns of seronegative women who receive milk from human milk banks are at risk of developing CMV disease. This can be minimized by limiting donor milk to CMV-negative donors or by appropriate pasteurization. Both primary and recurrent infections in pregnant women may result in congenital infections; however, the rate of transmission is much higher with primary infection (approximately 40% versus <1% with recurrent disease).

Because there is neither a vaccine for prevention of infection nor effective therapy for acute maternal infection, routine serologic screening of either women or neonates is of little benefit. Testing generally is limited to pregnant women in whom CMV exposure is suspected. Routine serologic testing of personnel in newborn nurseries is not recommended.

Although the presence of immunoglobulin M (IgM) CMV antibody is highly suggestive of primary maternal infection, false-positive and false-negative results occur. Establishing that seroconversion has occurred is the most accurate method for documenting primary maternal infection. Isolation of the virus or detection of CMV genome by polymerase chain reaction (PCR) from either amniotic fluid or fetal blood is the most sensitive test for detecting fetal infection. Fetal blood obtained by cordocentesis may be tested for CMV-specific IgM, but this test is less sensitive than culture or PCR. For an infected fetus, ultrasound abnormalities or cordocentesis to detect elevated hepatic enzymes, anemia, and thrombocytopenia may be prognostic of severe infection.

Unequivocal evidence of CMV infection in the neonate who has not been diagnosed in utero requires recovery of the virus within 3 weeks of birth. Later in infancy, differentiation between intrauterine and perinatal infection is difficult to determine.

Enteroviruses

Wild-type poliovirus infection has been eliminated from the Western Hemisphere. Other enteroviral infections (coxsackieviruses, echoviruses, and polioviruses) are common and are spread by fecal–oral and respiratory routes. Infection in the third trimester can trigger labor. Signs of maternal infection often are mild and nonspecific.

Neonates who acquire infection without maternal antibody are at risk for severe disease. Manifestations can include pneumonia, exanthems, aseptic meningitis, encephalitis, paralysis, hepatitis, conjunctivitis, myocarditis, and pericarditis.

Diagnosis is confirmed by recovery of the virus from swabs of the throat or the anus and samples of stool, spinal fluid, or blood. Polymerase chain reaction testing of spinal fluid is more sensitive than culture.

No specific therapy is commercially available. Hospitalized newborns should be managed with contact as well as standard precautions.

HEPATITIS A VIRUS

Hepatitis A virus (HAV) has little effect on pregnancy and rarely is transmitted perinatally. The risk of transplacental transmission to the fetus is negligible, and there is no evidence that the virus is a teratogen. The most common mode of transmission is by the fecal–oral route. Diagnosis is confirmed by the demonstration of anti-HAV IgM antibodies.

Vaccines for hepatitis A are highly effective and approved for use. Although vaccine safety in pregnancy has not been established, the risk to the developing fetus is theoretically low because the vaccine contains inactivated, purified viral proteins. Pregnant women with the following risk factors are candidates for vaccination: intravenous drug users, travelers to endemic regions, those living in communities with a high prevalence of hepatitis A, women who work with HAV-infected primates, women with either chronic liver disease or a liver transplant, and women with clotting disorders who receive clotting factor concentrate. Immunoglobulin is effective for both preexposure and postexposure prophylaxis and can be used during pregnancy.

In neonatal intensive care units, nosocomial outbreaks have been reported but are infrequent. Prevention of spread of the virus is based on contact precautions, with emphasis on careful handwashing. With appropriate hygienic precautions, breastfeeding is permissible. Although immunoglobulin has been administered to newborns in specific situations, the efficacy of this practice has not been established.

HEPATITIS B VIRUS

Hepatitis B virus (HBV) infection accounts for approximately 35% of reported cases of viral hepatitis. Although 85–90% of older children and adults experience complete resolution following an acute infection,

6–10% will develop a chronic infection and continue to manifest HBV surface antigen (HBsAg). Transmission of HBV from the woman to the neonate occurs primarily during delivery. Neonates born to women who are antigen positive are at risk of infection. Approximately 70–90% of infected neonates become chronic carriers of HBsAg.

MATERNAL INFECTION

Because historical information about risk factors identifies fewer than one half of chronic carriers, serologic testing for HBsAg is recommended for all pregnant women as part of routine prenatal care. Women who were not screened during pregnancy, those who are at high risk for infection (eg, intravenous drug users, women with recurrent sexually transmitted diseases [STDs]), and those with clinical hepatitis should be tested at the time of admission to the hospital.

Women who are HBsAg negative but who have risk factors for HBV infection should be offered vaccination during pregnancy. The adult dose of HBV vaccine is 10–20 µg (1 mL) injected into the deltoid muscle; intramuscular injection in the buttocks may not be as effective and is not recommended. A series of three doses is required; the second and third doses are given 1 and 6 months after the first dose. A two-dose schedule, administered at time zero and again 4 to 6 months later, is available for adolescents aged 11–15 years using the adult dose of a hepatitis B recombinant vaccine.

Hepatitis B vaccine is recommended for household contacts and sexual partners of chronic carriers of HBV (ie, those who are HBsAg positive) unless immunity has previously been demonstrated. Previously nonimmunized sexual partners of persons with acute HBV infection should receive a single dose of hepatitis B immune globulin (HBIG) and should begin an HBV vaccine series if they are serologically negative. Serologic testing to determine susceptibility, although not usually cost-effective and not recommended routinely, may be considered provided it does not delay or impede vaccine uptake.

Newborn Immunization

Universal HBV immunization is recommended for all neonates. Three intramuscular doses are required to provide effective protection (Table 9-1).

Table 9–1. Recommended Schedules for Hepatitis B Virus Immunoprophylaxis of Neonates to Prevent Perinatal Transmission*

Status	Dosing Schedule	Age
Neonates of HBsAg-positive women[†]	HBV vaccine 1	Birth (within 12 hours)
	HBIG (0.5 mL IM)	Birth (within 12 hours)
	HBV vaccine 2	1–2 months
	HBV vaccine 3	6 months
Neonates of HBsAg-negative women	HBV vaccine 1	Birth (preferably before hospital discharge) to 2 months
	HBV vaccine 2	1–2 months after dose 1
	HBV vaccine 3	6–18 months
Neonates born to women not screened for HBsAg before delivery	HBV vaccine 1	Birth (within 12 hours)
	HBIG	If the woman is subsequently found to be HBsAg positive, give 0.5 mL IM as soon as possible (no later than 1 week after birth)
	HBV vaccine 2	1–2 months
	HBV vaccine 3	6–18 months

Abbreviations: HBV, hepatitis B virus; HbsAg, hepatitis B surface antigen; HBIG, hepatitis B immune globulin; IM, intramuscularly.
*These recommendations may not apply to preterm neonates.
[†]Neonates of HBsAg-positive women should be vaccinated at age 6 months.
Used and modified with permission of the American Academy of Pediatrics, 2000 Red book: report of the Committee on Infectious Diseases, 25th ed, Copyright of the American Academy of Pediatrics, 2000.

For neonates born to HBsAg-negative women, the first dose of vaccine should be administered during the newborn period or by age 2 months; the second dose 1–2 months later; and the third dose by age 6–18 months. Alternatively, vaccine may be administered at 2-month intervals, concurrent with other childhood vaccines at ages 2, 4, and 6 months. Because of suboptimal immune response in some preterm neonates, the current American Academy of Pediatric (AAP) recommendation is to delay the start of hepatitis B immunization in low-risk preterm neonates, who weigh less than 2 kg at birth, until they reach 2 kg or until age 2 months. The appropriate dose (Table 9–2) can be given into the deltoid muscle or into the anterolateral thigh muscle of neonates.

Both term and preterm neonates born to women known to be HBsAg positive should be vaccinated shortly after delivery and should receive one dose of HBIG preferably within 12 hours of birth. Prophylaxis for exposed newborns can prevent perinatal HBV infection in approximately 95% of neonates when the three-dose immunization series is completed and HBIG is given within 12 hours after birth. The initial dose of HBV vaccine can be administered concurrently with HBIG but should be given at a different site. No special care of the neonate is indicated other than removal of maternal blood to avoid inoculation of the virus contaminating the skin. The second dose of vaccine should be administered at 1–2 months of chronologic age, regardless of the neonate's gestational age or birth weight. The third dose should be given at age 6 months. For preterm neonates who weigh less than 2 kg at birth, the initial vaccine dose is given at birth but is not counted in the required three-dose schedule; therefore, these infants receive four doses (birth, when weight reaches 2 kg or at age 2 months, 1–2 months later, and at age 6 months).

At 1–3 months after completion of the immunization schedule for newborns of HBsAg-positive women, testing is indicated to ensure response or to identify neonates who have become chronically infected. Breastfeeding of newborns by HBsAg-positive women poses no additional risk for the transmission of HBV.

Newborns of women whose HBsAg status is unknown should receive HBV vaccine within 12 hours of birth, in a dose appropriate for

Table 9–2. Recommended Doses of Hepatitis B Virus Vaccines in Neonates

Maternal Status	Vaccine Type	
	Recombivax HB	Energix-B
HBsAg-positive*	5 µg (0.5 mL)[†]	10 µg (0.5 mL)
HBsAg-negative	5 µg (0.5 mL)[†]	10 µg (0.5 mL)

Abbreviation: HbsAg, hepatitis B virus surface antigen.

*Hepatitis B immune globulin (0.5 mL) also should be given.

[†]Pediatric formulation

Used and modified with permission of the American Academy of Pediatrics, 2000 Red book: report of the Committee on Infectious Diseases, 25th ed, Copyright of the American Academy of Pediatrics, 2000.

neonates born to HBsAg-positive women. The woman's blood should be obtained for testing on admission. If the woman is subsequently found to be HBsAg positive, the neonate should receive HBIG as soon as possible (within 7 days of birth) and should receive the second and third doses of vaccine as recommended for neonates of HBsAg-positive women.

Hepatitis C Virus

Hepatitis C virus (HCV) is the principal cause of non-A, non-B hepatitis. Until the implementation of universal screening for HCV in donors of blood products, the virus accounted for as many as 95% of cases of posttransfusion hepatitis. The primary known route of transmission is parenteral exposure to blood and blood products from HCV-infected individuals. Sexual transmission among monogamous couples is uncommon as is transmission among family contacts. In most cases, no source can be identified.

Infection with HCV is diagnosed serologically by the presence of HCV antibodies or by detection of HCV RNA. Positive enzyme immunoassay antibody test results should be confirmed by additional testing with a more specific assay such as recombinant immunoblot assay, particularly when asymptomatic individuals are being tested. As many as 70% of patients with HCV infection develop chronic liver disease, and cirrhosis ultimately develops in 20–25% of these patients. Therefore, liver enzyme and function tests should be obtained in patients who are antibody positive.

Routine serologic testing during pregnancy for HCV infection is not recommended. Testing should be reserved for those whose history suggests an increased risk of infection, such as from blood transfusion, intravenous drug use, or occupational percutaneous or mucosal surface blood exposure.

Women who are infected with HCV should be advised that transmission of HCV by breastfeeding is possible but has not been documented. According to current guidelines of the U.S. Public Health

Service, maternal HCV infection is not a contraindication to breastfeeding. The decision to do so should be based on an informed discussion between the woman and her health care provider.

Maternal–fetal (vertical) transmission of HCV occurs at a rate of less than 10% (range, 0–25%). The risk of transmission, which correlates with maternal HCV RNA level, appears to be increased for women infected with the human immunodeficiency virus (HIV). Immune globulin manufactured in the United States does not contain antibodies to HCV and is unlikely to prevent infection following exposure. Immunoglobulin G and antiviral agents are not recommended for postexposure prophylaxis of neonates born to women with HCV. The natural history of perinatally acquired hepatitis C infection is the subject of ongoing studies. Children born to HCV-positive women should be tested for HCV infection. However, antibody testing should (in most cases) be deferred until at least age 12 months, when passively transferred maternal HCV antibodies have decreased below detectable levels. If earlier diagnosis of HCV infection is desired, PCR for HCV RNA may be performed at or before the neonate's well child visit at 1–2 months.

Herpes Simplex Virus

Treatment and Counseling During Pregnancy

The prevalence of infection with herpes simplex virus (HSV) has increased 30% in the past few decades. Most patients with unequivocal serologic evidence of infection do not have a positive history of genital ulcers. Nevertheless, all women and their partners should be asked about a history of genital HSV infection. A genital herpes infection is classified as primary when it occurs in a woman with no prior HSV infection (ie, seronegative to both HSV type 1 [HSV-1] and HSV type 2 [HSV-2]), nonprimary first episode when it occurs in a woman with a history of heterologous infection (eg, first HSV-2 infection in a woman with prior HSV-1 infection), and recurrent when it occurs in a woman with clinical or serologic evidence of prior genital herpes (of the same serotype).

Women with primary genital HSV lesions (symptomatic or asymptomatic) who deliver vaginally have a high risk (33–50%) of transmitting infection to their neonates. With recurrent disease, the risk of transmission during a vaginal delivery is much lower (< 2–5%). Women with nonprimary first infections have an intermediate risk of maternal to neonatal transmission. Distinguishing among primary, nonprimary first episode, and recurrent HSV infection in women on the basis of clinical findings is not accurate. Most newborns infected with HSV are delivered to women who have asymptomatic or unrecognized infections.

Studies of acyclovir use among pregnant women suggest that acyclovir treatment orally, near term, reduces the rate of abdominal delivery in women who have frequent recurrences or nonprimary first episode genital herpes because of a decrease in the incidence of active lesions at delivery. However, the Centers for Disease Control and Prevention (CDC) currently does not recommend routine administration of acyclovir to pregnant women who have a history of recurrent herpes. Acyclovir is indicated intravenously to treat maternal life-threatening HSV infection (eg, disseminated infection that includes encephalitis, pneumonitis, and hepatitis). Although long-term safety and efficacy of administering acyclovir systemically have not yet been established, no evidence has been found of any adverse effects on the fetus.

Couples should be educated about the natural history of genital HSV infection and should be advised that, if either partner is infected, they should abstain from sexual contact while lesions are present. To minimize the risk of transmission, use of condoms is recommended for asymptomatic HSV-infected individuals. Susceptible pregnant women should avoid sexual contact during the last 6–8 weeks of gestation if their partners have active genital HSV infections.

Obstetric Management

Women with a history of genital HSV infection should be questioned about recent symptoms and should undergo careful examination of the perineum before delivery. If no lesions are observed, neonates may be delivered vaginally.

Cesarean delivery is indicated for all women with active (primary and recurrent) genital HSV lesions at the time of delivery. In patients with active HSV infection and ruptured membranes at or near term, a cesarean delivery should be performed as soon as the necessary personnel and equipment can be readied. Local neonatal infection may result from the use of fetal scalp electrode monitoring in patients with a history of herpes, even when lesions are not present. However, if there are indications for fetal scalp monitoring, it may be appropriate in a woman who has a history of recurrent HSV and no active lesions.

Contact precautions (in addition to standard precautions) should be used for women with clinically evident or serologically confirmed primary genital HSV infection or nongenital HSV infection in the labor, delivery, and postpartum care areas. For recurrent mucocutaneous lesions, standard precautions are sufficient. Health care personnel and the woman herself should use gloves for direct contact with the infected area or with contaminated dressings, and meticulous handwashing is essential. The labor and delivery rooms require only routine, careful cleaning and disinfection before using the rooms for other patients.

Management of Exposed Newborns

Most neonatal infections are caused by HSV-2, although infection with HSV-1 also can occur. Most neonates who develop HSV infection acquire the infection during passage through the infected maternal lower genital tract, or by ascending infection to the fetus, sometimes even though membranes are apparently intact. Rare sources of neonatal infection include: 1) postnatal transmission from the parents, hospital personnel, or other close contact, most often from a nongenital infection (eg, mouth, hands, or around the breasts); and 2) postnatal transmission in the nursery from another infected neonate, probably from the hands of personnel attending the neonates.

Neonates born vaginally through infected birth canals require close observation because the transmission rate of HSV is as high as 50% for neonates of women with active primary genital herpes. Specimens for herpes cultures should be obtained at 24 to 48 hours after birth from urine, stool or rectum, mouth, and nasopharynx. Some experts recommend empiric treatment with acyclovir (20 mg/kg intravenously every 8 hours) pending results of cultures and clinical course although no data exist to support the efficacy of this approach. Other experts would await positive culture results or clinical manifestations of infection before starting acyclovir therapy. Parents and providers should be educated about the signs and symptoms of neonatal HSV infection, which include vesicular lesions of the skin, respiratory distress, seizures, or signs of sepsis. A neonate with any of these manifestations should be evaluated immediately for possible HSV infection. Specimens for HSV culture should be obtained from skin lesions, conjunctiva, nasopharynx, mouth, rectum, urine, blood buffy coat, and cerebrospinal fluid (CSF). Cerebrospinal fluid also should be studied by PCR. Acyclovir therapy should be initiated if any of the culture or PCR test results are positive or HSV infection is otherwise strongly suspected.

Neonates born vaginally (or by cesarean delivery if membranes have ruptured) to a women with active HSV lesions should be physically separated from other neonates and managed with contact precautions if they remain in the nursery during the incubation period; an isolation room is not essential. Alternatively, the neonate may stay with the woman in a private room after the woman has been instructed on proper preventive care to reduce postpartum transmission.

The risk of HSV infection is extremely low in neonates born to asymptomatic women with a history of recurrent genital herpes and in those born to symptomatic women by cesarean delivery before rupture of membranes. Special isolation precautions are not needed for these neonates. Neonates born by cesarean delivery to women with herpetic lesions with intact membranes should be cultured for HSV as recommended previously for neonates exposed by vaginal delivery, and they should be observed. The length of in-hospital observation is empirical and is based on risk factors, local resources, and access to adequate follow-up. Parents should be instructed to report early signs of infection. Antiviral therapy should be initiated if culture results from the neonate are positive or if HSV infection is strongly suspected for other reasons.

Early Diagnosis and Management of Disease in Neonates

Cultures obtained from the eye, mouth, or rectum of neonates born to women who are known or who are strongly suspected of being infected with HSV can assist in management decisions. A positive culture obtained 24–48 hours or more after delivery suggests HSV infection and is an indication for immediate institution of antiviral therapy, even in the absence of symptoms. Direct fluorescent antibody staining of scrapings of skin, eye, or mucus membrane lesions can provide a rapid diagnosis. Polymerase chain reaction is a sensitive method for detecting HSV DNA; it is useful for examining spinal fluid samples. Polymerase chain reaction is widely available, but quality control varies among laboratories.

The neonate should be physically segregated and managed with contact precautions for the duration of the illness; an isolation room is desirable. Personnel having contact with skin lesions or potentially infectious secretions should use gowns and gloves. Antiviral therapy is effective in the treatment of neonatal HSV infection and should be initiated if HSV is suspected. Neonates with HSV disease should be managed in a facility that provides subspecialty care and consultation. Five percent to ten percent of treated neonates will develop life-threatening recurrences requiring retreatment in the first month of life. Long-term suppressive acyclovir therapy to prevent relapses is effective but is associated with adverse drug reactions such as neutropenia and is, therefore, not routinely recommended.

Although HSV infection is more likely to occur at a site of skin trauma, no data indicate that the circumcision of male neonates who may have been exposed to HSV at birth should be postponed. It may be prudent, however, to delay circumcision for approximately 1 month in neonates at the highest risk of disease (eg, neonates delivered vaginally to women with active genital lesions).

Contact of Neonates with Herpes Simplex Virus-Infected Mothers

A woman with HSV infection should be taught about her infection and about hygienic measures to prevent postpartum transmission of the infection to her neonate. Before touching her newborn, the woman should wash her hands carefully and use a clean barrier to ensure that the neonate does not come into contact with lesions or potentially infectious material. If the woman has genital HSV infection, her newborn may room with her after she has been instructed in protective measures. Breastfeeding is permissible if the woman has no vesicular herpetic lesions in the breast area and all active cutaneous lesions are covered.

A woman with herpes labialis (cold sore) or stomatitis should not kiss or nuzzle her newborn until the lesions have cleared. Careful handwashing is important. She may wear a disposable surgical mask when she touches her newborn until the lesions have crusted and dried. Herpetic lesions on other skin sites should be covered. Direct contact of a newborn with other family members or friends who have active HSV infection should be avoided.

HUMAN IMMUNODEFICIENCY VIRUS

Etiology

Acquired immunodeficiency syndrome (AIDS) is caused by HIV type 1 (HIV-1) and, less commonly, HIV type 2 (HIV-2), a related virus that is extremely uncommon in the United States but is more common in West Africa.

Epidemiology

Human immunodeficiency virus has been isolated from blood (including lymphocytes, macrophages, and plasma), CSF, pleural fluid, human milk, semen, cervical secretions, saliva, urine, and tears. However, only blood, semen, cervical secretions, and human milk have been implicated epidemiologically in the transmission of infection.

Well-documented modes of HIV transmission in the United States are sexual contact (both heterosexual and homosexual), skin penetration by contaminated needles or other sharp instruments, and mother-to-neonate transmission before or near the time of birth and from breastfeeding. Infection with HIV continues to spread among women of childbearing age and is occurring increasingly in rural as well as urban areas. The predominant risk behavior is unprotected sexual intercourse. Before effective perinatal HIV interventions, the incidence of perinatal HIV infection has mirrored increases in STDs in women.

In the absence of any intervention, the risk of infection for a neonate born to an HIV-seropositive mother is approximately 25% (range 13–39%). The exact timing of transmission from an infected mother to her neonate is uncertain. Evidence suggests that in the absence of breastfeeding, 30% of transmission occurs before birth and 70% occurs around the time of delivery. Most prenatal transmission probably occurs close to delivery.

Management

Clear medical benefits are derived from pregnant women knowing their HIV serostatus. Demonstrated benefits include early diagnosis and treatment to delay active disease in women and significant reduction in perinatal transmission through early treatment with zidovudine (ZDV). Routine testing for all pregnant women is recommended. Ideally, this should follow counseling and informed consent. Extensive pretest counseling has been perceived as a barrier to routine prenatal testing. The American College of Obstetricians and Gynecologists (ACOG) and the American Academy of Pediatrics (AAP) have endorsed the recommendation of the Institute of Medicine for universal (routine) testing with "notification." Many states have laws governing the process of consent for testing. Universal testing with notification would conflict with some of those laws. Providers must comply with their states' laws. When maternal serostatus is unknown, HIV testing of the newborn remains important for diagnostic and therapeutic reasons.

The individual providing health care for the newborn should be informed of the mother's HIV serostatus to ensure appropriate care and testing. In some states, physicians are required to obtain the mother's written authorization before disclosing her HIV status to other health care providers who are not members of the woman's health care team, such as her neonate's health care provider. Health care providers who are not experienced in the care of pregnant HIV-infected women may want to refer to specialty care from providers who are knowledgeable in this area.

Prenatal and intrapartum administration of ZDV to HIV-infected pregnant women has been shown to reduce the rate of HIV transmission to newborns by 68%. In a large, multicenter randomized controlled trial, ZDV treatment of infected mothers, beginning with oral administration at 14–34 weeks of gestation, followed by intrapartum intravenous ZDV and postnatal oral treatment of the neonates for 6 weeks, reduced vertical transmission from 25.5% in the control group to 8.3%. No significant short-term side effects were observed from ZDV use other than mild, self-limited anemia in the neonates. These neonates have been followed for several years, and no untoward effects of ZDV have been observed. Although theoretical concerns about the prophylactic use of

ZDV remain, it is recommended that ZDV chemoprophylaxis be used to prevent perinatal transmission. The decision to use ZDV should be made by the patient only after discussing with her doctor the benefits for and potential risks to herself and her child. The U.S. Public Health Service Task Force recommends the following ZDV regimen for HIV-infected pregnant women and their newborns:

- Eligibility (therapy also should be discussed and considered with all HIV-infected pregnant women, even those who do not meet these criteria):
  — Pregnancy at 14–34 weeks of gestation
  — No antiretroviral therapy during the current pregnancy
  — No clinical indications for antenatal antiretroviral therapy
  — CD4 + T lymphocyte count of greater than 200 cells/mm^3 at the time of entry into the study
- Maternal treatment:
  —Antepartum—Oral administration of 100 mg of ZDV five times daily, initiated at 14–34 weeks of gestation and continued throughout the pregnancy
  —Intrapartum—Intravenous administration of ZDV in a 1-hour loading dose of 2 mg/kg of body weight, followed by a continuous infusion of 1 mg/kg of body weight per hour until delivery
- Neonatal treatment—Oral administration of ZDV to the newborn (ZDV syrup at 2 mg/kg of body weight per dose every 6 hours) for the first 6 weeks of life, beginning 8–12 hours after delivery

Because shorter-course ZDV therapy may be effective in reducing the transmission rate, ZDV prophylaxis should be offered to HIV-infected pregnant women whose gestation is beyond 34 weeks and to newborns whose mothers who did not receive ZDV.

Since the last edition of Guidelines, substantial advances have been made in the understanding of the pathogenesis of HIV-1 infection and in the treatment and monitoring of HIV-1 disease. Accordingly, advances have resulted in changes in standard antiretroviral therapy for HIV-1 infected adults. More aggressive combination drug regimens that maximally suppress viral replication are now recommended. Although there are considerations associated with pregnancy that may affect decisions regarding timing and choice of therapy, pregnancy is not a reason to defer such standard therapy. Offering antiretroviral therapy to HIV-1 infected women during pregnancy, either to treat HIV-1 infection or to reduce perinatal transmission or for both, should be accompanied by discussion of the known and unknown short-term and long-term benefits and risks of such therapy for infected women and their neonates. Standard antiretroviral therapy should be discussed with and offered to pregnant women infected with HIV-1. Additionally, to prevent perinatal transmission, ZDV chemoprophylaxis should be incorporated into the antiretroviral regimen. As noted previously, a substantial proportion of cases occur as a result of exposure to the virus during labor and delivery. Consistent results indicating a significant relationship between route of delivery and vertical transmission of HIV have now been published. In sum, this body of evidence indicates that cesarean delivery performed before the onset of labor and before the rupture of membranes ("scheduled cesarean delivery") does reduce the likelihood of vertical transmission of HIV (to approximately 2%) compared with either unscheduled cesarean delivery or vaginal delivery. This is true whether or not the patient is receiving ZDV therapy. There are not enough data to address the question of how long after the onset of labor or rupture of the membranes the benefit is lost. It is clear that the maternal morbidity is greater with cesarean delivery than vaginal delivery. Women infected with HIV, whose viral loads are greater than 1,000 copies/mL, should be offered scheduled cesarean delivery to further reduce the risk of vertical transmission of HIV beyond that achievable with ZDV prophylaxis alone. There is a gradient of benefit for the neonate to be gained from cesarean delivery, with the greatest benefit to be gained from scheduled procedures in women at highest risk for vertical transmission with relatively high plasma viral loads. There are insufficient data to demonstrate a benefit of cesarean delivery performed after the onset of labor or rupture of membranes.

Women with very low plasma viral loads (less than 1,000 copies/mL) were found to have a low risk of vertical transmission (less than 2%), even without routine use of scheduled cesarean delivery. There are not enough data to demonstrate a benefit of scheduled cesarean delivery for women with plasma viral loads of less than 1,000 copies/mL. The decision regarding route of delivery in these circumstances must be individualized. The patient's autonomy in making the decision regarding route of delivery must be respected.

Current recommendations for adults are that plasma viral load determinations should be done at "base-line" and every 3 months or following changes in therapy. Plasma viral load should be followed during pregnancy as well. Because of the rapid advances in this area, refer to the CDC (www.cdc.gov) and the HIV/AIDS Treatment Information Service (www.hivatis.org) for treatment recommendations.

Human immunodeficiency virus DNA has been detected in both the cellular and cell-free fractions of human breast milk, and breastfeeding has been implicated in the transmission of HIV infection. Women infected with HIV should be counseled not to breastfeed their babies and they should not donate to milk banks.

Serial testing for HIV should be performed on neonates born to seropositive mothers. Optimally, testing is performed within the first few days of life, at age 1 month, and again at age 4–6 months or later. Using virologic diagnostic techniques, such as HIV culture, PCR, and immune complex-dissociated p24 antigen, HIV infection can be diagnosed in 30–50% of infected neonates at birth and in nearly 100% of infected neonates by ages 4–6 months. Early identification of infected neonates is essential for adequate medical management. Antiretroviral therapy is indicated for most HIV-infected children. Whenever possible, enrollment into clinical trails should be encouraged. Therapeutic strategies are changing rapidly, primary care physicians are encouraged to participate in the care of HIV-infected children in consultation with specialists. Several web sites provide information regarding diagnosis and therapy (www.hivatis.rog, www.atis.org).

Pneumocystis carinii pneumonia can be an early complication of perinatally acquired HIV. *P. carinii* pneumonia prophylaxis should begin at age 4–6 weeks in all neonates born to HIV-infected women, regardless of the neonate's CD4 + T lymphocyte count.

If a neonate is found to be seropositive when the maternal serostatus is unknown, the health care provider for the child should ensure that this information and its significance is relayed to the mother. With her consent and possibly written authorization as required by state law, it also should be communicated to her health care provider.

Because HIV (as well as other viral agents, such as HBV) may be present in blood, vaginal secretions, amniotic fluid, and other fluids, standard precautions (previously "universal precautions") should be strictly followed during all vaginal and cesarean deliveries. Gloves should be used when handling the placenta or the neonate until blood and amniotic fluid have been removed from the neonate's skin.

After delivery, HIV-infected women can receive care in the postpartum care unit, with the use of standard precautions. Obstetric providers may need to refer the HIV-infected women to another health care provider for medical care after pregnancy. Few neonates with HIV infection show clinical evidence of infection in the first weeks after delivery. To minimize risk to health care personnel, routine standard precautions should be used. Prompt and careful removal of blood from the neonate's skin is important. There is no need for other special precautions or for isolation of the neonate with an HIV-infected mother; rooming-in is acceptable. Gloves should be worn for contact with blood or blood-containing fluids and for procedures that entail exposure to blood. Gloves are not required for prevention of HIV transmission while changing diapers.

HUMAN PAPILLOMAVIRUS

Genital warts caused by human papillomavirus (HPV) are common. Infection with certain types of HPV also appears to be related to the subsequent development of genital neoplasms. Cervical or vaginal HPV infections usually are asymptomatic. Studies using DNA diagnostic techniques detect the virus in up to 40% of sexually active young women. Pap tests are less useful for the diagnosis of subclinical cervical infection. Most genital HPV infections are sexually transmitted.

Genital HPV infections may be exacerbated during pregnancy. The papillary lesions may proliferate on the vulva and in the vagina, and lesions may become increasingly friable during pregnancy. Cryotherapy, laser therapy, and trichloroacetic acid may be used safely to treat genital HPV infection in pregnancy. Podophyllin, 5-fluorouracil, and interferon generally are not recommended during pregnancy because of concern that they may be toxic to the fetus.

The risk that a neonate born to a mother who has a genital HPV infection will develop subsequent laryngeal papillomatosis is very small. These lesions are thought to result from aspiration of infectious secretions during passage through the birth canal. The latent period may be several years before HPV lesions become clinically significant in children. Because the risk of respiratory papillomatosis is low, cesarean delivery is not recommended solely to protect the neonate from HPV infection. In women with extensive condylomata, however, cesarean delivery may be necessary because of poor vaginal or vulvar distensibility and the related increased likelihood of extensive vulvovaginal lacerations. Neonates born to mothers with HPV infection do not need to be managed with special precautions in the nursery.

HUMAN PARVOVIRUS

Parvovirus B19 is the agent that causes erythema infectiosum. Approximately one half of pregnant women are immune to parvovirus B19. When infection occurs during pregnancy, the incidence of fetal morbidity and mortality is low. However, parvovirus B19 can infect fetal erythroid precursors and cause anemia, which can lead to nonimmune hydrops and death. Most reported maternal infections that have resulted in fetal death occurred in the first half of pregnancy, and fetal death and spontaneous abortion usually have occurred 4–6 weeks after infection. Third-trimester maternal infections followed by the birth of anemic newborns have been described. Congenital anomalies caused by parvovirus have not been reported.

Because of widespread asymptomatic parvovirus infection in both adults and children, all women are at some risk of exposure, particularly those with school-aged children. Pregnant women who learn that they have been in contact with children who were either in the incubation period of erythema infectiosum or in an aplastic crisis should be counseled about the potential risk to the fetus and should be offered the option of serologic testing. Fetal ultrasound will detect hydrops, but the frequency with which serial measurements should be performed is not known. In some cases, maternal serum alpha-fetoprotein levels may be elevated by the presence of fetal hydrops. A hydropic fetus can be treated by intrauterine transfusion when severe anemia has been documented by cordocentesis, although spontaneous resolution may occur.

In view of the high prevalence of parvovirus B19, the low risk of ill effects to the fetus, and the fact that avoidance of child care or teaching can reduce but not eliminate the risk of infection, pregnant women should not be routinely excluded from workplaces where erythema infectiosum is present. Pregnant health care workers should be aware that patients with erythema infectiosum are most contagious in the week before the onset of illness and unlikely to be contagious after the onset of rash, while patients with an aplastic crisis remain contagious from before the onset of symptoms through the next week or even longer. Routine infection control practices such as handwashing, standard precautions, and droplet precautions reduce transmission.

RESPIRATORY SYNCYTIAL VIRUS

Respiratory syncytial virus (RSV) is a common cause of respiratory infection in infancy and the most common cause of hospitalization for lower respiratory illness in newborns. Preterm newborns and those with chronic lung disease or congenital heart disease (CHD) are at increased risk for severe RSV disease. Prophylaxis to prevent RSV in newborns at increased risk for severe disease, particularly those with chronic lung disease receiving medical management on a long-term basis, is available using either an intravenous RSV immune globulin (RSV-IGIV) preparation or an RSV intramuscular monoclonal antibody, palivizumab. Both preparations decrease the risk of severe RSV disease and hospitalization. No studies have been performed to directly compare the relative efficacy of the two products. Intravenous RSV-IG requires monthly infusions (750 mg/kg per dose) and palivizumab requires monthly intramuscular injections (15 mg/kg per dose) throughout the RSV season. Both preparations are costly. Palivizumab is not a human blood product and, therefore, is not associated with the risk of acquisition of bloodborne pathogens, a potential risk of RSV-IGIV. Newborns receiving RSV-IGIV prophylaxis (but not those receiving palivizumab) should have immunization with measles–mumps–rubella and varicella vaccines deferred for 9 months after the last dose. Currently available data do not support the need for supplemental doses of other childhood vaccines or changes in their time of administration. In the RSV-IGIV trial, immunoprophylaxis decreased the overall rate of hospitalization for non-RSV respiratory infections, whereas palivizumab did not. This may be of value for newborns younger than 6 months who are not eligible for influenza immunization as well as for newborns with severe pulmonary disease in whom all respiratory infections may be important. These products are contraindicated for use in children with CHD. The current AAP recommendations are:

1. Respiratory syncytial virus prophylaxis should be considered for newborns and young children younger than 2 years with chronic lung disease requiring medical management within 6 months before the RSV season. Those with more severe chronic lung disease may benefit from prophylaxis for two RSV seasons. Palivizumab is preferred for most high-risk children because of its ease of administration, safety, and effectiveness.

2. Newborns born at 32 weeks gestation or younger also may benefit from RSV prophylaxis. Newborns born at 28 weeks of gestation or younger may benefit from prophylaxis up to age 12 months, while those born at 29–32 weeks of gestation may benefit from prophylaxis up to age 6 months.

3. Given the large number of patients born between 32 and 35 weeks of gestation and the cost of the drug, the use of palivizumab and RSV IGIV in this population should be reserved for newborns with additional risk factors.

4. Palivizumab and RSV-IGIV are not licensed by the U.S. Food and Drug Administration for patients with CHD. Available data indicate that RSV-IGIV is contraindicated in patients with cyanotic CHD. However, patients with chronic lung disease, who were born preterm, or both, who meet the criteria in the first and second recommendations and who also have asymptomatic acyanotic CHD (eg, patent ductus arteriosus or ventricular septal defect) may benefit from prophylaxis.

5. Respiratory syncytial virus prophylaxis should be initiated at the onset of the RSV season and terminated at the end of the season. There is regional variation with regard to the time window of the RSV season, although in most areas of the United States, the season begins in October to December and ends in March to May. Providers should contact their local health departments or diagnostic laboratories to determine the optimal schedule.

6. Respiratory syncytial virus may be transmitted in the hospital setting and cause serious disease in higher-risk newborns. The major means to prevent RSV disease is strict observance of infection control practices, including identifying and cohorting RSV-infected patients.

A critical aspect of RSV prevention is parent education about the importance of avoiding exposure to and transmission of the virus. Preventive measures include limiting, when feasible, exposure to contagious settings, such as child care centers. The importance of handwashing should be emphasized in all settings, including the home, particularly during periods when contact with high-risk children who have a respiratory infection can occur.

RUBELLA

Prevention and Management During Pregnancy

Surveillance for susceptibility to rubella infection is essential in prenatal care. Each patient should be screened serologically at the first prenatal visit unless she is known to be immune by a previous serologic test.

Seropositive women do not need further testing, regardless of their subsequent history of exposure. If a seronegative pregnant woman is exposed to rubella or develops symptoms that suggest infection, she should be retested for antibody titers to establish whether infection has occurred. Specimens should be obtained as soon as possible after exposure, again 2 weeks later, and, if necessary, 4 weeks after exposure. Serum specimens from both acute and convalescent periods should be tested on the same day in the same laboratory; a negative test result in all samples indicates infection has not occurred while a positive test result in the second sample, but not the first (seroconversion), indicates recent infection. Detection of rubella-specific IgM antibodies usually indicates recent infection, but false positive results occur. Isolation of the virus from throat swabs establishes a diagnosis of acute rubella.

If rubella is diagnosed in a pregnant woman, the patient should be advised of the risks of fetal infection; the choice of pregnancy termination should be discussed. Structural malformation may be caused by infection during embryogenesis, and while fetal infection may occur throughout pregnancy, defects are rare when infection occurs after the 20th week of gestation. The overall risk of defects during the third trimester is probably no greater than that associated with uncomplicated pregnancies. If a woman chooses not to terminate her pregnancy, administration of immune globulin as soon as possible after exposure may be considered. However, no data demonstrate that immune globulin prevents fetal infection. The absence of clinical signs in a woman who has received immune globulin does not guarantee that infection has been prevented.

The rubella vaccine is a live attenuated virus and is highly effective with few side effects in rubella susceptible women of reproductive age. Women found to be susceptible during pregnancy should be offered vaccination postpartum and before discharge from the hospital. Breastfeeding is not a contradiction to receiving the rubella vaccine.

Rubella vaccination is not recommended during pregnancy and following immunization women should be advised to avoid conception for 1 month. However, a woman who conceives within 1 month of rubella vaccination or who is inadvertently vaccinated in early pregnancy should be counseled that the teratogenic risk to the fetus is theoretic. Although asymptomatic infection can occur, no case of congenital rubella syndrome has arisen from a woman given the current rubella vaccine (human diploid vaccine RA 27/3) during pregnancy. Therefore, receipt of the rubella vaccine during pregnancy is not an indication for interruption of pregnancy. The CDC has discontinued its registry of women vaccinated during pregnancy. However, all suspected cases of congenital rubella syndrome, whether caused by wild-type virus or vaccine virus infection, should continue to be reported to local and state health departments. There is no risk to a pregnant woman of having a child in her household vaccinated.

Neonatal Management

Neonates who show signs of congenital rubella infection or who were born to women known to have had rubella during pregnancy, including neonates with few or no obvious clinical manifestations at birth, should be managed with contact isolation, preferably in a private room. Care of the neonate should be provided only by personnel known to be immune to rubella. Efforts should be made to obtain viral cultures from the neonate and to document the infection. Neonates with congenital rubella should be considered contagious until age 1 year unless nasopharyngeal and urine cultures (after age 3 months) are repeatedly negative for the rubella virus.

VARICELLA–ZOSTER VIRUS

Women with varicella–zoster virus (VZV) infection (chickenpox) during pregnancy are no more likely to develop varicella pneumonia than are other adults, but varicella pneumonia is more severe during pregnancy. Therefore, pregnant women with VZV infection should be observed closely for pulmonary symptoms. Although no evidence indicates that maternal administration of VZV immune globulin (VZIG) after exposure reduces the rare occurrence of congenital varicella syndrome, postexposure prophylaxis with VZIG may prevent or ameliorate the illness in nonimmune pregnant women, as it does in other adults. The majority (70–90%) of women with a negative or uncertain history of varicella, are immune. A positive history of varicella is highly predictive of serologic immunity. A pregnant woman who has been exposed to VZV (through intimate or household contact) and who has no history of prior infection should be tested for immunity. If she is not immune, administration of VZIG should be considered within 96 hours of exposure. Varicella–zoster virus immune globulin is available from the American Red Cross Blood Services. If chickenpox is diagnosed during pregnancy, antiviral therapy with acyclovir should be considered.

First trimester varicella infections have been associated with an increased risk of spontaneous abortion. Second trimester varicella infections have been associated with a 2% risk of a congenital syndrome characterized by limb hypoplasia, cutaneous scars, chorioretinitis, cataracts, cortical atrophy, and microcephaly.

If the onset of clinical maternal infection occurs within 5 days before or 2 days after delivery (ie, before the development of maternal antibody, indicating that no VZV antibody has crossed the placenta), VZIG (125 U) should be administered to the neonate as soon as possible. Once VZIG is administered, the neonate can be isolated with the mother. Administration of VZIG is not indicated for healthy, term neonates exposed postnatally to VZV, including newborns of women whose rash developed more than 48 hours after delivery.

Extremely low-birth-weight (LBW) neonates (born at < 28 weeks of gestation or ≤1,000 g) who are exposed to VZV postnatally should receive VZIG (125 U) regardless of maternal history, because of the poor transfer of antibody across the placenta early in pregnancy. Hospitalized preterm neonates born at 28 weeks of gestation or later who are exposed postnatally to chickenpox and whose mothers have no history of chickenpox also should receive VZIG.

Hospitalized women with VZV infection must be kept under airborne and contact precautions. Hospitalized neonates born to women with active VZV infection should be isolated until age 21 days (if VZIG is not given) or until age 28 days (if VZIG is given). Hospitalized neonates who are exposed postnatally should be isolated from 8 to 21 days after onset of the rash in the index case. Neonates with VZV infection should be isolated in a private room, and airborne and contact precautions should be maintained for the duration of the illness. Neonates with congenital VZV infection acquired earlier in gestation do not require special precautions or isolation.

Live-attenuated VZV vaccine, licensed in 1995, is routinely recommended for susceptible children, beginning at age 12 months, and adolescents. Susceptible adults, particularly those in high-risk categories, also should be offered immunization. For adolescents and adults, the primary vaccination series consists of two doses administered subcutaneously 4–8 weeks apart.

Pregnant women should not be vaccinated and vaccinated women should be advised to avoid pregnancy for 1 month after each dose because of concern about possible fetal effects. Surveillance data to date of fetal outcomes after inadvertent vaccine exposures, however, have not found any cases of fetal varicella syndrome. A pregnant household member is not a contraindication to vaccination of a child.

Bacterial Infections

GROUP B STREPTOCOCCI

The proportion of pregnant women colonized with group B streptococci (GBS) ranges from approximately 10% to 30%, but the ability to isolate the organism can be intermittent. Although antepartum rectal or genital colonization usually is asymptomatic, GBS accounts for significant peripartum infection (eg, endometritis, amnionitis, and urinary tract infections).

Before adoption of national prevention guidelines, an estimated 7,600 episodes of GBS sepsis occurred annually in newborns (a rate of 1.8 per 1,000 live births) in the United States, with more than 300 deaths annually among neonates younger than 90 days. Invasive GBS disease in the newborn is primarily characterized by sepsis, pneumonia, and meningitis. Vertical transmission of GBS during labor or delivery may result in invasive infection in the newborn during the first week of life. Known as early-onset GBS infection, this constitutes approximately 80% of GBS disease in newborns. Late-onset GBS disease in the newborn also may occur as a result of vertical transmission or of nosocomial or community-acquired infection. In recent years, there have been reports of invasive GBS disease occurring beyond age 3 months (late, late-onset disease), usually in very LBW preterm neonates.

The risk of early-onset disease is increased by preterm birth (birth at <37 weeks of gestation), a prolonged interval (≥18 hours) between rupture of amniotic membranes and delivery, and clinically evident amnionitis (maternal temperature of ≥38°C [≥100.4°F]). Other factors associated with a higher risk of early-onset disease include GBS bacteriuria during pregnancy and previous delivery of a neonate with GBS disease.

In 1996, the CDC, ACOG, and AAP recommended adopting either a culture-based or a risk-based approach for the prevention of early-onset GBS disease. Using the risk-based approach, women with preterm labor (less than 37 weeks of gestation), preterm premature rupture of membranes (less than 37 weeks of gestation), rupture of membranes 18 hours or longer, previous birth of a child with GBS disease, or maternal fever during labor (≥38°C or 100.4°F) received intrapartum antibiotic prophylaxis. With both culture-based and risk-based approaches, women with GBS bacteriuria during their current pregnancy or women who previously delivered an infant with early-onset GBS disease were candidates for intrapartum antibiotic prophylaxis. The culture-based approach required obtaining a single swab from the lower vagina (introitus) and perianal area, placing the swab in transport media, and culturing in selective broth media. Use of prenatal cultures remote from term to identify women who are colonized with GBS at delivery may not be accurate, and the CDC, ACOG, and AAP recommended obtaining rectovaginal cultures at 35–37 weeks of gestation. All women with positive culture of GBS should be treated with intrapartum antibiotic prophylaxis.

Coinciding with active prevention efforts in the 1990s, the incidence of early-onset disease decreased by 70% to 0.5 cases per 1,000 live births in 1999. Projections derived from 1999 active surveillance data from the Active Bacterial Core Surveillance/Emerging Infections Program Network estimate that intrapartum antibiotics prevented nearly 4,500 early-onset cases and 225 deaths that year. Other countries that have adopted perinatal GBS prevention guidelines similar to the United States have seen comparable decreases in early-onset disease incidence. Recent estimates of early-onset disease incidence in the United States suggest a slight increase in incidence from 1999 to 2000, consistent with a plateau in the impact of prevention efforts.

Since publication of the last edition of Guidelines, new data have emerged comparing the risk-based and culture-based strategies for the prevention of early-onset GBS disease. Because of the rapidly evolving nature of this issue, the reader is referred to the web sites of the CDC (www.cdc.gov), ACOG (www.acog.org), and AAP (www.aap.org) for the latest recommendations on strategies to help prevent early-onset GBS infection in newborns.

LISTERIOSIS

The major cause of epidemic and sporadic listeriosis infections is foodborne transmission. Incriminated foods include unpasteurized milk, cheese, and other dairy products; undercooked poultry; and prepared meats, such as hot dogs, deli meats, and pâté. Asymptomatic fecal and vaginal carriage can result in sporadic neonatal disease, which can cause early-onset neonatal infections from transplacental or ascending intrauterine infection or from exposure during delivery.

Maternal infection has been associated with preterm delivery and other obstetric complications. Late-onset neonatal infection results from acquisition of the organism during passage through the birth canal or possibly from environmental sources.

Listeria monocytogenes can be recovered on blood agar media from cultures of usually sterile body sites (eg, blood, CSF). Special techniques may be needed to recover *L monocytogenes* from sites with mixed flora (eg, vagina, rectum). Gram staining of gastric aspirate or CSF from an infected newborn may demonstrate the organism. Because of morphologic similarity to diphtheroids and streptococci, a culture isolate of *L monocytogenes* mistakenly can be considered a contaminant or saprophyte.

Prompt diagnosis and antibiotic treatment of maternal listeriosis may prevent fetal or perinatal infection. *L monocytogenes* is highly sensitive to ampicillin, but there may be a synergistic benefit to ampicillin plus gentamicin. Culturing for *L monocytogenes* during a subsequent pregnancy has been proposed. However, there are no data on the value of such cultures.

Signs of listeriosis in the newborn vary widely and often are nonspecific. The clinical picture may be similar to that of GBS infection with early- and late-onset syndromes. Therapy with intravenous ampicillin and an aminoglycoside is recommended for neonatal infections.

GONORRHEA

Management in Pregnant Women

Gonorrhea occurs most commonly in individuals aged 15–29 years, and the highest reported incidence occurs in young men aged 20–24 years. In females, the highest rates are in adolescents aged 15–19 years. Risk factors include lower socioeconomic status, single status, early onset of sexual activity, multiple sexual partners, and substance use.

Pregnant women with risk factors for or symptoms of gonorrhea should be cultured for *Neisseria gonorrhoeae* at an early prenatal visit. A repeat culture should be obtained in the third trimester for women at increased risk for gonorrhea and other STDs. DNA tests also are available to detect *N gonorrhoeae*.

Because of the prevalence of penicillin-resistant *N gonorrhoeae*, an extended spectrum (third-generation) cephalosporin (ceftriaxone 125 mg intramuscularly or cefixime 400 mg orally) is recommended for treatment. Tetracyclines and fluoroquinolones are contraindicated in pregnancy. Women who cannot tolerate a cephalosporin should be administered a single 2-g dose of spectinomycin intramuscularly. Because concurrent infection with *Chlamydia trachomatis* is common, patients with gonococcal infections also should be treated for presumptive chlamydial infection and should be evaluated for co-infection with syphilis, HIV, and other STDs. Either erythromycin or amoxicillin is recommended for the treatment of presumptive or diagnosed *C trachomatis* infection during pregnancy. Azithromycin in a single dose (1 g) is an acceptable alternative to erythromycin for the treatment of *C trachomatis* infection in nonpregnant individuals, but well-controlled, adequate studies in pregnant women have not been performed. A test-of-cure is not routinely recommended in persons with uncomplicated gonorrhea, provided that symptoms resolve. All cases of gonorrhea must be reported to public health officials.

Neonatal Clinical Manifestations

Infection in the newborn usually involves the eyes. Antimicrobial prophylaxis immediately after delivery is recommended for all neonates. Topical 1% silver nitrate solution, 0.5% erythromycin ointment, 1% tetracycline ointment, and 2.5% povidone-iodine solution are considered equally effective in preventing gonococcal ophthalmia. An occasional case of gonococcal ophthalmia or disseminated gonococcal infection can occur in neonates born to women with gonococcal disease. Neonates born to women with active gonorrhea should receive a single dose of ceftriaxone, 125 mg, intravenously or intramuscularly; for LBW neonates, the dose is 25–50 mg/kg of body weight. Cefotaxime in a single dose (100 mg/kg given intravenously or intramuscularly) is an alternative. Single-dose systemic antibiotic therapy is effective treatment for gonococcal ophthalmia and prophylaxis for disseminated disease.

In addition to ophthalmia, neonatal disease includes scalp abscess, vaginitis, and systemic disease with bacteremia, arthritis, meningitis, or endocarditis. Neonates with clinical gonococcal disease should be hospitalized and cultures of blood, cerebrospinal fluid, eye discharge, or other sites of infection should be obtained. For neonates with positive cultures (ie, disseminated infection), the recommended antimicrobial therapy is ceftriaxone (25–50 mg/kg per day intravenously or intramuscularly, not to exceed 125 mg given in a single daily dose) or cefotaxime (50–100 mg/kg per day, divided into two doses given every 12 hours). Cefotaxime is preferred for neonates with hyperbilirubinemia. Duration of antibiotic treatment depends on the site of infection; a single dose is adequate for conjunctivitis while 7 days is recommended for disseminated infection and 10–14 days is recommended for meningitis. Infected neonates should be managed with standard precautions.

CHLAMYDIA

Chlamydia trachomatis is the most common sexually transmitted organism in the United States; it has been detected in the cervix of 2–13% of pregnant women and generally is found in 5% or more of women in all populations. Prevalence is highest (about 37%) in sexually active adolescent females. Unrecognized infection is common. Important risk factors for chlamydial infection include unmarried status, recent change in sexual partner or multiple concurrent partners, younger than 25 years, inner-city residence, history or presence of other STDs, and little or no prenatal care. Pregnant women at high risk for chlamydia should be screened for infection during the first prenatal care visit, and testing may be repeated at the third trimester.

Most infected women have few symptoms, but *C trachomatis* may cause urethritis and mucopurulent (nongonococcal) cervicitis. Chlamydial infection also is associated with postpartum endometritis and infertility. Infection may be transmitted from the genital tract of infected women to their neonates during birth; approximately 50% of neonates born to infected women become colonized with *C trachomatis*. Purulent conjunctivitis develops a few days to several weeks after delivery in 25–50% of neonates who acquire *C trachomatis* infection, and neonatal pneumonia occurs in 5–20%. The diagnosis of *C trachomatis* infection is based on a cell culture, direct fluorescent antibody staining, enzyme immunoassay, DNA probe, or PCR.

Treatment should be administered to women who have known *C trachomatis* infection (ie, with mucopurulent cervicitis) or whose neonates are infected. Women whose sexual partners have nongonococcal urethritis or epididymitis are presumed to be infected and also should be treated. Simultaneous treatment of partners is an important component of the therapeutic regimen. Doxycycline and ofloxacin are contraindicated in pregnancy and only limited data are available on the safety and efficacy of azithromycin in pregnant women. Recommended regimens for treating *C trachomatis* infection in pregnant women include erythromycin base 500 mg orally four times daily for 7 days. Alternative regimens in pregnant women include erythromycin base (250 mg orally four times daily for 14 days), erythromycin ethylsuccinate (800 mg orally four times daily for 7 days), erythromycin ethylsuccinate (400 mg orally four times daily for 14 days), or azithromycin (1 g orally in a single dose). Note that erythromycin estolate is contraindicated during pregnancy because of drug related hepatotoxicity. Preliminary data indicate that azithromycin may be safe and effective but are not sufficient to recommend the routine use of azithromycin in pregnant women. Amoxicillin (500 mg orally three times daily for 7 to 10 days) is an alternative but less effective therapy for women who can not tolerate erythromycin. Repeat testing, preferably by culture, 3 weeks after completion of erythromycin or amoxicillin treatment regimens may be considered.

Neonates born to women known to have untreated chlamydial infection should be evaluated and monitored for development of disease. Chlamydial infections in the neonate generally are mild and responsive to antimicrobial therapy. Prophylactic cesarean delivery is not warranted. Routine instillation of topical erythromycin or tetracycline into the conjunctival sac of the neonate shortly after birth has not been proved to prevent neonatal conjunctivitis or other infections caused by *C trachomatis*. Neonates with chlamydial conjunctivitis or chlamydial pneumonia should be treated with oral erythromycin for 14 days. If hospitalized, patients should be managed with standard precautions. Recent evidence shows an association between infantile hypertrophic pyloric stenosis and orally administered erythromycin in infants younger than 6 weeks.

Tuberculosis

Screening

Once considered rare in the United States, the incidence of tuberculosis has increased considerably in women of childbearing age. In endemic areas, the incidence of tuberculosis may approach 0.1% of pregnant women. All pregnant women who are at high risk for tuberculosis should be screened with a Mantoux skin test with purified protein derivative (PPD) when they begin receiving prenatal care. High-risk factors for tuberculosis include:

- Human immunodeficiency virus infection
- Close contact with individuals known or suspected to have tuberculosis
- Medical risk factors known to increase risk of disease (eg, lymphoma, diabetes mellitus, chronic renal failure, immunosuppression)
- Birth in a country with a high prevalence of tuberculosis
- Medically underserved status
- Low socioeconomic status
- Alcohol addiction
- Intravenous drug use
- Residence in a long-term care facility (eg, correctional institutions, mental institutions, nursing homes and facilities)
- Health care professionals working in facilities where the risk of exposure to *Mycobacterium tuberculosis* is increased

Definitions and Diagnosis

Latent tuberculosis infection is defined by a positive tuberculin skin test in an individual with no physical findings of disease and either a normal chest X-ray or only granuloma or calcification in the lung parenchyma or regional lymph nodes or both. The purpose of treating latent tuberculosis infection is to prevent progression to disease. Tuberculosis disease is diagnosed in an individual with infection in whom signs, symptoms, positive cultures, or radiographic manifestations of *M tuberculosis* are apparent.

Isolation of *M tuberculosis* by culture from early morning gastric aspirate, sputum, pleural fluid, or other body fluids establishes the diagnosis of active disease. *M tuberculosis* is slow growing, usually requiring 2–10 weeks for isolation from cultured materials. Smears to demonstrate acid-fast bacilli should be performed on sputum and body fluids.

Management During Pregnancy

Treatment regimens for tuberculosis are based on the presence or absence of active disease, primarily determined by chest X-ray and sputum culture and, in the absence of active disease, the likelihood of progressing to disease. The risk of progression to active disease is highest in the 2 years after seroconversion to positive PPD. For this reason, the recommended medication in women known to have converted within the previous 2 years but with no evidence of active disease is isoniazid (300 mg per day) starting after the first trimester and continuing for 9 months. For HIV-infected women, the duration of isoniazid therapy is 12 months.

Pregnant women should be skin tested only if they have a specific risk factor for latent tuberculosis infection or active tuberculosis. When the skin test is positive, the time of seroconversion usually is not known. If a chest X-ray is normal, some experts prefer to delay treatment until after delivery because pregnancy itself does not increase risk for progression to disease and because of an increased risk of hepatotoxicity during pregnancy and immediately postpartum. Other experts recommend treatment with careful monitoring for hepatitis. All pregnant women receiving isoniazid also should take pyridoxine.

If a pregnant woman is diagnosed with active disease (by positive cultures or by compatible clinical or X-ray findings), prompt multidrug therapy is recommended to protect both the woman and the fetus. Isoniazid and rifampin, supplemented by ethambutol if isoniazid drug resistance is suspected, are currently recommended drugs. Pyrazinamide is frequently used in a three- or four-drug regimen, but safety data in pregnancy have not been published. Therapy is continued for at least 6 months for drug-susceptible disease.

Neonatal Management

Because tuberculosis usually is transmitted by inhalation of droplet nuclei produced by an adult or adolescent with infectious primary tuberculosis, acquisition of *M tuberculosis* by newborns generally occurs only after delivery. Infection can occur before birth as a result of hematogenous dissemination, which seeds the placenta; as a result of infected amniotic fluid in utero; or at the time of delivery as a result of fetal aspiration of tubercle bacilli in women with tuberculosis endometritis. On the rare occasions in which congenital tuberculosis is suspected, diagnostic evaluations and treatment of the neonate and the mother should be initiated promptly.

Management of a newborn whose mother (or other household contact) is suspected of having tuberculosis is based on individual considerations. Whenever possible, separation of the mother (or contact) and the neonate should be minimized. Differing circumstances and resulting recommendations include:

- The mother (or household contact) has a negative X-ray—If the mother is asymptomatic, no separation of the mother and the neonate is required. The mother usually is a candidate for treatment of latent tuberculosis infection. The newborn needs no special evaluation or therapy. Because the positive tuberculin test could be a marker of an unrecognized case of contagious tuberculosis within the household, other household members should have Mantoux skin tests with PPD and further evaluation.

- The mother (or household contact) has an abnormal chest X-ray—If the X-ray is abnormal, the mother and the neonate should be separated until the mother has been evaluated and, if active tuberculosis disease is found, until she is receiving antituberculosis therapy. Other household members should have Mantoux skin test with PPD and further evaluation.

- The mother (or household contact) has an abnormal chest roentgenogram but no evidence of active disease—If the mother's chest roentgenogram is abnormal but the history, physical examination, sputum smear, and roentgenogram indicate no evidence of active disease, the neonate can be assumed to be at low risk of *M tuberculosis* infection. The radiographic abnormality in this circumstance is probably because of another cause or because of a quiescent focus of tuberculosis. In the latter case, the mother may develop contagious, active tuberculosis, if untreated, and should receive appropriate therapy, if not previously treated. She and her neonate should receive follow-up care. Other household members should have a Mantoux skin test with PPD and further evaluation.

- The mother (or household contact) has clinical or radiographic evidence of active, possibly contagious tuberculosis—The mother (or household contact) should be reported immediately to the public health department so that investigation of all household members can be performed within several days. All contacts should have a tuberculin skin test, chest roentgenogram, and physical examination. The neonate should be evaluated for congenital tuberculosis and should be tested for HIV infection. The mother and the neonate should be separated until both are receiving appropriate therapy and the mother is deemed to be noncontagious. If the infant is receiving isoniazid, separation is not necessary. Other household members should have skin testing and further evaluation.

If congenital tuberculosis is excluded, isoniazid is given until the neonate is age 3–4 months, at which time the Mantoux skin test with PPD should be repeated. If the skin test is positive, the child should be reassessed for tuberculosis. If disease is not present, isoniazid should be continued for a total of at least 9 months; HIV-infected children should be treated for 12 months. If the skin test is negative and the mother and other family members with tuberculosis have good adherence and response to treatment and are no longer infectious, isoniazid may be discontinued. The neonate should be evaluated at monthly intervals during treatment.

If the mother (or household contact) has disease caused by multiple-drug-resistant *M tuberculosis* or has poor adherence to treatment and directly observed therapy is not possible, the neonate should be separated from the ill family member and bacillus Calmette–Guérin (BCG) vaccination may be considered for the neonate. Because the response to the vaccine in neonates may be delayed and inadequate for prevention of tuberculosis, directly observed therapy of the affected household contact is preferred.

Untoward effects of isoniazid therapy in newborns are rare. The incidence of hepatitis during isoniazid therapy is so low in otherwise healthy neonates that routine determination of serum aminotransferase concentrations is not recommended. The maternal use of isoniazid is considered to be compatible with breastfeeding. Breastfeeding is considered safe during maternal antituberculosis therapy as long as the neonate is not concurrently taking oral antituberculosis therapy. (If both the mother and the neonate are taking antituberculosis therapy, excessive drug concentrations may occur in the neonate.) Breastfed neonates of women taking isoniazid therapy should receive a multivitamin supplement, including pyridoxine. Drugs in breast milk should not be considered effective treatment or prophylaxis of the neonate.

Bacillus Calmette–Guérin vaccine is a live vaccine prepared from attenuated strains of *Mycobacterium bovis*. Although BCG is recommended by the Expanded Programme on Immunization of the World Health Organization and is widely used throughout the world, BCG use in the United States is limited to selected circumstances. Bacillus Calmette–Guérin vaccine should be considered only for uninfected neonates and children who are at high risk of intimate and prolonged exposure to patients with persistently infectious pulmonary tuberculosis, who cannot be removed from the source of exposure, and who cannot be placed on long-term preventive therapy. The vaccine also should be considered for neonates who are continuously exposed to patients infected with *M tuberculosis* that is resistant to isoniazid and rifampin and who cannot be removed from the source of exposure.

Spirochetal Infections

Syphilis

Syphilis persists in the United States; rates of infection are highest in urban areas and the rural South. All pregnant women should be serologically screened for syphilis as early as possible in pregnancy and again at delivery (as well as after exposure to an infected partner). Because false-negative serologic tests may occur in early primary infection and infection after the first prenatal visit is possible, patients who are considered to be at high risk for syphilis or who are from areas of high prevalence should be retested at the beginning of the third trimester.

The specificity of serologic testing is high if both a nontreponemal screening test (Venereal Disease Research Laboratory [VDRL] or Rapid Plasma Reagin [RPR] test) and a subsequent treponemal serologic test are reactive. Microscopic dark-field and histologic examinations for spirochetes are most reliable when lesions are present.

Congenital syphilis is most often acquired through hematogenous transplacental infection of the fetus, although direct contact of the neonate with infectious lesions during or after delivery also can result in infection. Transplacental infection can occur throughout pregnancy and at any stage of maternal infection.

Treatment for Pregnant Women

Pregnant women with syphilis should be treated with a penicillin regimen appropriate to the stage of infection. Women who are allergic to penicillin should be desensitized and then treated with the drug. Tetracycline and doxycycline are contraindicated during pregnancy. Erythromycin is suboptimal because poor transplacental passage or poor patient compliance may result in failure to cure infection in the fetus.

Women with syphilis should be queried about substance use, especially cocaine. Results of the maternal serologic tests and treatment, if given, should be recorded in the neonate's medical record or be made available to the neonate's pediatrician.

Evaluation of Newborns for Congenital Infection

No newborn should leave any hospital without determination of the syphilis serologic status of his or her mother. A neonate should be evaluated for congenital syphilis if he or she is born to a mother with a positive treponemal test result who has one or more of the following conditions:

- Syphilis and HIV infection
- Untreated or inadequately treated syphilis
- Syphilis during pregnancy treated with a nonpenicillin regimen and inadequate regimen, such as erythromycin

- Syphilis during pregnancy treated with an appropriate penicillin regimen that failed to produce the expected decrease in nontreponemal antibody titer after therapy
- Syphilis treated less than 1 month before delivery (because treatment failures occur and the efficacy of treatment cannot be assumed)
- Syphilis treatment not documented
- Syphilis treated before pregnancy but with insufficient serologic follow-up during pregnancy to assess the response to treatment and current infection status

Neonates born to women with any of the preceding conditions should be evaluated for syphilis. This evaluation should include:

- Physical examination
- Quantitative nontreponemal and a treponemal serologic test for syphilis on the infant's serum sample
- Cerebrospinal fluid evaluation, including a VDRL
- Long-bone X-ray (unless the diagnosis has been otherwise established)
- If available, determination of antitreponemal IgM antibody by a testing method recognized by the CDC, either as a standard or provisional method
- Complete blood cell and platelet counts
- Other clinically indicated tests (eg, chest X-ray)
- Pathologic examination of the placenta or umbilical cord, if available, also is recommended

The VDRL or RPR test is commonly used to evaluate newborns for congenital infection with *Treponema pallidum*. For testing, serum from the neonate is preferred to umbilical cord blood because the latter can produce false-positive and false-negative results.

A diagnosis of congenital syphilis is frequently difficult to establish because clinical evidence of infection may not be apparent at birth and serologic test results may be equivocal or difficult to interpret. A reactive serologic test for syphilis (eg, VDRL, RPR, or fluorescent treponemal antibody absorption test) on neonatal blood does not necessarily indicate that the neonate is infected. If the reaction is caused only by passively transferred maternal antibody, the neonate's VDRL titer usually is lower than the mother's and reverts to negative in 4–6 months. A positive fluorescent treponemal antibody absorption test caused by passively transferred antibody may take up to 1 year to become negative. A persistently reactive serologic test result for syphilis suggests infection, and an increasing titer is almost diagnostic.

Clinical symptoms of early congenital syphilis frequently are absent or nonspecific. Long-bone X-rays may be useful in establishing a diagnosis in neonates with suspected or proved congenital syphilis.

Moist, open syphilitic lesions are infectious. Standard precautions are sufficient for neonates with suspected or proved congenital syphilis. Health care personnel and parents should wear gloves when handling the neonate until antibiotic therapy has been administered for at least 24 hours. Individuals in intimate contact with the neonate before isolation precautions and treatment were instituted should be examined for the presence of lesions 2–3 weeks later and tested serologically for infection.

Parenteral penicillin G remains the preferred therapy for syphilis at any stage. Treatment of neonates with congenital syphilis is summarized in Table 9–3. Cases of syphilis must be reported to the public health authorities.

Lyme Disease

Lyme disease is caused by a spirochete *(Borrelia burgdorferi)* transmitted by deer ticks. Early stages of the disease are characterized by a distinctive bull's-eye skin lesion (erythema migrans) that occurs in 60–80% of patients, and nonspecific, flulike symptoms. Untreated disease can result in neurologic or cardiac manifestations within 4–6 weeks after the onset of early signs and symptoms. A late manifestation of Lyme disease is arthritis, usually intermittent inflammatory arthritis of a large joint. Untreated patients can develop joint involvement ranging from mild to moderate arthralgia to chronic destructive joint disease. No definitive early diagnostic tests, including serology, are commercially available. Patients in the later stages of Lyme disease usually will be seropositive, but false-positive and false-negative tests are common.

Table 9–3. Recommended Treatment of Neonates (≤4 Weeks) with Proven or Possible Congenital Syphilis

Clinical Status of Newborn	Antimicrobial Therapy
Proven or highly probable disease	Aqueous crystalline penicillin G 100,000 to 150,000 U/kg/d (administered bid 50,000/dose IV in the first week of life, and tid in the second to fourth week of life) for 10 days* OR Procaine penicillin G 50,000 U/kg/d IM in a single dose for 10 d*
Asymptomatic, normal CSF, CBC, platelet count, and radiographic examination when maternal treatment is:	
—None, inadequate penicillin treatment†, undocumented, failed, or reinfected	Aqueous crystalline penicillin G, IV, dosing as above, for 10–14 days* OR Clinical, serologic follow-up and benzathine penicillin G, 50,000 U/kg IM, single dose
—Adequate but given <1 month before delivery, the mother's response to treatment is not demonstrated by a fourfold decrease in titer of a nontreponemal serologic test, or erythromycin therapy	Clinical, serologic follow-up and benzathine penicillin G, 50,000 U/kg IM, single dose‡

Abbreviations: CSF, cerebrospinal fluid; CBC, complete blood cell count; IM, intramuscularly; IV, intravenously.

*If more than 1 day of therapy is missed, the entire course should be restarted.

†Inadequate dose, sequential serologic tests do not demonstrate a fourfold or greater decrease in a nontreponemal antibody titer

‡Some experts recommend aqueous crystalline penicillin G, as for proven or highly probable disease. Other experts would follow the neonate without giving antibiotic therapy if both clinical and serologic follow-up can be ensured.

Used and modified with permission of the American Academy of Pediatrics, 2000 Red book: report of the Committee on Infectious Diseases, 25th ed, Copyright of the American Academy of Pediatrics, 2000.

Suspicion of early maternal infection is based on a history of exposure to tick bites, the presence of the distinctive skin lesion, and nonspecific, flulike symptoms. Adequately treated patients may never develop antibodies to spirochetes.

Spirochetes can cross the placenta and, in rare cases, have been found in the tissues of stillborn fetuses. However, the frequency and significance of fetal infection is unknown. Although malformations, intrauterine fetal death, preterm birth, and rash in the newborn have occurred in association with infection in the pregnant woman, a causal relationship has not been established. Current data do not support counseling for pregnancy termination. No evidence exists that Lyme disease can be transmitted via breast milk. The neonate's health care provider should be informed when maternal disease is suspected.

Recommended treatment of suspected early disease in pregnant women is the same as for nonpregnant women—amoxicillin, 500 mg three times per day for 2–3 weeks. For women who are allergic to penicillin, erythromycin is recommended for 2–3 weeks. For patients who are unable to tolerate erythromycin, cefuroxime axetil is an alternative for patients with immediate and anaphylactic hypersensitivity to penicillin who have undergone penicillin desensitization.

The best preventive measure is to avoid heavily wooded areas. If entrance into such areas is necessary, long-sleeved shirts and long pants tucked in at the ankle are helpful. Prophylactic antibiotic therapy for deer tick bites is not routinely recommended.

Parasitic Infections

MALARIA

Although malaria is mainly confined to tropical areas of Africa, Asia, and Latin America, international travel and migration have made malaria a disease to consider in developed countries. The classic symptoms are high fever with chills, rigors, sweats, and headache.

Malaria infection may be more severe in pregnant women and also may increase the risk of adverse outcomes of pregnancy, including spontaneous abortion, stillbirth, preterm birth, and LBW. Because of the risk to both the woman and the fetus, and because no chemoprophylactic regimen is completely effective, pregnant women (or women likely to become pregnant) should avoid travel to malaria endemic areas. If travel to a malaria endemic area is necessary, appropriate consultation should be sought for chemoprophylaxis recommendations based on the malaria species and drug resistance patterns prevalent in that area.

Congenital malaria is rare. Signs and symptoms resemble those of neonatal sepsis.

Definitive diagnosis (of the mother and the neonate) relies on identification of the parasite on stained blood films. Both thick and thin films should be examined. Treatment of infection is based on the infecting species, possible drug resistance, and severity of disease. If malaria is a diagnostic consideration in a pregnant woman or newborn, consultation with appropriate specialists is recommended for optimal patient management.

TOXOPLASMOSIS

Toxoplasmosis is a protozoan infection caused by *Toxoplasma gondii*. As many as one third of women in the United States have antibodies to this organism. Infection is acquired from eating infected raw or poorly cooked meat and from exposure to oocysts in the stools of infected domestic cats. Infected women generally are asymptomatic.

Although congenital infection is more common after maternal infection in the third trimester, the sequelae from first-trimester fetal infection are more severe. Congenital infection may result in chorioretinitis, hydrocephaly, microcephaly, and intracranial calcifications. Neonates of women who are infected with both HIV and *T gondii* should be evaluated for congenital toxoplasmosis.

The diagnosis of maternal infection is based on serologic antibody testing. Routine screening of pregnant women is not indicated, except in the presence of HIV infection. Because the presence of antibodies before pregnancy indicates immunity, the appropriate time to test for immunity to toxoplasmosis in women at risk is before conception. Demonstration of seroconversion is the best method of confirming the diagnosis of acute infection. A significant increase in IgG titer in paired samples taken 2–4 weeks apart (tested simultaneously) or the presence of *T gondii*-specific IgM most often indicates recent or current infection.

Although the presence of antitoxoplasma IgM antibodies is suggestive of acute infection, such IgM antibodies may persist for several months. In addition, with commercially available kits, there often are false-positive results. Before making treatment recommendations, it is recommended that confirmation of increased antitoxoplasma IgM antibodies be obtained in a reference laboratory.

A definitive diagnosis of congenital toxoplasmosis can be made prenatally by: 1) detecting the parasite in fetal blood or amniotic fluid, or 2) documenting antitoxoplasma IgM and IgA antibodies in fetal blood. The parasite can be isolated by mouse inoculation or detected by PCR in a reference laboratory. If the diagnosis is suspected (but unconfirmed) at the time of birth, ophthalmologic, auditory, and neurologic examinations should be performed. *T gondii* may be isolated from the placenta, umbilical cord, or neonate's peripheral blood by mouse inoculation or PCR. Congenital toxoplasmosis can be diagnosed serologically by the detection of antitoxoplasma-specific IgM or IgA antibodies or by the persistence of antitoxoplasma IgG beyond age 12 months.

Therapy of infected mothers with spiramycin (available through the U.S. Food and Drug Administration) may reduce the incidence of fetal infection but will not prevent sequelae in the fetus if congenital infection does occur. The combination of pyrimethamine and sulfadiazine should be considered if the mother acquires infection during the third trimester, although the efficacy of such therapy has not been proved. In one study, routine neonatal screening for toxoplasmosis with early treatment of infected neonates decreased the frequency of long-term sequelae. However, routine neonatal screening for toxoplasmosis currently is not recommended in the United States.

For neonates with both symptomatic and asymptomatic congenital toxoplasmosis, pyrimethamine and sulfadiazine (supplemented with folinic acid) are recommended. The duration of therapy is prolonged (1 year) and has been shown to improve outcome. Neonates with congenital toxoplasmosis should be managed in consultation with infectious disease specialists.

Bibliography

1998 guidelines for the treatment of sexually transmitted diseases. Centers for Disease Control and Prevention. MMWR Recomm Rep 1998;47(RR-1):1–111.

Adoption of hospital policies for prevention of perinatal group B streptococcal disease—United States, 1997. MMWR Morb Mortal Wkly Rep 1998;47: 665–70.

American Academy of Pediatrics. Pickering LK, editor. 2000 Red book: report of the Committee on Infectious Diseases. 25th ed. Elk Grove Village (IL): AAP; 2000.

American Academy of Pediatrics, American College of Obstetricians and Gynecologists. Joint statement on human immunodeficiency virus screening. ACOG Statement of Policy 75. Elk Grove Village (IL): AAP; Washington, DC: ACOG; 1999.

American College of Obstetricians and Gynecologists. Management of herpes in pregnancy. ACOG Practice Bulletin 8. Washington, DC: ACOG; 1999.

American College of Obstetricians and Gynecologists. Perinatal viral and parasitic infections. ACOG Practice Bulletin 20. Washington, DC: ACOG; 2000.

American College of Obstetricians and Gynecologists. Prevention of early-onset group B streptococcal disease in newborns. ACOG Committee Opinion 173. Washington, DC: ACOG; 1996.

American College of Obstetricians and Gynecologists. Scheduled cesarean delivery and the prevention of vertical transmission of HIV infection. ACOG Committee Opinion 234. Washington, DC: ACOG; 2000.

American College of Obstetricians and Gynecologists. Viral hepatitis in pregnancy. ACOG Educational Bulletin 248. Washington, DC: ACOG, 1998.

Centers for Disease Control. Rubella. In: Epidemiology and prevention of vaccine-preventable diseases. 7th ed. Atlanta (GA): CDC; 2002. p.124–38.

Human milk, breastfeeding, and transmission of human immunodeficiency virus in the United States. American Academy of Pediatrics, Committee on Pediatric AIDS. Pediatrics 1995;96:977–9.

Perinatal human immunodeficiency virus testing. American Academy of Pediatrics Provisional Committee on Pediatric AIDS. Pediatrics 1995;95:303–7.

Prevention of perinatal group B streptococcal disease: a public health perspective. Centers for Disease Control and Prevention. MMWR Recomm Rep 1996; 45(RR-7):1–24.

Prevention of respiratory syncytial virus infections: indications for the use of palivizumab and update on the use of RSV-IGIV. American Academy of Pediatrics Committee on Infectious Diseases and Committee on Fetus and Newborn. Pediatrics 1998;102:1211–16.

Public Health Service Task Force recommendations for the use of antiretroviral drugs in pregnant women infected with HIV-1 for maternal health and for reducing perinatal HIV-1 transmission in the United States. Centers for Disease Control and Prevention. MMWR Recomm Rep 1998;47 RR-2):1–20.

Recommendations of the U.S. Public Health Service Task Force on the use of zidovudine to reduce perinatal transmission of human immunodeficiency virus. Centers for Disease Control and Prevention. MMWR Recomm Rep 1994;43(RR-11):1-20.

Respiratory syncytial virus immune globulin intravenous: indications for use. American Academy of Pediatrics Committee on Infectious Diseases and Committee on Fetus and Newborn. Pediatrics 1997;99:645-50.

Revised guidelines for prevention of early-onset group B streptococcal (GBS) infection. American Academy of Pediatrics Committee on Infectious Diseases and Committee on Fetus and Newborn. Pediatrics 1997;99:489-96.

Schuchat A. Group B streptococcus. Lancet 1999;353:51-6.

Targeted tuberculin testing and treatment of latent tuberculosis infection. The official statement of the American Thoracic Society was adopted by the ATS Board of Directors, July 1999. This is a Joint Statement of the American Thoracic Society (ATS) and the Centers for Disease Control and Prevention (CDC). This statement was endorsed by the Council of the Infectious Diseases Society of America. (ISDA), September 1999, and the sections of this statement. Am J Respir Crit Care Med 2000;161:S221-47.

Update on timing of hepatitis B vaccination for premature infants and for children with lapsed immunization. American Academy of Pediatrics, Committee on Infectious Diseases. Pediatrics 1994;94:403-4.

CHAPTER 10

Infection Control

The mother–newborn dyad usually is free of significant infectious processes. However, colonization of the neonate by organisms acquired throughout the delivery process can occur. When exposed to certain organisms, the outcome may be devastating for the neonate, the mother, or both. Many neonatal infections that occur in intensive care units are caused by pathogens acquired from the hospital environment, ie, nosocomial infections.

Surveillance for Nosocomial Infection

The infection control committee of each hospital should work with perinatal care personnel to establish workable definitions of nosocomial infection for surveillance purposes. For obstetric patients, a nosocomial infection can be defined broadly as one that is neither present nor incubating when the patient is admitted to the hospital. Therefore, many cases of endometritis or urinary tract infection that occur postpartum are nosocomial, even though the causative organisms may be endogenous to the female genital tract.

Nosocomial infection in the neonate is defined as an infection that develops after 48 hours after delivery, albeit many of these are caused by organisms acquired from the woman rather than from the hospital environment. This definition should be applied consistently to allow uniform reporting and analysis of nosocomial infections.

Obstetric and nursery personnel should cooperate with hospital infection control personnel in conducting and reviewing the results of surveillance programs for nosocomial infections. This type of monitoring provides information about any unusual problems or clusters of infection, the risks associated with certain procedures or techniques, and the success of specific preventive measures. It also can provide temporal trends, allow comparison with other nurseries using this standard definition, and provide feedback to responsible personnel in the nursery.

Prevention of infections requires a multifaceted approach. This includes meticulous patient care techniques, and the use of antibiotics to reduce the potential for disrupting the balance of colonizing flora and promoting antimicrobial resistant organisms

Prevention and Control of Infections

Nursery Admission Policies

Newborns transferred from a nursery at another hospital usually are not admitted to the normal newborn nursery but rather to intensive care nursery areas. Standard precautions should be taken to prevent the transmission of colonizing organisms from infants in one nursery to those in another. Neonates may be moved safely from one nursery area to another under usual circumstances. Neonates should be approached as though they harbored colonies of unique flora that should not be transmitted to any other neonate. To promote appropriate continuity of care, some neonates may need to be readmitted to the nursery a few days after being discharged. Newborns with suspected infectious diseases should not be readmitted to the normal newborn nursery but can be admitted to specialized areas where additional precautions (airborne, contact, droplet) can be provided to control the risks to other newborns.

Routine culturing of neonates' respiratory or gastrointestinal tract or skin for surveillance purposes is not recommended, but cultures from lesions or sites of infection are recommended to identify the etiology. When clusters of infections caused by a single strain of bacteria are noted, appropriate personnel should be notified. Routine surveillance cultures can be useful for outbreak definition and control.

Usually only clinically apparent infections should be recorded in the surveillance data during an outbreak of infection. However, it is important to document organisms responsible for colonization of all neonates so that appropriate isolation and cohorting procedures can be undertaken.

Both obstetric and nursery personnel are involved in providing perinatal care. Therefore, precise communication between these groups about infectious diseases is essential. Nursery personnel should be notified in advance of the birth of a neonate who may have a congenital or perinatal infection or of a mother who is known to be infected with, or a chronic carrier of, an organism (eg, *Salmonella* species, human immunodeficiency virus [HIV], hepatitis B virus [HBV], hepatitis C virus, or herpes simplex virus).

Standard Precautions

The Centers for Disease Control and Prevention (CDC) recommends that standard precautions should be used consistently for all patients. The concept of standard precautions intends to prevent transmission of bloodborne pathogens and recognize the importance of all body fluids, secretions, excretions, and contaminated items in the transmission of nosocomial pathogens. These precautions apply to: 1) blood; 2) all body fluids, secretions, and excretions except sweat; 3) nonintact skin; and 4) mucous membranes. Standard precautions include handwashing; gloves (in addition to handwashing); masks, eye protection, and face shields; and nonsterile gowns.

Disposal of contaminated equipment or materials should always be accomplished using standard precautions and careful handwashing. Instruments should not be shared and each newborn's bedside should be considered a separate clean environment.

The federal Occupational Safety and Health Administration (OSHA) has issued regulations designed to minimize the transmission of HIV, HBV, and other potentially infectious organisms in the workplace. The OSHA guidelines are extensively discussed in Appendix F. The regulations apply to all employees in physicians' offices, hospitals, medical laboratories, and other health care facilities where workers could be reasonably anticipated to come into contact with blood and other potentially infectious material. The OSHA regulations require employers to implement an exposure control plan to minimize employees' exposure to bloodborne and infectious pathogens. The plan must contain the following components:

- Personal protective equipment for employees exposed to blood and other body fluids
- Housekeeping requirements
- Provision of HBV vaccination to employees
- Postexposure evaluation and follow-up procedures
- Employee training
- Use of warning labels
- Recordkeeping requirements
- Adoption of certain work practice controls (eg, handwashing facilities, disposal of contaminated needles, handling and storage of specimens, and efforts at establishing needleless blood drawing systems)

These requirements are enforced by OSHA or, in the case of states with OSHA-approved comparable job safety and health plans, by state agencies. Violations are punishable by fines.

Health Standards for Personnel

Obstetric and nursery personnel, as well as others who have significant contact with newborns, should be as free of transmissible infectious diseases as possible. Each hospital should establish written policies and procedures for assessing the health of personnel assigned to perinatal care services, restricting their contact with patients when necessary, maintaining their health records, and reporting any illness that they may have. These policies and procedures should address screening for immunity to measles, rubella, mumps, varicella–zoster virus, HBV, pertussis, tetanus, diptheria, and tuberculosis. The frequency and need for screening employees should be determined by local epidemiologic data. Personnel with active tuberculosis should be restricted from patient contact until adequate treatment has occurred and noninfective status verified. All susceptible, nonpregnant hospital personnel should be offered immunization against rubella, varicella–zoster virus, and HBV. Offering annual influenza immunization to nursery personnel is strongly encouraged.

Ideally, individuals with a respiratory, cutaneous, mucocutaneous, or gastrointestinal infection should not have direct contact with neonates. Personnel with exudative skin lesions or weeping dermatitis should refrain from all direct patient care and should not handle patient care equipment until the condition resolves. Personnel in contact with neonates should report personal infections, inability to wash hands (eg, because of casts or braces), and other conditions to their immediate supervisors and should be medically examined to determine suitability for patient contact. Decisions regarding the exclusion of staff members from obstetric and nursery areas should be made on an individual basis. Employee health policies should be worded and applied in a way to ensure that personnel feel free to report infectious problems without fear of income loss.

Transmission of herpes simplex virus from infected personnel to neonates in newborn nurseries is rare. Personnel with cold sores who have direct contact with newborns should cover their lesions and carefully observe handwashing policies. Transmission of herpes simplex virus infection from personnel with genital lesions is not likely. Personnel with herpetic hand infections (herpetic whitlow) should not participate in patient care until the lesions have healed.

Personnel in neonatal units are likely to be exposed to infants excreting cytomegalovirus. Acquisition of cytomegalovirus infection from infants is prevented by compliance with Standard Precautions. Women of childbearing age who work in neonatal units should be counseled about the relatively low risk of exposure should they become pregnant. A routine program of serologic testing of obstetric and nursery hospital employees for immunity to cytomegalovirus is not recommended.

When possible, personnel assigned to obstetric or newborn areas should not be moved between or from other assigned areas of the hospital. Employee education regarding Standard Precautions and other proper infection control techniques should occur regularly. All personnel should be required to strictly follow established infection control procedures.

Handwashing

Health care personnel should be alert to the potential for contamination and practice meticulous techniques to prevent acquisition of pathogens from infected patients. Handwashing before and after each patient contact remains the single most important routine practice in the control of nosocomial infections. Additional policies and procedures are required for critically ill neonates (see the CDC web site, www.cdc/nidod/hip/Guide/guide.htm).

Before handling neonates for the first time on a work shift, personnel should scrub their hands and arms to a point above the elbow with an antiseptic soap. After 3 minutes of washing, the hands should be rinsed thoroughly and dried with paper towels.

A 10-second wash without a brush, but with soap and vigorous rubbing, is required before and after handling each neonate and after touching objects whether or not gloves are worn. Handwashing facilities and materials must be easily accessible. Handwashing is required even when gloves have been worn. Handwashing should occur before and immediately following removal of gloves. Personnel should remove rings, watches, and bracelets before washing their hands and entering the obstetric or nursery areas. Fingernails should be trimmed short, and no false fingernails or opaque polish should be permitted. Clear nail polish on natural nails appears to have no detrimental effect although dark colors may obscure the subungual space and reduce the likelihood of careful cleaning. Antiseptic preparations should be used for scrubbing before entering the nursery, before and after providing care, before performing invasive procedures, and after touching secretions, blood, or equipment.

For routine handwashing, bactericidal soap and water may be sufficient. The bactericidal agents most useful for handwashing in the nursery are chlorhexidine gluconate (4%) and iodophor preparations; both are active against a broad-spectrum of gram-positive and gram-negative organisms. Iodophor preparations often are more drying to the skin. Hexachlorophene-based preparations may be especially useful during nursery outbreaks of *Staphylococcus aureus* infection, but they are not recommended for routine handwashing.

All antiseptic or bactericidal soaps are sensitizing or irritating to the skin, and some individuals may need to use plain soap or mild detergents. Liquid soap dispensers and their contents can become contaminated. This problem can be avoided by using disposable brushes or pads that contain an antiseptic handwashing agent. Alcohol-containing foams and gel satisfactorily kill bacteria when applied to clean hands and require 15 seconds to 2 minutes of contact (in accordance with manufacturers' recommendations). However, alcohol-containing products are not appropriate for cleaning physically soiled hands.

Exposure of Health Care Professionals to Human Immunodeficiency Virus

Health care workers who have had percutaneous or mucous membrane exposure to blood or bloody secretions from an HIV-infected woman or HIV-exposed or HIV-infected newborn must be given medical evaluation and follow-up as prescribed in the OSHA regulations on occupational exposure to bloodborne pathogens. Human immunodeficiency virus infection and evaluation is discussed in Chapter 9.

Dress Codes

Each hospital should establish dress codes for regular and part-time personnel who enter the labor, delivery, and nursery areas. Sterile, long-sleeved gowns should be worn by all personnel who have direct contact with the sterile field during vaginal deliveries, obstetric surgical procedures, and surgical procedures in the nursery. When personnel leave the operative room and while they are in the hospital, surgical scrub suits should be covered. Hospital policies regarding sterile areas should be established and maintained.

Some hospitals have approved more flexible dress codes for personnel who work in birthing rooms; however, the CDC recommends that all health care workers who perform or assist in deliveries wear gloves, gowns, surgical masks, caps, shoe covers, and eye protection during the procedure. Wearing aprons or gowns made of impervious material during cesarean delivery may provide additional protection. Gloves should be worn when handling the placenta or the neonate until blood and amniotic fluid have been removed from the neonate's skin. Hands should be washed immediately before gloving and after gloves are removed or when skin surfaces are contaminated with blood.

Recent studies have demonstrated that cover gowns are not necessary for regular personnel in the nursery or neonatal intensive care unit, as long as handwashing is strictly enforced. When a neonate is held outside the bassinet by nursing or other neonatal intensive care unit personnel, a long-sleeved gown should be worn over the clothing and either discarded after use or maintained for use exclusively in the care of that neonate. If one gown is used for each neonate, the gowns should be changed regularly.

Caps, beard bags, and masks should be worn during certain surgical procedures, including umbilical vessel catheterization. Long hair should be restrained so that it does not touch the neonate or equipment during patient examinations or treatments. High-efficiency, disposable masks should be used, but even these masks remain effective for only a few hours. Masks should be worn so that they cover both the nose and the mouth, and they should be discarded as soon as they are removed from the nose and mouth.

Sterile gloves should be used during deliveries and all invasive procedures performed in either the obstetric or the nursery area. Disposable, nonsterile gloves may be useful in the care of patients in isolation or in the performance of procedures that may result in contamination of the hands.

Obstetric Considerations

The areas where cesarean deliveries and tubal ligations are performed are operating rooms and are subject to all policies pertaining to such facilities. Therefore, all persons present should wear appropriate operating room attire. For those close to the sterile surgical field, this attire includes clean scrub clothing, sterile operating room gowns, caps, masks, eye protection, gloves, and shoe covers. For those not involved with the surgical field, a sterile operating room gown is not required, but caps, masks, and shoe covers should be worn. The surgical field should be prepared and draped according to standard recommendations.

Shaving, if needed, should be performed within 2 hours of the procedure. Clipping hair very close to the skin is preferred to shaving.

Intrauterine pressure catheters (for monitoring contractions or for amnioinfusion) or internal fetal electrodes (for fetal heart rate monitoring) should be inserted and maintained in accordance with standard sterile techniques. All fluids used should be sterile. To minimize the chance of contamination, the packing of the devices should be opened only at the time of their use and proper sterile techniques should be followed during their handling and insertion. Whenever possible, disposable items are preferable.

NEONATAL CONSIDERATIONS

Invasive Procedures

Percutaneous placement of peripheral arterial or venous cannulas is associated with a lower risk of infection in neonates than is surgical placement. The cannulas should be removed promptly if signs of device-associated infection occur. A safe maximal duration of cannulation for intravascular catheters has not been established; the risks and benefits should be assessed daily for each neonate. Intravascular catheters should not be used or left in place unless they are clearly indicated for medical management. Each unit should have a written policy on the procedures governing the use of these catheters.

Arterial cannulas are an ideal pressure-monitoring device in a closed system, but often they also are used for obtaining blood samples. These samples should be obtained aseptically, with precautions to avoid contamination of the system and with the realization that the risk of cannula infection is increased.

Total parenteral nutrition generally is safe but has been associated with infection, including bacteremia and fungemia. A multidisciplinary team approach involving pharmacists, nurses, and physicians is strongly recommended to reduce the incidence of infections and other complications. Meticulous attention should be given to aseptic insertion and maintenance of the cannula and to aseptic techniques of fluid administration. All parenteral nutrition fluids should be mixed in a central pharmacy, under a laminar flow hood. Because lipid emulsions are especially susceptible to contamination with a wide variety of bacteria and fungi that can proliferate to high concentrations within hours, particular caution must be taken in the storage and administration of these emulsions. Unit-dose amounts may be delivered from the pharmacy. Opened bottles must be discarded no later than 24 hours after the seal has been broken. Intravenous tubing, stopcocks, and flush syringes should be changed (using sterile technique) on a regular basis and no less frequently than every 72 hours. If an increased incidence of infection is noted, tubing should be changed more frequently.

Intravascular Solutions

The hospital pharmacy should establish a system to ensure a satisfactory and safe means of providing sterile, unpreserved fluids to the nursery areas. The CDC has no recommendations for the duration of infusion (hang time) of nonlipid-containing parenteral-nutrition fluids. Infusion of lipid-containing parenteral-nutrition fluids should be completed in 24 hours and 12 hours if lipid is given alone.

Solutions with benzyl alcohol are contraindicated in neonates because their use may lead to severe metabolic acidosis, encephalopathy, or death. When the fluid administered is to contain heparin, it should be added to the fluid in the hospital pharmacy whenever possible. Flush solutions should be kept at room temperature no longer than 8 hours before being used or discarded. They should be labeled clearly with the time of opening or preparation.

Antibiotics

The efficacy of antibiotics used for prophylaxis in newborns has not been documented. Prophylaxis is strongly discouraged except for specific indication (eg, ophthalmia neonatorum). The relative frequencies of documented infections in neonates, etiologic agents, and patterns of antimicrobial susceptibility should be monitored by the infection control committee. The most well-tolerated, narrow spectrum and effective antibiotic regimens should be selected after analysis of these data. The indiscriminate and nonjudicious use of either systemic or topical antibiotics promotes the emergence of resistant strains of bacteria, making subsequent therapy for clinical infections more difficult and dangerous.

Women with Postpartum Infections

The neonate need not be isolated from a mother with a postpartum infection in most circumstances. Women with abscesses or infected or draining wounds should have appropriate cover dressings. If it is not possible to cover the infected or draining wound completely, the infant should be placed in a separate room. Gloves and, if necessary, gowns should be worn by staff during all contact with infected patients.

Mothers with communicable diseases (eg, group A streptococci, active tuberculosis, varicella) that are likely to be transmitted to the newborn should be separated from the newborn until the infection is no longer communicable, based on the natural history of the infection and the effectiveness of therapy in eliminating contagion. A mother with postpartum fever that is not due to a specific communicable cause can be allowed to feed and care for her newborn. With the exception of specific infections (see "Contraindications to Breastfeeding" in Chapter 7), breastfeeding is rarely contraindicated in maternal infection. Criteria for allowing mothers to handle neonates include:

- She feels well enough to handle the neonate.
- She washes her hands thoroughly under supervision.
- She wears a clean gown.
- She avoids contact of the neonate with contaminated clothes, linen, dressings, or pads.

A woman with a respiratory tract infection should be made aware that the infection can be transmitted not only by droplets but also by hands and fomites. Therefore, she should practice strict handwashing techniques and appropriately handle or dispose of contaminated tissues and any other items that may have come in contact with infectious secretions. If needed, she can wear a surgical mask to reduce the chance of droplet spread to her neonate.

Postpartum women who are infected with nonobstetric-related communicable diseases should be treated according to the precautions and isolation techniques required by the specific disease. If the required guidelines cannot be followed safely in the obstetric unit, the patient should be transferred to the appropriate unit where such care can be provided.

Cohorts

During epidemics, a comprehensive program of infection control is required. Even if an intensive investigation is not indicated, the results of the control measures should be evaluated to ensure that they have been effective and the problem has been resolved. Because many infections become apparent only after neonates leave the hospital, each hospital should establish procedures to be used during a suspected or confirmed epidemic for disease surveillance of recently discharged neonates. The hospital infection control personnel and appropriate public health officials should be notified promptly about suspected or confirmed epidemics.

Neonates with overt infection and those who are colonized should be identified rapidly and placed in cohorts—separate areas where newborns with similar exposures or illnesses receive care. If rapid identification of these neonates is not possible, separate cohorts should be established for neonates with disease, those who have been exposed, those who have not been exposed, and those who are newly admitted. The success of cohort programs depends largely on the willingness and ability of nursery and ancillary personnel to adhere strictly to the cohort system and to follow established practices.

Neonates with Infections

The housing of an infected neonate or one suspected of being infected depends on the overall condition of the neonate and the type of care required, the available space and facilities, the nurse-to-patient ratio, and the size and type of the neonatal care service. Other factors to be considered include the type of infection, the clinical manifestations, the source and possible modes of its transmission, and the number of colonized or infected neonates.

ISOLATION

In many instances (notable exceptions are neonatal varicella–zoster virus infection or epidemics of bacterial infection), it is unnecessary to isolate infected neonates if certain criteria are met:

1. Sufficient nursing and medical staff are on duty to provide comprehensive care

2. Sufficient space is provided for a 4–6-ft aisle between neonatal stations
3. Two or more sinks for handwashing are available in each nursery room or area
4. Continuing instruction is provided about the ways in which infections spread

If these criteria are not met, an isolation room with separate scrub facilities is necessary. Physical separation with assignment of separate health care personnel for each area is best. In 1996, the CDC recommended new isolation guidelines for hospitalized patients. These guidelines suggest standard precautions for care of all patients regardless of diagnosis and Transmission-Based Precautions for patients who are infected or colonized with pathogens that are spread by airborne, droplet, or contact routes. Isolation categories, with examples, are listed in Table 10–1.

Forced-air incubators provide adequate isolation for infected neonates. Although these incubators filter incoming air, they do not filter the air that is discharged into the nursery. They are, therefore, satisfactory for limited protective isolation of neonates, but they should not be relied on to prevent transmission of microorganisms from infected neonates to others.

When an isolation room is deemed necessary, blinds, windows, and other structural items must allow for ease of regular cleaning of this room. An intercom should be provided. Air from this room should be exhausted to the outside and not to the rest of the nursery.

Gastroenteritis, Abscess, Viral Respiratory Infection, or Cutaneous Infection

Contact precautions should be observed when treating patients with viral respiratory infection, gastroenteritis, cutaneous infections, or draining lesions of abscesses that cannot be contained adequately by a dressing. All personnel should use gowns and disposable gloves when providing direct patient care. Contaminated items should be properly discarded and gowns and gloves should be discarded before leaving the room. The environment may be heavily contaminated with the infecting microorganism, and these organisms often are transmitted on the hands

Table 10–1. Isolation Categories

Isolation Category	Private Room	Hand-washing	Mask	Gown	Gloves	Examples
Standard	No	Yes	Yes*	Yes	Yes	Possible exposure to blood, all body fluids, or secretions and excretions
Contact	Yes Cohort (if private room not available)	Yes	No	Yes	Yes	Multidrug-resistant bacteria, RSV, rotavirus, cutaneous HSV, varicella (also see Airborne)
Droplet	Yes Cohort (if private room not available)	Yes	Yes	No	No	Pertussis, rubella, mumps, parvovirus B19, respiratory viruses, bacterial meningitis
Airborne	Yes Negative air-pressure ventilation	Yes	Yes	No	No	Varicella (also see Contact), measles, tuberculosis

Abbreviations: HSV, herpes simplex virus; RSV, respiratory syncytial virus
*During procedures or activities likely to generate splashes or sprays
Used and modified with permission of the American Academy of Pediatrics, 2000 Red book: report of the Committee on Infectious Diseases, 25th ed, Copyright of the American Academy of Pediatrics, 2000.

of personnel to other neonates. If more than one neonate is infected, a cohort approach should be taken.

Congenital Infections

Standard precautions are adequate isolation procedures for most congenital infections with the exceptions of congenital rubella that requires droplet isolation or suspected herpetic infection that will require contact isolation.

Viral Infections

Many viruses, such as respiratory syncytial virus, coxsackieviruses, or echoviruses, spread rapidly among neonates and personnel in a nursery. Such viral infections can be serious in neonates, sometimes resulting in death. Because neonates may shed selected viruses after their clinical illness has been resolved, they become reservoirs of infection. It is believed that the enteroviruses and respiratory syncytial virus are transmitted predominantly by direct or indirect contact by the hands of personnel that become contaminated with virus-containing secretions or with contaminated environmental surfaces or fomites. Contact isolation is required to prevent this type of spread.

Neonates usually are ineffective disseminators of infectious bacterial or viral aerosols. Neonates with confirmed or possible infections caused by a viral agent that could be transmitted by the airborne route should be separated from other neonates by: 1) transfer from the nursery area; 2) rooming-in with the mother; or 3) enclosure of all other neonates in the area in incubators.

Environmental Control

The physician in charge and the nursing supervisor of the obstetric and nursery areas should work with infection control personnel and other appropriate groups (eg, representatives of the respiratory therapy service, central supply, and housekeeping) to establish an environmental control program for the labor, delivery, and nursery areas. This program should include specific procedures in a written policy manual for cleaning and disinfection or sterilization of patient care areas, equipment, and supplies. Consultation for specific details and problems is essential. Nursing supervisors should ensure that these procedures are carried out correctly.

METHODS OF STERILIZATION AND DISINFECTION

All medical and hospital personnel should understand the difference between sterilization and disinfection. Sterilization is the destruction of all microorganisms, including spores. Disinfection is simply a reduction in the number of contaminating microorganisms. High-level disinfection is the elimination or destruction of all microorganisms except spores. Cleaning is the physical removal of organic material or soil, including microorganisms, from objects.

Devices that enter tissue or the vascular system should be sterile. For neonates, devices that come into contact with mucous membranes or that have prolonged or intimate contact with skin also should be sterile. Much of the equipment required in perinatal care areas, however, can be used safely if it is satisfactorily cleaned and disinfected; clean, dry surfaces do not support the growth of microorganisms.

It is sometimes necessary to decontaminate equipment before it is cleaned and sterilized or disinfected to allow processing without exposing personnel to hazardous microbes. The equipment must be cleaned thoroughly to remove all blood, tissue, secretions, food, and other residue. Without thorough cleaning, no method of sterilization or disinfection can be effective. Furthermore, some chemical disinfectants are inactivated by organic materials.

Sterilization

Methods of sterilization include steam autoclaving, dry heat, and gaseous (ethylene oxide) or liquid chemical (eg, 2% glutaraldehyde) techniques. The preferred method of sterilization is steam autoclaving, because this is the least expensive method and provides the greatest margin of safety. Some equipment may be damaged by steam, however, and must be sterilized by another method. The ideal method for sterilization must be established for each piece of equipment.

Equipment made of material that absorbs ethylene oxide usually requires 8–12 hours of aeration after sterilization with ethylene oxide before it can be used again. Ethylene oxide sterilization of supplies or equipment should be preceded by a comprehensive review of data on the aeration time required for each material to be processed and the extent to which toxicity standards have been established. An ethylene oxide sterilization plan requires the presence of sufficient backup equipment to allow time for aeration.

Equipment that cannot be sterilized with steam or ethylene oxide may be satisfactorily sterilized after cleaning by immersion for 10 hours in acetic acid liquid sterilant or 2% glutaraldehyde or other acceptable liquid sporicide. This immersion should be followed by three rinses with sterile water (or tap water with at least 10 mg of hypochlorite per liter), thorough drying, and packaging in sterile wrappers.

High-Level Disinfection

Equipment that does not need to be sterilized may be subjected to high-level disinfection. Both hot-water pasteurization and chemical disinfection are satisfactory. Pasteurization of equipment requires immersing it in water at 80–85°C (176–185°F) for 15 minutes or 75°C (167°F) for 30 minutes. After air drying (preferably in a cabinet with heated, filtered air), disinfected items should be aseptically wrapped and stored until needed. Although spores are not eradicated by this method, bacterial and viral decontamination is adequate. The original reports of the equipment manufacturer should be consulted for a list of any parts or materials that may be warped or damaged at these temperatures.

The choice of liquid chemicals for high-level disinfection depends on the type of equipment to be disinfected. In many instances, immersion of the equipment for 20 minutes in 2% glutaraldehyde, followed by three rinses with sterile water (or tap water with at least 10 mg of hypochlorite per liter) and thorough drying is satisfactory.

CLEANING AND DISINFECTING NONCRITICAL SURFACES

Selection of Disinfectants

Although numerous disinfectants are available, no single agent or preparation is ideal for all purposes. Consideration should be given to the agent and its special use, as well as to the types of organisms likely to be contaminating the object that is to be disinfected. Special attention should be given to the recommended concentration of each disinfectant and to its time of exposure. Unnecessary exposure of neonates to disinfectants should be avoided, and strict adherence to manufacturers' recommendations is essential.

Quaternary ammonias, chlorine compounds, and phenolic compounds are satisfactory disinfectants. Sodium hypochlorite has been suggested for disinfection of HIV-exposed surfaces. Use of any of these substances should be limited to disinfectant–detergent products registered by the U.S. Environmental Protection Agency and recommended by the manufacturer for nursery surfaces with which neonates have contact. Information about specific label claims of commercial germicides can be obtained from this agency or from the Association for Professionals in Infection Control and Epidemiology.

General Housekeeping

The following order of cleaning is recommended:

1. Patient areas
2. Accessory areas
3. Adjacent halls

It is not known whether floor bacteria are a source of nosocomial infection, but regular cleaning prevents the accumulation of pathogenic bacteria. Disinfectant–detergents have been shown to be more effective than soap and water alone in cleaning floors, although hospital floors are rapidly recontaminated after disinfection. Available disinfectant–detergents may differ in effectiveness.

During the cleaning process, dust should not be dispersed into the air. Removal of dust by a dry vacuum machine, followed by wet vacuuming, is effective in cleaning and disinfecting hospital floors. Once dust has been removed, scrubbing with a mop and a disinfectant–detergent solution should be sufficient to clean and disinfect floors. Mop heads should be machine laundered and thoroughly dried daily.

Standard types of portable vacuum cleaners should not be used in nurseries or delivery areas because particulate matter and microbial contamination in the room may be disturbed and distributed by the exhaust jet. Vacuum cleaners that discharge outside the patient care area (ie, central vacuum cleaning systems or portable vacuums) should be used so that only the cleaning wand, floor tool, and high-efficiency, particulate air-filtered vacuum hose are brought into the patient care area.

Cabinet counters, work surfaces, and similar horizontal areas may be subject to heavy contamination during routine use. These areas should be cleaned once per day and between patient use with a disinfectant–detergent and clean cloths; friction cleaning is important to ensure physical removal of dirt and contaminating microorganisms. Surfaces that are contaminated by patient specimens or accidental spills should be carefully cleaned and disinfected.

Walls, windows, and storage shelves may be reservoirs of pathogenic microorganisms if grossly soiled or if dust and dirt are allowed to accumulate. These areas and similar noncritical surfaces should be scrubbed periodically with a disinfectant–detergent solution as part of the general housekeeping program.

Faucet aerators may be useful to reduce water splashing in sinks, but they are notoriously susceptible to contamination with a variety of hydrophilic bacteria. For this reason, removing aerators permanently may be preferred to periodic cleaning and disinfection. Sinks should have backsplashes to prevent the retention of pooling water, a source of bacterial growth. Sinks should be scrubbed clean daily with a disinfectant–detergent; drain traps should not need routine cleaning or disinfection.

Written policies should be established for the removal and disposal of solid wastes. Sturdy plastic liners should be used in trash receptacles; these liners should be sealed before they are removed from the trash receptacles. In patient care areas, trash receptacles should be cleaned and disinfected regularly. Infectious material requires special handling and disposal.

Special housekeeping personnel should be assigned to clean the nursery. If the nursery is small, they also may be assigned to work in the obstetric areas or other clean areas of the hospital. The nursery should be cleaned daily at an appropriate time. Intensive care nurseries should ideally be cleaned when traffic is minimal, if possible.

CLEANING AND DISINFECTING PATIENT CARE EQUIPMENT

Incubators, Open Care Units, and Bassinets

After a neonate has been discharged, the care unit used by that neonate should be thoroughly cleaned and disinfected. A disinfectant–detergent registered by the U.S. Environmental Protection Agency is recommended for this purpose. Manufacturers' directions for use of a disinfectant–detergent should be followed carefully. A bassinet or incubator should never be cleaned when occupied. Newborns who remain in the nursery for an extended period should be transferred periodically to a different, disinfected unit.

When a care unit is being cleaned and disinfected, all detachable parts should be removed and scrubbed meticulously. If the incubator has a fan, it should be cleaned and disinfected; the manufacturer's instructions should be followed to avoid equipment damage. The air filter should be maintained as recommended by the manufacturer. Mattresses should be replaced when the surface covering is broken, because such a break precludes effective disinfection or sterilization. Mattresses may be sterilized by heat or gas. Portholes and porthole cuffs and sleeves are easily contaminated, often heavily; cuffs should be replaced on a regular schedule or cleaned and disinfected frequently with freshly prepared mild soap or quaternary ammonium disinfectant–detergent solutions. Incubators not in use should be thoroughly dried by running the incubator hot without water in the reservoir for 24 hours after disinfection.

Evaporative humidifiers in incubators usually do not produce contaminated aerosols, but contaminated water reservoirs may be responsible for direct rather than airborne transmission of infection. Reservoirs should be filled with sterile water only, and they should be drained and refilled with sterile water every 24 hours. In many areas of the United States and in hospitals with a central ventilation system, environmental humidity levels may be sufficiently high to eliminate the need for additional humidification in most cases, and water reservoirs may be left dry. If humidification is necessary, a source of humidity external to the incubator may be preferable to incubator humidifiers. An external humidifier can be changed daily and the equipment sent for cleaning and sterilization or disinfection.

Nebulizers, Water Traps, and Respiratory Support Equipment

Nebulizers and attached tubing should be replaced by clean, sterile equipment (or equipment that has been subjected to high-level disinfection) in accordance with established hospital policy. Failure to replace tubing may result in contamination of freshly cleaned equipment. Water traps also should be replaced regularly by autoclaved or disinfected equipment. Only sterile water should be used for nebulizers or water traps; residual water should be discarded when these containers are refilled. Water condensed in tubing loops should be removed and discarded and should not be allowed to reflux into the container.

Other Equipment

Cleaning and disinfection or sterilization of equipment should be performed between patients. Equipment that is used for only one patient should be replaced, cleaned, and disinfected or sterilized according to an established schedule. Disposable equipment should be replaced with approximately the same frequency as reusable equipment is recycled. Disposable equipment should never be reused.

Resuscitators, face masks, laryngoscopes, eye speculums, and other items used in direct contact with neonates should be dismantled, thoroughly cleaned, and sterilized, if possible. Alternately, the equipment may be subjected to high-level disinfection with liquid chemicals or by pasteurization. Equipment such as tubing for respiratory or oxygen therapy should be either sterilized or discarded after use. Stethoscopes and similar types of diagnostic instruments should be wiped with iodophor or alcohol before use, unless they are used for individual patients or the instruments become contaminated between uses. Mouth-controlled suctioning should not be used. Standard precautions should be used when any type of suctioning is performed.

Neonatal Linen

Procedures for laundering, making up packs, and delivering linen to the nursery should be established by the medical, nursing, laundry, and administrative staffs of the hospital. Each delivery of clean linen should contain sufficient linen for at least one 8-hour shift. Linen should be cleaned and transported in covered carts to the nursery areas. Autoclaving linen has not been shown to be effective in preventing infections in normal newborn nurseries or intensive care areas. No new garments or linen should be used for neonates without prior laundering.

An established procedure for the disposal of soiled linen should be strictly followed. Chutes for the transfer of soiled linen from patient care areas to the laundry are not acceptable unless they are under negative air pressure. Soiled linen should be discarded into impervious plastic bags placed in hampers that are easy to clean and disinfect. Soiled diapers should be placed in special diaper receptacles immediately after removal from the neonate; they should never be rinsed in the nursery. All personnel should be aware that handling dirty diapers with bare hands can result in heavy contamination and transient colonization of the hands with microorganisms that cannot be easily eliminated with handwashing and can be readily transmitted to the next neonate for whom they provide care.

Plastic bags of soiled diapers (reusable or disposable) and other linen should be sealed and removed from the nursery at least every 8 hours. Individuals who collect the bags of soiled diapers or linen need not enter the nursery if all bags are placed outside the nursery. Sealed bags of reusable, soiled nursery linens should be taken to the laundry at least twice each day; sealed bags of disposable diapers also should be taken away at least twice per day.

Laundering

Diapers and other nursery linens should be washed separately from other hospital linen and with products used to retain softness. Acidification neutralizes the alkalis used in the washing process and is responsible for the greatest bacterial destruction. Standard precautions should be taken in handling linen soiled with blood. Chlorine bleach should be used for any items that are contaminated with blood.

The chemicals trichlorocarbanilide or the sodium salt of pentachlorophenol should not be used in hospital laundering because they may be harmful. To avoid the hazards associated with the use of such chemicals or enzymes in the hospital laundry, the physician in charge should be aware of all agents in use and should be informed before any changes are made in laundry chemicals or procedures. Therefore, caution should be exercised when new laundry or cleaning agents are introduced into the nursery or when procedures are changed.

Bibliography

American Academy of Pediatrics. Pickering LK, editor. 2000 Red book: report of the Committee on Infectious Diseases. 25th ed. Elk Grove Village (IL): AAP; 2000.

Garner JS. Guideline for isolation precautions in hospitals. Part I. Evolution of isolation practices; Hospital Infection Control Practices Advisory Committee. Am J Infect Control 1996;24:24–31.

Garner JS. Guideline for isolation precautions in hospitals. The Hospital Infection Control Practices Advisory Committee. Infect Control Hosp Epidemiol 1996;17:53–80.

Larson EL. APIC guideline for handwashing and hand antisepsis in health care settings. Am J Infect Control 1995;23:251–69.

Moolenaar RL, Crutcher JM, San Joaquin VH, Sewell LV, Hutwagner LC, Carson LA, et al. A prolonged outbreak of Pseudomonas aeruginosa in a neonatal intensive care unit: did staff fingernails play a role in disease transmission? Infect Control Hosp Epidemiol 2000;21:80–5.

Update: provisional Public Health Service recommendations for chemoprophylaxis after occupational exposure to HIV. MMWR Morb Mortal Wkly Rep 1996;45:468–80.

ACOG Antepartum Record and Discharge/Postpartum Form

DATE _____

NAME _____
      LAST   FIRST   MIDDLE

ID # _____ HOSPITAL OF DELIVERY _____

NEWBORN'S PHYSICIAN _____ REFERRED BY _____

FINAL EDD _____   PRIMARY PROVIDER/GROUP _____

BIRTH DATE	AGE	RACE	MARITAL STATUS S M W D SEP	ADDRESS		
MONTH DAY YEAR						
OCCUPATION		EDUCATION (LAST GRADE COMPLETED)		ZIP	PHONE	(H) (O)
LANGUAGE				INSURANCE CARRIER/MEDICAID #		
HUSBAND/DOMESTIC PARTNER			PHONE	POLICY #		
FATHER OF BABY			PHONE	EMERGENCY CONTACT		PHONE

TOTAL PREG	FULL TERM	PREMATURE	AB. INDUCED	AB. SPONTANEOUS	ECTOPICS	MULTIPLE BIRTHS	LIVING

MENSTRUAL HISTORY

LMP ☐ DEFINITE ☐ APPROXIMATE (MONTH KNOWN)   MENSES MONTHLY ☐ YES ☐ NO   FREQUENCY: Q _____ DAYS   MENARCHE _____ (AGE ONSET)

      ☐ UNKNOWN   ☐ NORMAL AMOUNT/DURATION   PRIOR MENSES _____ DATE   ON BCP AT CONCEPT ☐ YES ☐ NO   hCG + ___/___/___

      ☐ FINAL _____

PAST PREGNANCIES (LAST SIX)

DATE MONTH/ YEAR	GA WEEKS	LENGTH OF LABOR	BIRTH WEIGHT	SEX M/F	TYPE DELIVERY	ANES.	PLACE OF DELIVERY	PRETERM LABOR YES/NO	COMMENTS/ COMPLICATIONS

MEDICAL HISTORY

	O Neg. + Pos.	DETAIL POSITIVE REMARKS INCLUDE DATE & TREATMENT			O Neg. + Pos.	DETAIL POSITIVE REMARKS INCLUDE DATE & TREATMENT
1. DIABETES			17. D (RH) SENSITIZED			
2. HYPERTENSION			18. PULMONARY (TB, ASTHMA)			
3. HEART DISEASE			19. SEASONAL ALLERGIES			
4. AUTOIMMUNE DISORDER			20. DRUG/LATEX ALLERGIES/ REACTIONS			
5. KIDNEY DISEASE/UTI						
6. NEUROLOGIC/EPILEPSY			21. BREAST			
7. PSYCHIATRIC			22. GYN SURGERY			
8. DEPRESSION/POSTPARTUM DEPRESSION			23. OPERATIONS/ HOSPITALIZATIONS (YEAR & REASON)			
9. HEPATITIS/LIVER DISEASE						
10. VARICOSITIES/PHLEBITIS						
11. THYROID DYSFUNCTION			24. ANESTHETIC COMPLICATIONS			
12. TRAUMA/VIOLENCE			25. HISTORY OF ABNORMAL PAP			
13. HISTORY OF BLOOD TRANSFUS.	AMT/DAY PREPREG	AMT/DAY PREG	# YEARS USE	26. UTERINE ANOMALY/DES		
				27. INFERTILITY		
14. TOBACCO				28. RELEVANT FAMILY HISTORY		
15. ALCOHOL						
16. ILLICIT/RECREATIONAL DRUGS				29. OTHER		

COMMENTS _____

ACOG ANTEPARTUM RECORD (FORM A)

Patient Addressograph

SYMPTOMS SINCE LMP

GENETIC SCREENING/TERATOLOGY COUNSELING
INCLUDES PATIENT, BABY'S FATHER, OR ANYONE IN EITHER FAMILY WITH:

	YES	NO		YES	NO
1. PATIENT'S AGE ≥ 35 YEARS AS OF ESTIMATED DATE OF DELIVERY			12. HUNTINGTON'S CHOREA		
2. THALASSEMIA (ITALIAN, GREEK, MEDITERRANEAN, OR ASIAN BACKGROUND); MCV <80			13. MENTAL RETARDATION/AUTISM		
3. NEURAL TUBE DEFECT (MENINGOMYELOCELE, SPINA BIFIDA, OR ANENCEPHALY)			IF YES, WAS PERSON TESTED FOR FRAGILE X?		
			14. OTHER INHERITED GENETIC OR CHROMOSOMAL DISORDER		
4. CONGENITAL HEART DEFECT			15. MATERNAL METABOLIC DISORDER (EG, TYPE 1 DIABETES, PKU)		
5. DOWN SYNDROME			16. PATIENT OR BABY'S FATHER HAD A CHILD WITH BIRTH DEFECTS, NOT LISTED ABOVE		
6. TAY-SACHS (EG, JEWISH, CAJUN, FRENCH CANADIAN)					
7. CANAVAN DISEASE			17. RECURRENT PREGNANCY LOSS, OR A STILLBIRTH		
8. SICKLE CELL DISEASE OR TRAIT (AFRICAN)			18. MEDICATIONS (INCLUDING SUPPLEMENTS, VITAMINS, HERBS OR OTC DRUGS)/ILLICIT/RECREATIONAL DRUGS/ALCOHOL SINCE LAST MENSTRUAL PERIOD		
9. HEMOPHILIA OR OTHER BLOOD DISORDERS					
10. MUSCULAR DYSTROPHY			IF YES, AGENT(S) AND STRENGTH/DOSAGE		
11. CYSTIC FIBROSIS			19. ANY OTHER		

COMMENTS/COUNSELING _____

INFECTION HISTORY	YES	NO		YES	NO
1. LIVE WITH SOMEONE WITH TB OR EXPOSED TO TB			4. HISTORY OF STD, GONORRHEA, CHLAMYDIA, HPV, SYPHILIS		
2. PATIENT OR PARTNER HAS HISTORY OF GENITAL HERPES					
3. RASH OR VIRAL ILLNESS SINCE LAST MENSTRUAL PERIOD			5. OTHER (See Comments)		

COMMENTS _____

INTERVIEWER'S SIGNATURE _____

INITIAL PHYSICAL EXAMINATION

DATE ___ / ___ / ___   HEIGHT _____   BP _____

1. HEENT	☐ NORMAL	☐ ABNORMAL	12. VULVA	☐ NORMAL	☐ CONDYLOMA	☐ LESIONS
2. FUNDI	☐ NORMAL	☐ ABNORMAL	13. VAGINA	☐ NORMAL	☐ INFLAMMATION	☐ DISCHARGE
3. TEETH	☐ NORMAL	☐ ABNORMAL	14. CERVIX	☐ NORMAL	☐ INFLAMMATION	☐ LESIONS
4. THYROID	☐ NORMAL	☐ ABNORMAL	15. UTERUS SIZE	___ WEEKS		☐ FIBROIDS
5. BREASTS	☐ NORMAL	☐ ABNORMAL	16. ADNEXA	☐ NORMAL	☐ MASS	
6. LUNGS	☐ NORMAL	☐ ABNORMAL	17. RECTUM	☐ NORMAL	☐ ABNORMAL	
7. HEART	☐ NORMAL	☐ ABNORMAL	18. DIAGONAL CONJUGATE	☐ REACHED	☐ NO	___ CM
8. ABDOMEN	☐ NORMAL	☐ ABNORMAL	19. SPINES	☐ AVERAGE	☐ PROMINENT	☐ BLUNT
9. EXTREMITIES	☐ NORMAL	☐ ABNORMAL	20. SACRUM	☐ CONCAVE	☐ STRAIGHT	☐ ANTERIOR
10. SKIN	☐ NORMAL	☐ ABNORMAL	21. SUBPUBIC ARCH	☐ NORMAL	☐ WIDE	☐ NARROW
11. LYMPH NODES	☐ NORMAL	☐ ABNORMAL	22. GYNECOID PELVIC TYPE	☐ YES	☐ NO	

COMMENTS (Number and explain abnormals) _____

EXAM BY _____

ACOG ANTEPARTUM RECORD (FORM B)

Patient Addressograph

NAME _____
    LAST   FIRST   MIDDLE

DRUG ALLERGY	LATEX ALLERGY		
IS BLOOD TRANSFUSION ACCEPTABLE IN AN EMERGENCY? ☐ YES ☐ NO	ANESTHESIA CONSULT PLANNED ☐ YES ☐ NO		

PROBLEMS/PLANS

1. _____
2. _____
3. _____
4. _____
5. _____
6. _____

MEDICATION LIST   Start date   Stop date

1. _____ ___/___/___ ___/___/___
2. _____ ___/___/___ ___/___/___
3. _____ ___/___/___ ___/___/___
4. _____ ___/___/___ ___/___/___
5. _____ ___/___/___ ___/___/___
6. _____ ___/___/___ ___/___/___

EDD CONFIRMATION

INITIAL EDD			
LMP	___/___/___	=	EDD ___/___/___
INITIAL EXAM	___/___/___	= ___ WKS = EDD ___/___/___	
ULTRASOUND	___/___/___	= ___ WKS = EDD ___/___/___	
INITIAL EDD	___/___/___	INITIALED BY _____	

18–20-WEEK EDD UPDATE

QUICKENING	___/___/___	+22 WKS = ___/___/___
FUNDAL HT. AT UMBIL.	___/___/___	+20 WKS = ___/___/___
ULTRASOUND	___/___/___	= ___ WKS = ___/___/___
FINAL EDD	___/___/___	INITIALED BY _____

PREPREGNANCY WEIGHT _____

WEEKS GEST. (BEST EST.)	FUNDAL HEIGHT (CM)	PRESENTATION	FHR	FETAL MOVEMENT	PRETERM LABOR SIGNS/SYMPTOMS +=PRESENT 0=ABSENT	CERVIX EXAM (DIL./EFF./STA.) ULTRASOUND LENGTH	BLOOD PRESSURE	WEIGHT	URINE (ALBUMIN/GLUCOSE)	NEXT APPOINTMENT	PROVIDER (INITIALS)	COMMENTS

PROBLEMS _____

COMMENTS _____

ACOG ANTEPARTUM RECORD (FORM C)

Patient Addressograph

LABORATORY AND EDUCATION

INITIAL LABS	DATE	RESULT	REVIEWED
BLOOD TYPE	/ /	A B AB O	
D (Rh) TYPE	/ /		
ANTIBODY SCREEN	/ /		
HCT/HGB	/ /	_____ % _____ g/dL	
PAP TEST	/ /	NORMAL/ABNORMAL/_____	
RUBELLA	/ /		
VDRL	/ /		
URINE CULTURE/SCREEN	/ /		
HBsAg	/ /		
HIV COUNSELING/TESTING*	/ /	POS NEG. DECLINED	

OPTIONAL LABS	DATE	RESULT	
HGB ELECTROPHORESIS	/ /	AA AS SS AC SC AF A_2	
PPD	/ /		
CHLAMYDIA	/ /		
GONORRHEA	/ /		
GENETIC SCREENING TESTS (SEE FORM B)	/ /		
OTHER			

8–18-WEEK LABS (WHEN INDICATED/ELECTED)	DATE	RESULT	
ULTRASOUND	/ /		
MSAFP/MULTIPLE MARKERS	/ /		
AMNIO/CVS	/ /		
KARYOTYPE	/ /	46, XX OR 46, XY/OTHER_____	
AMNIOTIC FLUID (AFP)	/ /	NORMAL_____ ABNORMAL_____	

24–28-WEEK LABS (WHEN INDICATED)	DATE	RESULT	
HCT/HGB	/ /	_____ % _____ g/dL	
DIABETES SCREEN	/ /	1 HOUR_____	
GTT (IF SCREEN ABNORMAL)	/ /	____FBS ____1 HOUR	
		____2 HOUR ____3 HOUR	
D (Rh) ANTIBODY SCREEN	/ /		
ANTI-D IMMUNE GLOBULIN (RhIG) GIVEN (28 WKS)	/ /	SIGNATURE _____	

32–36-WEEK LABS (WHEN INDICATED)	DATE	RESULT	
HCT/HGB (RECOMMENDED)	/ /	_____ % _____ g/dL	
ULTRASOUND	/ /		
VDRL	/ /		
GONORRHEA	/ /		
CHLAMYDIA	/ /		
GROUP B STREP IF USING CULTURE STRATEGY N/A IF USING RISK STRATEGY. (35–37 WKS)	/ /		

COMMENTS/ADDITIONAL LABS

*Check state requirements before recording results.

PROVIDER SIGNATURE (AS REQUIRED)_____

ACOG ANTEPARTUM RECORD (FORM D)

NAME _____
      LAST   FIRST   MIDDLE

PLANS/EDUCATION
(COUNSELED ☐)—BY TRIMESTER. INITIAL AND DATE WHEN DISCUSSED.

	COMPLETED	NEED FOR FURTHER DISCUSSION
FIRST TRIMESTER		
☐ HIV AND OTHER ROUTINE PRENATAL TESTS		
☐ RISK FACTORS IDENTIFIED BY PRENATAL HISTORY		
☐ ANTICIPATED COURSE OF PRENATAL CARE		
☐ NUTRITION AND WEIGHT GAIN COUNSELING		
☐ TOXOPLASMOSIS PRECAUTIONS (CATS/RAW MEAT)		
☐ SEXUAL ACTIVITY		
☐ EXERCISE		
☐ ENVIRONMENTAL/WORK HAZARDS		
☐ TRAVEL		
☐ TOBACCO (ASK, ADVISE, ASSESS, ASSIST, AND ARRANGE)		
☐ ALCOHOL		
☐ ILLICIT/RECREATIONAL DRUGS		
☐ USE OF ANY MEDICATIONS (INCLUDING SUPPLEMENTS, VITAMINS, HERBS, OR OTC DRUGS)		
☐ INDICATIONS FOR ULTRASOUND		
☐ DOMESTIC VIOLENCE		
☐ SEAT BELT USE		
☐ CHILDBIRTH CLASSES/HOSPITAL FACILITIES		
SECOND TRIMESTER		
☐ SIGNS AND SYMPTOMS OF PRETERM LABOR		
☐ ABNORMAL LAB VALUES		
☐ INFLUENZA VACCINE		
☐ SELECTING A PEDIATRICIAN		
☐ POSTPARTUM FAMILY PLANNING/TUBAL STERILIZATION		
THIRD TRIMESTER		
☐ ANESTHESIA/ANALGESIA PLANS		
☐ FETAL MOVEMENT MONITORING		
☐ LABOR SIGNS		
☐ VBAC COUNSELING		
☐ SIGNS AND SYMPTOMS OF PREGNANCY-INDUCED HYPERTENSION		
☐ POSTTERM COUNSELING		
☐ CIRCUMCISION		
☐ BREAST OR BOTTLE FEEDING		
☐ POSTPARTUM DEPRESSION		
☐ NEWBORN CAR SEAT		
☐ FAMILY MEDICAL LEAVE OR DISABILITY FORMS		
REQUESTS		

	DATE	INITIALS
TUBAL STERILIZATION CONSENT SIGNED	__/__/__	_____
HISTORY AND PHYSICAL HAS BEEN SENT TO HOSPITAL, IF APPLICABLE	__/__/__	_____

ACOG ANTEPARTUM RECORD (FORM E)

Plans/Education Notes

_____
_____
_____
_____
_____
_____
_____
_____
_____
_____
_____
_____
_____
_____
_____
_____
_____
_____
_____
_____
_____
_____
_____
_____
_____
_____
_____
_____
_____
_____
_____
_____
_____

ACOG ANTEPARTUM RECORD (FORM E, *continued*)

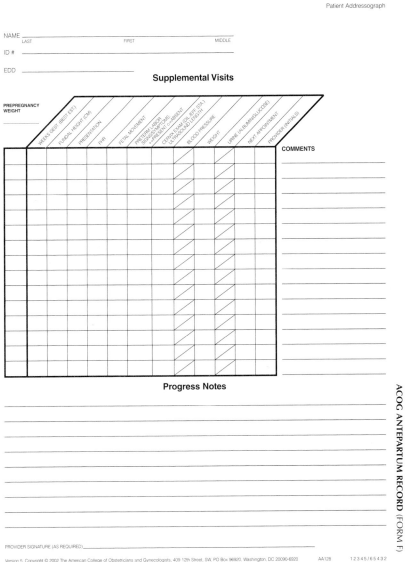

Patient Addressograph

NAME _____
    LAST   FIRST   MIDDLE

ID # _____

EDD _____

Supplemental Visits

PREPREGNANCY
WEIGHT
_____

WEEKS GEST. (BEST EST.)
FUNDAL HEIGHT (CM)
PRESENTATION
FHR
FETAL MOVEMENT
PRETERM LABOR SIGNS/SYMPTOMS
CERVIX EXAM (DIL/EFF/STA.) + PRESENT or ABSENT
ULTRASOUND LENGTH
BLOOD PRESSURE
WEIGHT
URINE (ALBUMIN/GLUCOSE)
NEXT APPOINTMENT
PROVIDER (INITIALS)

COMMENTS

Progress Notes

PROVIDER SIGNATURE (AS REQUIRED) _____

ACOG ANTEPARTUM RECORD (FORM F)

NAME _____
     LAST   FIRST   MIDDLE

ID # _____

Progress Notes

PROVIDER SIGNATURE (AS REQUIRED) _____

ACOG ANTEPARTUM RECORD (FORM G)

DISCHARGE/POSTPARTUM FORM

DELIVERY DATE _____   HOSPITAL _____

DISCHARGE DATE _____

DELIVERY INFORMATION

DELIVERY AT_____WEEKS

☐ VAGINAL   ☐ CESAREAN   TUBAL STERILIZATION ☐ YES ☐ NO
  ☐ SVD   ☐ PRIMARY (For_____)   NOTES _____
  ☐ VACUUM   ☐ REPEAT - ELECTIVE   _____
  ☐ FORCEPS   ☐ REPEAT - UNSUCCESSFUL VBAC _____
  ☐ EPISIOTOMY ☐ INCISION   _____
  ☐ LACERATIONS ☐ LOW TRANSVERSE   _____
  ☐ VBAC   ☐ LOW VERTICAL   _____
               ☐ CLASSICAL   DELIVERED BY_____

LABOR
☐ NONE
☐ SPONTANEOUS
☐ INDUCED
☐ AUGMENTED

ANESTHESIA
☐ NONE
☐ LOCAL/PUDENDAL
☐ EPIDURAL
☐ SPINAL
☐ GENERAL
☐ OTHER

POSTPARTUM INFORMATION

COMPLICATIONS

☐ NONE   ☐ HEMORRHAGE   ☐ INFECTION   ☐ HYPERTENSION   ☐ OTHER _____

DISCHARGE INFORMATION

NEONATAL INFORMATION

NAME OF BABY_____

SEX
☐ FEMALE   ☐ MALE
       CIRCUMCISION
            ☐ YES ☐ NO

BIRTH WEIGHT _____

DISPOSITION
☐ HOME WITH MOTHER ☐ IN HOSPITAL
☐ TRANSFER   ☐ NEONATAL DEATH
☐ STILLBIRTH   ☐ OTHER

COMPLICATIONS/ANOMALIES _____
_____
_____
_____

PEDIATRICIAN _____

MATERNAL INFORMATION

HGB/HCT LEVEL _____

MEDICATIONS _____
_____

FEEDING METHOD   ☐ BREAST   ☐ BOTTLE

CONTRACEPTIVE METHOD (IF APPLICABLE) _____
_____

DIAGNOSTIC STUDIES PENDING _____
_____
_____

SECONDARY DIAGNOSIS/PREEXISTING CONDITIONS
☐ ASTHMA   ☐ HYPERTENSION
☐ DIABETES ☐ OTHER _____

IMMUNIZATIONS GIVEN
☐ ANTI-D IMMUNE GLOBULIN
☐ RUBELLA
☐ OTHER _____
_____
_____

FOLLOW-UP APPT
DATE _____
LOCATION _____
OTHER _____
_____
_____
_____

INTERIM CONTACTS

DATE	COMMENT

PROVIDER SIGNATURE (AS REQUIRED)_____

POSTPARTUM VISIT

DATE _____

LAB STUDIES REQUESTED _____

_____

HGB/HCT _____ LAST PAP TEST _____

FEEDING METHOD _____

CONTRACEPTIVE METHOD _____

POSTPARTUM DEPRESSION SCREENING _____

INTIMATE PARTNER VIOLENCE SCREENING _____

INTERIM HISTORY

_____

_____

_____

_____

PHYSICAL EXAM

BP _____   WT _____

BREASTS   ☐ NORMAL _____

ABDOMEN   ☐ NORMAL _____

EXTERNAL GENITALS   ☐ NORMAL _____

VAGINA   ☐ NORMAL _____

CERVIX   ☐ NORMAL _____

UTERUS   ☐ NORMAL _____

ADNEXA   ☐ NORMAL _____

RECTAL-VAGINAL   ☐ NORMAL _____

PAP TEST   ☐ YES   ☐ NO

COMMENT

_____

_____

_____

_____

_____

_____

_____

_____

_____

_____

_____

_____

_____

_____

_____

_____

_____

_____

_____

_____

ALLERGIES _____

MEDICATIONS/CONTRACEPTION _____

_____

☐ DISPENSED

INTERVAL CARE RECOMMENDATIONS

FOR GENERAL HEALTH PROMOTION _____

_____

_____

_____

_____

_____

_____

FOR REPRODUCTIVE HEALTH PROMOTION _____

_____

_____

_____

_____

RETURN VISIT _____

REFERRALS _____

_____

EXAMINED BY _____

PROVIDER SIGNATURE (AS REQUIRED) _____

Early Pregnancy Risk Identification for Consultation

Risk Factor	Recommended Consultation*
Medical history and conditions	
Asthma	
Symptomatic on medication	Obstetrician–gynecologist
Severe (multiple hospitalizations)	MFM subspecialist
Cardiac disease	
Cyanotic, prior MI, aortic stenosis, pulmonary hypertension, Marfan syndrome, prosthetic valve, AHA Class II or greater	MFM subspecialist
Other	Obstetrician–gynecologist
Diabetes mellitus	
Class A–C	Obstetrician–gynecologist
Class D or greater	MFM subspecialist
Drug and alcohol use	Obstetrician–gynecologist
Epilepsy (on medication)	Obstetrician–gynecologist
Family history of genetic problems (Down syndrome, Tay–Sachs disease, PKU)	MFM subspecialist
Hemoglobinopathy (SS, SC, S-thal)	MFM subspecialist
Hypertension	
Chronic, with renal or heart disease	MFM subspecialist
Chronic, without renal or heart disease	Obstetrician–gynecologist
Prior pulmonary embolus or deep vein thrombosis	Obstetrician–gynecologist
Psychiatric illness	Obstetrician–gynecologist
Pulmonary disease	
Severe obstructive or restrictive	MFM subspecialist
Moderate	Obstetrician–gynecologist

(continued)

Early Pregnancy Risk Identification for Consultation *(continued)*

Risk Factor	Recommended Consultation*
Renal disease	
Chronic, creatinine ≥3 with or without hypertension	MFM subspecialist
Chronic, other	Obstetrician–gynecologist
Requirement for prolonged anticoagulation	MFM subspecialist
Severe systemic disease	MFM subspecialist
Obstetric history and conditions	
Age ≥35 at delivery	Obstetrician–gynecologist
Cesarean delivery, prior classical or vertical incision	Obstetrician–gynecologist
Incompetent cervix	Obstetrician–gynecologist
Prior fetal structural or chromosomal abnormality	MFM subspecialist
Prior neonatal death	Obstetrician–gynecologist
Prior fetal death	Obstetrician–gynecologist
Prior preterm delivery or preterm PROM	Obstetrician–gynecologist
Prior low birth weight (<2,500 g)	Obstetrician–gynecologist
Second-trimester pregnancy loss	Obstetrician–gynecologist
Uterine leiomyomata or malformation	Obstetrician–gynecologist
Initial laboratory tests	
HIV	
Symptomatic or low CD4 count	MFM subspecialist
Other	Obstetrician–gynecologist
CDE (Rh) or other blood group isoimmunization (excluding ABO, Lewis)	MFM subspecialist
Initial examination—condylomata (extensive, covering vulva or vaginal opening)	Obstetrician–gynecologist

Abbreviations: MFM, maternal–fetal medicine; MI, myocardial infarction; AHA, American Heart Association; PKU, phenylketonuria; PROM, premature rupture of membranes; HIV, human immunodeficiency virus.

*At the time of consultation, continued patient care should be determined to be by collaboration with the referring care provider or by transfer of care.

Modified from March of Dimes Birth Defects Foundation, Committee on Perinatal Health. Toward improving the outcome of pregnancy: the 90s and beyond. White Plains, New York: March of Dimes Birth Defects Foundation, 1993.

Ongoing Pregnancy Risk Identification for Consultation

Risk Factor	Recommended Consultation*
Medical history and conditions	
Drug/alcohol use	Obstetrician–gynecologist
Proteinuria (≥2+ by catheter sample, unexplained by urinary tract infection)	Obstetrician–gynecologist
Pyelonephritis	Obstetrician–gynecologist
Severe systemic disease that adversely affects pregnancy	MFM subspecialist
Obstetric history and conditions	
Blood pressure elevation (diastolic ≥90 mm Hg), no proteinuria	Obstetrician–gynecologist
Fetal growth restriction suspected	Obstetrician–gynecologist
Fetal abnormality suspected by ultrasonography	
Anencephaly	Obstetrician–gynecologist
Other	MFM subspecialist
Fetal demise	Obstetrician–gynecologist
Gestational age 41 weeks (to be seen by 42 weeks)	Obstetrician–gynecologist
Gestational diabetes mellitus	Obstetrician–gynecologist
Herpes, active lesions 36 weeks	Obstetrician–gynecologist
Hydramnios by ultrasonography	Obstetrician–gynecologist
Hyperemesis, persisting beyond first trimester	Obstetrician–gynecologist
Multiple gestation	Obstetrician–gynecologist
Oligohydramnios by ultrasonography	Obstetrician–gynecologist
Preterm labor, threatened, <37 weeks	Obstetrician–gynecologist
Premature rupture of membranes	Obstetrician–gynecologist
Vaginal bleeding ≥14 weeks	Obstetrician–gynecologist

(continued)

Ongoing Pregnancy Risk Identification for Consultation *(continued)*

Risk Factor	Recommended Consultation*
Examination and laboratory findings	
Abnormal MSAFP (low or high)	Obstetrician–gynecologist
Abnormal Pap test result	Obstetrician–gynecologist
Anemia (Hct <28%, unresponsive to iron therapy)	Obstetrician–gynecologist
Condylomata (extensive, covering labia and vaginal opening)	Obstetrician–gynecologist
HIV	
Symptomatic or low CD4 count	MFM subspecialist
Other	Obstetrician–gynecologist
CDE (Rh) or other blood group isoimmunization (excluding ABO, Lewis)	MFM subspecialist

Abbreviations: MFM, maternal–fetal medicine; MSAFP, maternal serum alpha-fetoprotein; Hct, hematocrit; HIV, human immunodeficiency virus.

*At the time of consultation, continued patient care should be determined to be by collaboration with the referring care provider or by transfer of care.

Modified from March of Dimes Birth Defects Foundation, Committee on Perinatal Health. Toward improving the outcome of pregnancy: the 90s and beyond. White Plains, New York: March of Dimes Birth Defects Foundation, 1993.

Federal Requirements for Patient Screening and Transfer

In 1986, the United States Congress first enacted legal requirements specifying how Medicare-participating hospitals with emergency services must handle individuals with emergency medical conditions or women who are in labor. Since then, the patient screening and transfer law has undergone numerous refinements and revisions. Physicians should expect that this law will continue to evolve and that there will be additional modifications to it in the future.

Requirements for an Appropriate Medical Screening Examination

Federal law requires that all Medicare-participating hospitals with emergency services must provide an "appropriate medical screening examination" for any individual who comes to the emergency department for medical treatment or examination to determine whether the patient has an emergency medical condition. This examination must be made within the capability of the hospital's emergency department, including ancillary services routinely available to the emergency department. For example, "[i]f a hospital has a department of obstetrics and gynecology, the hospital is responsible for adopting procedures under which the staff and resources of that department are available to treat a woman in labor who comes to its emergency department."

Medical screening examinations also must "...be conducted by individuals determined qualified by hospital by-laws or rules and regulations." Therefore, it is up to a hospital to designate who is a "qualified medical person" to provide an appropriate medical screening examination. The law does not require that physicians perform all screening examinations. Therefore, a hospital can determine under what circumstances a physician is required to provide medical screening and when screening can be done by a nonphysician.

Determining Whether a Patient Has an Emergency Medical Condition

The legal definition of "emergency medical condition" is not the same as the medical one. Under the law, it is defined as:

A medical condition manifesting itself by acute symptoms of sufficient severity (including severe pain, psychiatric disturbances and/or symptoms of substance abuse) such that the absence of immediate attention could reasonably be expected to result in—

(A) Placing the health of the individual (or, with respect to a pregnant woman, the health of the woman or her unborn child) in serious jeopardy;

(B) Serious impairment to bodily functions; or

(C) Serious dysfunction of any bodily organ or part.

It is important to note that, in the case of a pregnant woman who comes to a hospital emergency room, the health of the fetus also must be considered in determining whether an "emergency medical condition" exists.

Special Determination of Emergency Medical Conditions for Pregnant Women

The definition of an emergency medical condition also makes specific reference to a pregnant woman who is having contractions. It provides that an emergency medical condition exists if a pregnant woman is having contractions and "...there is inadequate time to effect a safe transfer to another hospital before delivery; or that transfer may pose a threat to the health or safety of the woman or the unborn child." An emergency medical condition does not exist, even when a woman is having contractions, as long as there is adequate time to effect a safe transfer before delivery and the transfer will not pose a threat to the health or safety of the mother or the fetus.

Labor is defined as:

...the process of childbirth beginning with the latent phase of labor or early phase of labor and continuing through delivery of the placenta. A woman experiencing contractions is in true labor unless a physician certifies that after a reasonable time of observation the woman is in false labor.

Under this definition, a physician must certify that a woman is in false labor before she can be released.

Patients with Emergency Medical Conditions

Once a patient comes to an emergency room, is appropriately screened, and is determined to have an emergency medical condition, the physician may:

1. Treat the patient and stabilize her condition
2. Transfer the patient to another medical facility in accordance with specific procedures outlined below

In situations in which a pregnant woman is in true labor, her condition will be considered stabilized once the child and the placenta are delivered.

Patients Can Refuse to Consent to Treatment

If a patient refuses to consent to treatment, the hospital has fulfilled its obligations under the law. If a patient refuses to consent to treatment, however, the following steps must be taken:

1. The patient must be informed of the risks and benefits of the examination or treatment or both.

2. The medical record must contain a description of the examination and treatment that was refused by the patient.

3. The hospital must take all reasonable steps to secure the patient's written informed refusal. The written document must indicate that the person has been informed of the risks and benefits of the examination or treatment or both.

Procedures for Transferring a Patient to Another Medical Facility

In general, a patient who meets the criteria of an emergency medical condition may not be transferred until he or she is stabilized. There are, however, some exceptions to this prohibition.

The patient may request a transfer, in writing, after being informed of the hospital's obligations under the law and the risks of transfer. The unstabilized patient's written request for transfer must indicate the reasons for the request and that the patient is aware of the risks and benefits of transfer.

An unstabilized patient also may be transferred if a physician signs a written certification that:

...based upon the information available at the time of transfer, the medical benefits reasonably expected from the provision of appropriate medical treatment at another medical facility outweigh the increased risks to the individual or, in the case of a woman in labor, to the woman or the unborn child, from being transferred.

The certification must contain a summary of the risks and benefits of transfer.

If a physician is not physically present in the emergency department at the time of the transfer of a patient, a qualified medical person can sign the certification described previously after consulting with a physician who authorizes the transfer. The physician must countersign the certification as contemporaneously as possible.

Patients Can Refuse to Consent to Transfer

If the hospital offers to transfer a patient, in accordance with the appropriate procedures, and the patient refuses to consent to transfer, the hospital also has fulfilled its obligations under the law. When a patient refuses to consent to the transfer, the hospital must take the following steps:

1. The patient must be informed of the risks and benefits of the transfer.

2. The medical record must contain a description of the proposed transfer that was refused by the patient.

3. The hospital must take all reasonable steps to secure the patient's written informed refusal. The written document must indicate that the person has been informed of the risks and benefits of the transfer and the reasons for the patient's refusal.

Additional Requirements of the Transferring and Receiving Hospitals

The transferring hospital must comply with the following requirements to ensure that the transfer was appropriate:

1. The receiving hospital must have space and qualified personnel to treat the patient and must have agreed to accept the transfer. A hospital with specialized capabilities, such as a neonatal intensive care unit, may not refuse to accept patients if space is available.

2. The transferring hospital must minimize the risks to the patient's health, and the transfer must be executed through the use of qualified personnel and transportation equipment.

3. The transferring hospital must send to the receiving hospital all medical records related to the emergency condition that are available at the time of transfer. These records include available history, records related to the emergency medical condition, observations of

signs or symptoms, preliminary diagnosis, results of diagnostic studies or telephone reports of the studies, treatment provided, results of any tests and informed written consent or certification, and the name of any on-call physician who has refused or failed to appear within a reasonable time to provide necessary stabilizing treatment. Other records not yet available must be sent as soon as possible.

General Requirements

The following general requirements should be met:

1. Medical records related to transfers must be retained by both the transferring and receiving hospitals for 5 years from the date of the transfer.

2. Hospitals are required to report to the Centers for Medicare and Medicaid Services or the state survey agency within 72 hours from the time of the transfer any time they have reason to believe they may have received a patient who was transferred in an unstable medical condition.

3. Hospitals are required to post signs in areas such as entrances, admitting areas, waiting rooms, and emergency departments with respect to their obligations under the patient screening and transfer law.

4. Hospitals also are required to post signs stating whether the hospital participates in the Medicaid program under a state-approved plan. This requirement applies to all hospitals, not only those that participate in Medicare.

5. Hospitals must keep a list of physicians who are on call after the initial examination to provide treatment to stabilize a patient with an emergency medical condition.

6. Hospitals must keep a central log of all individuals who come to the emergency department seeking assistance and the result of each individual's visit.

7. A hospital may not delay providing appropriate medical screening to inquire about payment method or insurance status.

Enforcement and Penalties

Physicians and hospitals violating these federal requirements for patient screening and transfer are subject to civil monetary penalties of up to $50,000 for each violation and to termination from the Medicare program. Hospitals are prohibited from penalizing physicians who report violations of the law or who refuse to transfer an individual with an unstabilized emergency medical condition.

Standard Terminology for Reporting of Reproductive Health Statistics in the United States*

The adoption of standard definitions and reporting requirements for reproductive health statistics will provide an improved basis for standardization and uniformity in the design, implementation, and evaluation of intervention strategies. The reduction of maternal and infant mortality and the improvement of the health of our nation's women and infants are the ultimate goals. The collection and analysis of reliable statistical data are an essential part of in-depth investigations and incorporate case finding, individual review, and analysis of risk factors. These studies could then yield valuable clinical information for practitioners, aiding them in improved case management for high-risk patients, which would result in decreased morbidity and mortality.

Both the collection and the use of statistics have been hampered by lack of understanding of differences in definitions, statistical tabulations, and reporting requirements among state, national, and international bodies. Misapplication and misinterpretation of data may lead to erroneous comparisons and conclusions. For example, specific requirements for reporting of fetal deaths often have been misinterpreted as implying a weight or gestational age for viability. Distinctions can and should be made among: 1) the definition of an event, 2) the reporting requirements for the event, and 3) the statistical tabulation and interpretation of the data. The definition indicates the meaning of a term (eg,

*Different states use different birth weight and gestational age criteria to define fetal death. The Committee on Obstetric Practice of the American College of Obstetricians and Gynecologists recommends that perinatal mortality statistics be based on a gestational weight of 500 g.

live birth, fetal death, or *maternal death*). A reporting requirement is that part of the defined event for which reporting is mandatory or desired. Statistical tabulations connote the presentation of data for the purpose of analysis and interpretation of existing and future conditions. The data should be collected in a manner that will allow them to be presented in different ways for different users. Adjustments should be made for variations in reporting before comparisons among data are attempted.

If information is collected and presented in a standardized manner, comparisons between the new data and the data obtained by previous reporting requirements can be delineated clearly and can contribute to improved public understanding of reproductive health statistics. For ease in assimilating this information, it is divided into three sections: 1) definitions, 2) statistical tabulations, and 3) reporting requirements and recommendations. Some of the definitions and recommendations are a departure from those currently or historically accepted; however, these recommendations were agreed on by the interorganizational group that was brought together to review terminology related to reproductive health issues.

Definitions

Live birth: The complete expulsion or extraction from the mother of a product of human conception, irrespective of the duration of pregnancy, which, after such expulsion or extraction, breathes or shows any other evidence of life, such as beating of the heart, pulsation of the umbilical cord, or definite movement of voluntary muscles, whether or not the umbilical cord has been cut or the placenta is attached. Heartbeats are to be distinguished from transient cardiac contractions; respirations are to be distinguished from fleeting respiratory efforts or gasps.

Birth weight: The weight of a neonate determined immediately after delivery or as soon thereafter as feasible. It should be expressed to the nearest gram.

Gestational age: The number of weeks that have elapsed between the first day of the last normal menstrual period (not the presumed time of conception) and the date of delivery, irrespective of whether the gestation results in a live birth or a fetal death.

Neonate:

Low birth weight—Any neonate, regardless of gestational age, whose weight at birth is less than 2,500 g.

Preterm*—Any neonate whose birth occurs through the end of the last day of the 37th week (259th day) following the onset of the last menstrual period.

Term—Any neonate whose birth occurs from the beginning of the first day (260th day) of the 38th week through the end of the last day of the 42nd week (294th day) following the onset of the last menstrual period.

Postterm—Any neonate whose birth occurs from the beginning of the first day (295th day) of the 43rd week following the onset of the last menstrual period.

Fetal death: Death before the complete expulsion or extraction from the mother of a product of human conception, fetus and placenta, irrespective of the duration of pregnancy; the death is indicated by the fact that, after such expulsion or extraction, the fetus does not breathe or show any other evidence of life, such as beating of the heart, pulsation of the umbilical cord, or definite movement of voluntary muscles. Heartbeats are to be distinguished from transient cardiac contractions; respirations are to be distinguished from fleeting respiratory efforts or gasps. This definition excludes induced termination of pregnancy.

Neonatal death: Death of a liveborn neonate before the neonate becomes age 28 days (up to and including 27 days, 23 hours, and 59 minutes from the moment of birth).

---

*These definitions are for statistical purposes and are not intended to affect clinical management. Appropriate assessment of fetal maturity for purposes of clinical management is delineated in Chapter 4.

Statisticians making a determination of the status of a neonate, namely preterm or term, should define preterm as less than 259 days and term as 259 days to less than 294 days to ensure comparable calculations with the medical community. Statisticians, by formula, subtract the date of the first day of the last menstrual period from the date of birth, whereas physicians include the first day, thus accounting for the difference.

Infant death: Any death at any time from birth up to, but not including, 1 year of age (364 days, 23 hours, and 59 minutes from the moment of birth).

*Maternal death:** The death of a woman from any cause related to or aggravated by pregnancy or its management (regardless of the duration or site of pregnancy), but not from accidental or incidental causes.

Direct obstetric death—The death of a woman resulting from obstetric complications of pregnancy, labor, or the puerperium; from interventions, omissions, or treatment; or from a chain of events resulting from any of these.

Indirect obstetric death—The death of a woman resulting from a previously existing disease or a disease that developed during pregnancy, labor, or the puerperium that did not have direct obstetric causes, although the physiologic effects of pregnancy were partially responsible for the death.

In 1987, the Centers for Disease Control and Prevention (CDC) collaborated with the Maternal Mortality Special Interest Group of the American College of Obstetricians and Gynecologists (ACOG), the Association of Vital Records and Health Statistics, and state and local health departments to initiate the National Pregnancy Mortality Surveillance System. The CDC/ACOG Maternal Mortality Study Group introduced two new terms, which are being used by the CDC and increasingly by some states and researchers. The study group differentiates between pregnancy-associated and pregnancy-related deaths.

Pregnancy-associated death: The death of any woman, from any cause, while pregnant or within 1 calendar year of termination of pregnancy, regardless of the duration and the site of pregnancy.

Pregnancy-related death: A pregnancy-associated death resulting from: 1) complications of the pregnancy itself, 2) the chain of events initiated by the pregnancy that led to death, or 3) aggravation of an unre-

---

*Death occurring to a woman during pregnancy or after its termination from causes not related to the pregnancy or to its complications or management is not considered a maternal death. Nonmaternal deaths may result from accidental causes (eg, auto accident or gunshot wound) or incidental causes (eg, concurrent malignancy).

lated condition by the physiologic or pharmacologic effects of the pregnancy that subsequently caused death.

Induced termination of pregnancy: The purposeful interruption of an intrauterine pregnancy with the intention other than to produce a liveborn infant, and which does not result in a live birth. This definition excludes management of prolonged retention of products of conception following fetal death.

Statistical Tabulations

Statistical tabulations for vital events related to pregnancy provide the medical and statistical community with valuable information on reproductive health and generate data on trends apparent in this country and worldwide. This information often is disaggregated and used to examine specific events over time or within selected geographic locations. In informing the public about health issues, media sources often report various statistical measures. Heightened public interest in health-related issues makes it essential that the medical community understand and have the capacity to interpret these statistics.

The following explanations of statistical tabulations are intended to provide the reader with a better understanding of the measures used for events related to reproduction.

Rate: A measure of the frequency of some event in relation to a unit of population during a specified time period, such as a year; events in the numerator of the rate occur to individuals in the denominator. Rates express the risk of the event in the specified population during a particular time. Rates generally are expressed as units of population in the denominator (eg, per 1,000, per 100,000). For example, the 1982 teenage birth rate was 52.9 live births per 1,000 women aged 15–19 years.

Ratios: A term that expresses a relationship of one element to a different element (where the numerator is not necessarily a subset of the denominator). A ratio generally is expressed per 1,000 of the denominator element. For example, the sex ratio of live births for 1982 was 1,051 males per 1,000 females.

In the formulae that follow, *period* refers to a calendar year.

Live Birth Measures

These measures are designed to show the rate at which childbearing is occurring in the population. The *crude birth rate*, which relates the total number of births to the total population, indicates the impact of fertility on population growth. The *general fertility rate* is a more specific measure of fertility because it relates the number of births to the population at risk, namely, women of childbearing age (assumed to be ages 15–44 years). An even more specific set of rates, the *age-specific birth rate*, relates the number of births to women of specific ages directly to the total number of women in that age group. Formulae for these measures are:

$$\text{Crude birth rate} = \frac{\text{Number of live births to women of all ages during a calendar year} \times 1{,}000}{\text{Total estimated mid-year population}}$$

$$\text{General fertility rate} = \frac{\text{Number of live births to women of all ages during a calendar year} \times 1{,}000}{\text{Estimated mid-year population of women aged 15–44 years}}$$

$$\text{General pregnancy rate} = \frac{\text{Number of live births + number of fetal deaths + number of induced terminations of pregnancy during a calendar year} \times 1{,}000}{\text{Estimated mid-year population of women aged 15–44 years}}$$

$$\text{Age-specific birth rate} = \frac{\text{Number of live births to women in a specific age group during a calendar year} \times 1{,}000}{\text{Estimated mid-year population of women in same age group}}$$

$$\text{Total fertility rate} = \text{The sum of age-specific birth rates of women at each age group 10–14 through 45–49.}$$

Five-year age groups are used; therefore, the sum is multiplied by 5. This rate also can be computed by using single years of age.

Because the birth weight of the infant is included on the birth certificate, it is possible to tabulate and focus an analysis on selected groups of live births, for example, those weighing 500 g or more. Births can be tabulated by where they occur. Therefore, they can be shown by place of occurrence, by place of residence, and by kind of setting of delivery, such as at a hospital or home. Most tabulations of vital statistics are routinely calculated by place of residence of the mother, but they could be tabulated on another basis as well. What is essential, however, is that the classification be the same for all events under consideration for a specific measure.

FETAL MORTALITY MEASURES

The population at risk for fetal mortality is the number of live births plus the number of fetal deaths in a year. Fetal death indices indicate the magnitude of late pregnancy losses.

It is recognized that most states report fetal deaths on the basis of gestational age. However, birth weight can be more accurately measured than can gestational age. Therefore, it is recommended that states adopt minimum reporting requirements of fetal deaths based on and labeled as specific birth weight rather than gestational age (see "Fetal Death" under "Reporting Requirements and Recommendations," as follows). In addition, statistical tabulations of fetal deaths should include, at a minimum, fetal deaths of 500 g or more.

It is recognized that states will not be able to immediately translate data from gestational age to weight, and, for comparative purposes, it may be desirable to know fetal death rates for various gestational periods. Therefore, the collection of both weight and gestational age is recommended to allow for these comparisons. When calculating fetal death rates based on gestational age, the number of weeks or more of stated or presumed gestation can be substituted for weight in the previous formulae.

$$\text{Fetal death rate} = \frac{\text{Number of fetal deaths } (x \text{ weight or more}) \text{ during a period} \times 1,000}{\text{Number of fetal deaths } (x \text{ weight or more}) + \text{number of live births during the same period}}$$

$$\text{Fetal death ratio} = \frac{\begin{array}{c}\text{Number of fetal deaths} \\ (x \text{ weight or more) during a period} \times 1{,}000\end{array}}{\begin{array}{c}\text{Number of live births} \\ \text{during the same period}\end{array}}$$

Perinatal Mortality Measures

Indices of perinatal mortality combine fetal deaths and live births with only brief survival (up to a few days or weeks) on the assumption that similar factors are associated with these losses. The population at risk is the total number of live births plus fetal deaths, or alternatively, the number of live births. Perinatal mortality indices can vary as to age of the fetus and the infant who is included in the particular tabulation. However, the concept itself cuts across all the calculations.

It is recommended that perinatal mortality measures be based on and labeled with specific weight rather than gestational age (see "Reporting Requirements and Recommendations," as follows).

$$\text{Perinatal mortality rate} = \frac{\begin{array}{c}\text{Number of infant deaths of less than} \\ x \text{ days} + \text{number of fetal deaths} \\ \text{(with stated or presumed weight} \\ \text{of } y \text{ or more) during the same period} \times 1{,}000\end{array}}{\begin{array}{c}\text{Number of live births} \\ \text{during the same period}\end{array}}$$

It is recognized that states will not be able to immediately translate data from gestational age to weight, and for purposes of comparability, knowledge of gestational age (based on last menstrual period) may be required and should be collected. When perinatal death rates based on gestational age are calculated, the number of weeks of a stated or presumed gestational age can be substituted for weight in the formulae. When comparisons based on gestational age are desired, the generally accepted breakdown is:

- Perinatal period I includes infant deaths occurring at less than 7 days and fetal deaths with a stated or presumed period of gestation of 28 weeks or more.

- Perinatal period II includes infant deaths occurring at less than 28 days and fetal deaths with a stated or presumed period of gestation of 20 weeks or more.

- Perinatal period III includes infant deaths occurring at less than 7 days and fetal deaths with a stated or presumed gestation of 20 weeks or more.

Perinatal measures can be specific for race and other characteristics. Perinatal events can be tabulated by where they occur. Therefore, they can be shown by place of occurrence, by place of residence, and by place of delivery, such as at a hospital or home. Most tabulations of vital statistics are routinely calculated by place of residence of the woman, but they could be tabulated by place of occurrence. What is essential, however, is that the classification be the same for all events under consideration for a specific measure.

Indices of infant mortality are designed to show the likelihood that live births with certain characteristics will survive the first year of life or, conversely, will die during the first year of life. For infant mortality, the "population at risk" is approximated by live births that occur in a calendar year. One can compare the infant mortality rate of different population groups, such as that between white and black infants. Interest sometimes focuses on two different periods in the first year of an infant's life, such as the very early period when the infant is younger than 28 days (up through 27 days, 23 hours, and 59 minutes from the moment of birth), called the neonatal period; and the later period starting at the end of the 28th day up to, but not including, age 1 year (364 days, 23 hours, and 59 minutes), called the postneonatal period. Accordingly, two indices reflect these differences, namely, the neonatal mortality rate and the postneonatal mortality rate. The neonatal period can be divided further for statistical tabulations:

- Neonatal period I is from the moment of birth through 23 hours and 59 minutes.

- Neonatal period II starts at the end of the 24th hour of life through 6 days, 23 hours, and 59 minutes.

- Neonatal period III starts at the end of the 7th day of life through 27 days, 23 hours, and 59 minutes.

The denominator for the postneonatal mortality rate also can be calculated by subtracting the number of neonatal deaths from the number of live births. This denominator more accurately defines the population at risk of death in the postneonatal period. In addition, it should be noted that infant deaths can be broken down into birth weight categories, if desired, for comparative purposes when birth and death records are linked (see "Reporting Requirements and Recommendations," as follows).

$$\text{Infant mortality rate} = \frac{\text{Number of infant deaths (neonatal and postneonatal) during a period} \times 1{,}000}{\text{Number of live births during the same period}}$$

$$\text{Neonatal mortality rate} = \frac{\text{Number of neonatal deaths during a period} \times 1{,}000}{\text{Number of live births during the same period}}$$

$$\text{Postneonatal mortality rate} = \frac{\text{Number of postneonatal deaths during a period} \times 1{,}000}{\text{Number of live births during the same period}}$$

MATERNAL MORTALITY MEASURES

Measures of maternal mortality are designed to indicate the likelihood that a pregnant woman will die from complications of pregnancy, childbirth, or the puerperium. Accordingly, the population at risk is an approximation of the population of pregnant women in a year; the approximation usually is taken to be the number of live births. Maternal mortality can be examined in terms of characteristics of the woman, such as age, race, and cause of death. The maternal mortality rate measures the risk of death from deliveries and complications of pregnancy, childbirth, and the puerperium.

The group exposed to risk consists of all women who have been pregnant at some time during the period. Therefore, the population at risk should theoretically include all fetal deaths (reported and unreported), all induced terminations of pregnancy, and all live births. Because most states do not require the reporting of all fetal deaths and a large number of states still do not require reporting of induced terminations of pregnancy, the entire population at risk cannot be included in the denominator. Therefore, the total number of live births has become the generally accepted denominator. It is recommended that when complete ascertainment of the denominator (ie, the number of pregnant women) is achieved, a modified maternal mortality rate should be defined, in addition to the traditional rate. The rate is most frequently expressed per 100,000 live births:

$$\text{Maternal mortality rate} = \frac{\text{Number of deaths attributed to maternal conditions during a period} \times 100{,}000}{\text{Number of live births during the same period}}$$

Death rates for specified maternal causes are computed by restricting the numerator to the specified cause. The maternal mortality rates specific for race and age groups are computed by appropriately restricting both the numerator and the denominator to the specified group. Caution should be used in interpreting rates in small geographic areas; it may not be possible to generate race- and age-specific rates.

For statistical comparisons with the World Health Organization (WHO), it is recommended that two tabulations of statistics be prepared: 1) maternal deaths within 42 days of the end of pregnancy (WHO); and 2) maternal deaths with no time limitation for comparison within the United States.

The CDC uses the following statistical measures of pregnancy-related mortality:

$$\text{Pregnancy mortality ratio} = \frac{\text{Number of pregnancy-related deaths during a period} \times 100{,}000}{\text{Number of live births during the same period}}$$

$$\text{Pregnancy mortality rate} = \frac{\text{Number of pregnancy-related deaths during a period} \times 100{,}000}{\text{Number of pregnancies (live births, fetal deaths, induced and spontaneous abortions, ectopic pregnancies, and molar pregnancies)}}$$

MEASURES OF INDUCED TERMINATION OF PREGNANCY

Measures of induced pregnancy termination parallel those of fetal deaths but refer to "induced" events. The population at risk for induced termination of pregnancy is taken to be live births in a year, which is used as a surrogate measure of pregnancies. Because this is not actually the total population at risk, this measure generally is considered to be a ratio.

$$\text{Induced termination of pregnancy ratio I} = \frac{\text{Number of induced terminations occurring during a period} \times 1{,}000}{\text{Number of live births occurring during the same period}}$$

Another measure is one that, by also including an estimate of pregnancies that do not result in live births, more closely approximates the population at risk:

$$\text{Induced termination of pregnancy ratio II} = \frac{\text{Number of induced terminations occurring during a period} \times 1{,}000}{\text{Number of induced terminations of pregnancies + live births + reported fetal deaths during the same period}}$$

Still a third measure is a rate that provides information on the probability that a woman of a certain age or race will have an induced termination of pregnancy:

$$\text{Induced termination of pregnancy rate} = \frac{\text{Number of induced terminations occurring during a period} \times 1{,}000}{\text{Female population aged 15–44 years}}$$

Sometimes indices for induced termination are specific for certain characteristics of the woman; that is, they can refer to women of particular age or race groups.

Reporting Requirements and Recommendations

Reporting requirements for vital events related to reproductive health enable the collection of data that are essential to the calculation of statistical tabulations to examine trends and changes at the local, state, and national levels. The data used in statistical tabulations may be only a portion of those collected, because of the need for consistency in a tabulation and because of the variations in reporting requirements from state to state. For instance, although a few states require that all fetal deaths, regardless of length of gestation, be reported, statistical tabulations of fetal death rates by the National Center for Health Statistics use only those fetal deaths occurring at 20 weeks or more of gestation.

Live Birth

It generally is recognized that all states report all live births, as defined in the definitions section of this document. It is recommended that all live births be reported, regardless of birth weight, length of gestation, or survival time.

Fetal Death

Reporting requirements for fetal deaths now vary from state to state. At present, most states require reporting of fetal deaths by gestational age. It generally is recognized that birth weight can be measured more accurately than can gestational age. The 1977 revision of the *Model State Vital Statistics Act and Regulations* recommends reporting of all spontaneous losses occurring at 20 weeks or more of gestation or weighing 350 g or more. It must be emphasized that a specific birth weight criterion for reporting of fetal deaths does not imply a point of viability and should be chosen instead for its feasibility in collecting useful data.

Current statistical tabulations of fetal deaths include, at a minimum, fetal deaths at 500 g or more. Furthermore, 27 states have adopted the requirement of reporting deaths of more than 20 weeks of gestation. Therefore, it is recommended that all state fetal death report forms include birth weight and gestational age.

PERINATAL MORTALITY

Perinatal mortality indices generally combine fetal deaths and live births that survive only briefly (up to a few days or weeks). Because reporting requirements of fetal deaths vary from state to state, perinatal mortality reporting also will vary (see definitions of perinatal periods in "Perinatal Mortality Measures" in this appendix).

As with fetal deaths, it is recommended that perinatal mortality be weight specific. However, for purposes of comparability, knowledge of gestational age (based on last menstrual period) should be collected.

INFANT MORTALITY

All states require that all infant deaths (neonatal plus postneonatal), as defined in the section "Definitions" in this document, be reported. Infant deaths by birth weight are not routinely available for the United States as a whole because birth weight information is not collected on the death certificate. However, because birth weight is reported on the birth certificate, it is possible to obtain information on infant deaths by birth weight by linking together the birth certificate and the death certificate for the same infant. At present, most states link birth and death certificates. A national linked birth certificate and infant death certificate file is now available.

In addition, it is recommended that infant death reports include the exact interval from birth rather than categories such as "neonatal" or "postneonatal." This, too, will allow for more specific age-related death analyses.

MATERNAL MORTALITY

Every state is required to report all maternal deaths. Because annual deaths attributed to maternal mortality is approximately only 300, emphasis must be placed on in-depth investigations. Case finding, together with individual review and analysis of risk factors contributing to maternal deaths, is of the highest importance. Collection of data regarding these rare events is critical, when combined, as it should be, with educational review by those closest to the case, usually the obstetrician–gynecologists in the hospital and the surrounding region. Such analysis can yield clinical information about risk factors associated with, for example, detection and treatment of ectopic pregnancies or with anesthesia. This clinical information can then be gathered and exchanged to help practitioners identify risk factors that contribute to maternal death and associated conditions.

The CDC/ACOG Maternal Mortality Study Group also has designed a new system of classifying pregnancy-related deaths after review of the case. This system differentiates between the immediate and underlying causes of death as stated on the death certificate, associated obstetric and medical conditions or complications, and the outcome of pregnancy. For example, if a woman died of a hemorrhage that resulted from a ruptured ectopic pregnancy, the immediate cause of death would be classified as "hemorrhage," the associated obstetric condition would be classified as "ruptured fallopian tube," and the outcome of pregnancy would be "ectopic pregnancy." This classification scheme allows analysis of the chain of events that led to the death.

Induced Termination of Pregnancy

The United States has no national system for reporting induced termination of pregnancy. State health departments vary greatly in their approaches to the compilation of these data, from compiling no data to: 1) periodically requesting hospitals, clinics, and physicians performing the procedures to voluntarily report total number of procedures performed; 2) requiring (by legislative or regulatory authority) hospitals, clinics, and physicians to periodically report aggregate level data on number or number and characteristics of procedures; or 3) requiring (by legal or regulatory authority) hospitals, clinics, and physicians to periodically report individual data on each procedure performed.

Since 1969, the CDC Division of Reproductive Health has published an annual Abortion Surveillance Report based on data provided from state health departments, when available, and from data voluntarily provided to the CDC from hospitals and clinics in states with no data available from health departments. In addition to information on the number and characteristics of induced terminations of pregnancy, the Abortion Surveillance Report contains information from the CDC abortion mortality surveillance, which was begun with the cooperation of state health departments in 1972. Investigation and review of each related death by epidemiologists in the Division of Reproductive Health result in improved detailed nosological identification of abortion mortality by type of risk.*

Since 1977, the National Center for Health Statistics has analyzed the induced terminations of pregnancy occurring in up to 13 states in which individual reports of induced termination are submitted to state vital registration offices. In addition, the Alan Guttmacher Institute, a private organization, publishes information on induced termination that it obtains from a nationwide survey of providers of induced termination.

Collecting information on the number of induced terminations of pregnancy, the characteristics of women having such procedures, and the number and characteristics of all deaths related to induced termination of pregnancy would be extremely valuable in identifying and evaluating risk factors for specific population groups and for the public in general. By gathering these data, studies could be instituted with practitioners. Knowing the outcomes could further the body of knowledge and ultimately reduce the risks.

Therefore, state health departments are urged to compile statistics on induced termination of pregnancy to evaluate and improve the quality of their data. Furthermore, state health departments that do not compile such statistics are urged to explore mechanisms for initiating their collection.

---

*The CDC Abortion Surveillance Report includes information on events categorized by the CDC as abortions (legal, illegal, and spontaneous). Although this terminology predates the recommendations in this document and is at variance with the definition herein, it has been commonly used and understood to include induced termination of pregnancy.

RATES OF VAGINAL BIRTHS AFTER CESAREAN DELIVERY

Two methods for defining VBAC rates are proposed:

1. $\text{VBAC rate} = \dfrac{\text{Total number of VBACs}}{\begin{array}{c}\text{Total number of women with prior cesarean}\\ \text{deliveries, including women who were}\\ \text{candidates for a trial of labor but declined and}\\ \text{women who were not candidates}\end{array}} \times 100$

2. $\begin{array}{c}\text{Trial of labor}\\ \text{success rate}\end{array} = \dfrac{\text{VBAC}}{\begin{array}{c}\text{Number of women who had a}\\ \text{trial of labor after cesarean delivery}\end{array}} \times 100$

Clearly, these rates are interrelated. However, calculations based on the rates as defined allow a more accurate comparison of practice between providers and between institutions.

CURRENT REPORTING REQUIREMENTS

The following general fetal death reporting requirements, as of March 1991, should be brought into conformity with the recommendations in this report:

Gestation of ≥20 weeks

Alabama	Iowa	Oklahoma
Alaska	Maryland*	Oregon*
Arizona*	Minnesota	Texas
California	Montana	Utah
Connecticut	Nebraska	Vermont*
Delaware	Nevada	Washington
Florida	New Jersey	West Virginia
Guam	North Carolina	Wyoming
Illinois	North Dakota	
Indiana	Ohio	

*Modifiers apply.

Gestation of ≥20 weeks or birth weight of ≥500 g:
District of Columbia

Gestation of ≥20 weeks or birth weight of ≥350 g:

Idaho	Massachusetts	New Hampshire
Kentucky	Mississippi	South Carolina
Louisiana	Missouri	Wisconsin

Birth weight of >350 g:
Kansas

Gestation of ≥20 weeks or birth weight of ≥400 g:
Michigan

Birth weight of ≥500 g:
New Mexico
South Dakota
Tennessee*

Gestation of ≥5 months:
Puerto Rico

Gestation of ≥16 weeks:
Pennsylvania

All products of human conception:

American Samoa	Maine	Rhode Island
Arkansas	New York City	Virginia
Colorado	New York State	Virgin Islands
Georgia	Northern Mariana	Hawaii Islands

*Modifiers apply.

Occupational Safety and Health Administration Regulations on Occupational Exposure to Bloodborne Pathogens*

In 1970, the U.S. Congress enacted the Occupational Safety and Health Act to protect workers from unsafe and unhealthy conditions in the workplace. To oversee this effort, the law also created the Occupational Safety and Health Administration (OSHA) within the U.S. Department of Labor. The Occupational Safety and Health Administration has the responsibility for developing and implementing job safety and health standards and regulations. Its standards and regulations apply to all employers and employees. To promote and ensure compliance with its standards, OSHA has the authority to conduct unannounced workplace inspections. It also maintains a reporting and record-keeping system to monitor job-related injuries and illnesses. Failure to comply with OSHA standards may result in the assessment of civil or criminal penalties.

In December 1991, OSHA issued new regulations on occupational exposure to bloodborne pathogens that are designed to minimize the transmission of human immunodeficiency virus (HIV), hepatitis B virus (HBV), and other potentially infectious materials in the workplace. The regulations cover all employees in physician offices, hospitals, medical laboratories, and other health care facilities where workers could be "reasonably anticipated" as a result of performing their job duties to

---

*Modified from Kaminetzky HA, Rutledge P. OSHA regulations and medical practice. Prim Care Update Ob/Gyn 1995;2:143–9.

come into contact with blood and other potentially infectious materials. The regulations were revised, effective April 2001, to comply with the Needlestick Safety and Prevention Act of 2000.

Approved State Plans

Under the federal law that created OSHA, states are encouraged to develop and operate—under OSHA guidance—state job safety and health plans. Currently, 23 states and 2 territories have OSHA-approved plans, which require them to provide standards and enforcement programs that are at least as effective as the federal standards. They are:

Alaska	Michigan	Tennessee
Arizona	Minnesota	Utah
California	Nevada	Vermont
Connecticut*	New Mexico	Virgin Islands
Hawaii	New York*	Virginia
Indiana	North Carolina	Washington
Iowa	Oregon	Wyoming
Kentucky	Puerto Rico	
Maryland	South Carolina	

A list of these state OSHA offices is available on the OSHA website at www.osha.gov/oshdir/states.html; call the number listed to receive a copy of the state's standards on occupational exposure to bloodborne pathogens. In Connecticut and New York, the state plans cover state and local government employees only; the private sector is covered by the federal OSHA standard. In addition, states with an OSHA-approved state plan must comply with the federal OSHA standard.

Complying with the Regulations

Exposure Control Plan

To comply with the regulations, health care employers are required to prepare a written "Exposure Control Plan" designed to eliminate or min-

*The state OSHA plan covers state and local government employees only.

imize employee exposure to bloodborne pathogens. This plan must list all job classifications in which employees are likely to be exposed to infectious materials and the relevant tasks and procedures performed by these employees. Infectious materials include blood, semen, vaginal secretions, peritoneal fluid, amniotic fluid, any body fluid visibly contaminated with blood, all body fluids in which it is impossible to differentiate between the body fluids, any unfixed human tissue or organ (living or dead), as well as HIV-containing cell or tissue cultures, organ cultures, and HIV- or HBV-containing culture medium or other solutions.

Under the plan, employers are required to adopt universal precautions, engineering and work practice controls, and personal protective equipment requirements. Employers must also establish a schedule for implementing:

- Housekeeping requirements
- Employee training and record-keeping requirements
- Hepatitis B virus vaccination for employees and postexposure evaluation and follow-up procedures
- Communication of hazards

A detailed discussion of each of these requirements follows. The plan must be accessible to employees and made available to OSHA on request. The Exposure Control Plan must be reviewed annually and updated to reflect changes in technology that eliminate or reduce exposure to bloodborne pathogens. The employer must document this annual consideration and the use of appropriate effective safer medical procedures and devices that are commercially available. In designing and reviewing the Exposure Compliance Plan, the employer must solicit input from nonmanagerial employees who are potentially exposed to injuries from contaminated sharps. Employers must document, in the Exposure Control Plan, how they received input from employees.

Mandatory Universal Precautions

The regulations require that universal precautions must be used to prevent contact with blood or other potentially infectious materials. It is OSHA's intention to follow the Centers for Disease Control and

Prevention guidelines on universal precautions. As defined by the Centers for Disease Control and Prevention, the concept of universal precautions requires the employer and employee to assume that blood and other body fluids are infectious and must be handled accordingly.

Engineering and Work Practice Controls

Specific engineering and work practice controls for the workplace must be implemented and examined for effectiveness on a regular schedule. These controls include the following guidelines:

1. Employers are required to provide handwashing facilities that are readily accessible to employees; when this is not feasible, employees must be provided with an antiseptic hand cleanser with clean cloth or paper towels or antiseptic towelettes. It is the employer's responsibility to ensure that employees wash their hands immediately after gloves and other protective garments are removed.

2. Contaminated needles and other contaminated sharp objects shall not be bent, recapped, or removed unless the employer can demonstrate that no alternative is feasible or that a specific medical procedure requires such action. Shearing or breaking of contaminated needles is prohibited. Recapping or needle removal must be accomplished by a mechanical device or a one-handed technique. Contaminated reusable sharp objects shall be placed in appropriate containers until properly reprocessed; these containers must be puncture resistant, leakproof, and labeled or color coded in accordance with the regulations for easy identification.

3. Eating, drinking, smoking, applying cosmetics or lip balm, and handling contact lenses are prohibited in work areas where there is a reasonable likelihood of exposure to potentially infectious materials.

4. Food and drink must not be kept in refrigerators, freezers, shelves, cabinets, or on countertops where blood or other potentially infectious materials are present.

5. All procedures involving blood or other infectious materials shall be performed in a manner to minimize splashing, spraying, spattering, and creating droplets; mouth pipetting or suctioning of blood or other potentially infectious materials is prohibited.

6. Specimens of blood or other potentially infectious materials must be placed in closed containers that prevent leakage during collection, handling, processing, storage, transport, or shipping; containers must be labeled or color coded in accordance with the regulations for easy identification. However, when a facility uses universal precautions in the handling of all specimens, the required labeling or color coding of specimens is not necessary as long as containers are recognizable as containing specimens; this exemption applies only while the specimens and containers remain in the facility. If outside contamination of the primary container occurs, it must be placed within a second container that is leakproof, puncture resistant, and labeled or color coded accordingly.

7. Equipment that could be contaminated with blood or other infectious materials must be examined before servicing or shipping and shall be decontaminated as necessary, unless the employer can demonstrate that decontamination of the equipment or parts of the equipment is not feasible. A label must be attached to the equipment stating which parts remain contaminated. The employer must ensure that this information is conveyed to all affected employees, the servicing representative, and/or the manufacturer before handling, servicing, or shipping so that the necessary precautions will be taken.

PERSONAL PROTECTIVE EQUIPMENT

The regulations also stress the importance of appropriate personal protective equipment that employers are required to provide at no cost to employees whose job duties expose them to blood and other infectious materials. Appropriate personal protective equipment includes but is not limited to gloves, gowns, laboratory coats, face shields or masks, eye protection, mouthpieces, resuscitation bags, pocket masks, or other ventilation devices. As defined by OSHA, personal protective equipment is considered "appropriate" if it prevents blood or other potentially infectious materials from reaching an employee's work clothes and skin, eyes, mouth, or other mucous membranes under normal conditions of use.

Employers must ensure that the employee uses appropriate personal protective equipment unless the employer can demonstrate that the employee temporarily declined to use the equipment, when under rare and extraordinary circumstances, it was the employee's professional judgment that use of personal protective equipment would have prevented the delivery of health care services or would have posed an increased hazard to the safety of the worker or co-worker. When an employee makes this judgment, the circumstances shall be investigated and documented to determine whether changes can be made to prevent such situations in the future.

Personal protective equipment in the appropriate sizes must be accessible at the worksite or issued to employees. The employer shall provide for laundering and disposal of personal protective equipment, as well as repair and replace this equipment when necessary to maintain its effectiveness, at no cost to the employee. If a garment(s) is penetrated by blood or other infectious materials, it must be removed immediately or as soon as feasible. All personal protective equipment must be removed before leaving the work area, whereupon it shall be placed in a designated area or storage container for washing or disposal.

Gloves must be worn when it can reasonably be anticipated that the employee may have hand contact with blood, other potentially infectious materials, mucous membranes, and nonintact skin; when performing vascular access procedures; and when handling or touching contaminated surfaces. Disposable gloves shall be replaced as soon as practical when contaminated or when torn or punctured; they shall not be washed or decontaminated for reuse. Utility gloves may be decontaminated for reuse but must be discarded if a glove is cracked, peeling, torn, punctured, or shows other signs of deterioration.

Masks in combination with goggles or protective eye shields must be worn whenever splashes, spray, spatter, or droplets of blood may be created and eye, nose, or mouth contamination can reasonably be anticipated. Gowns and other protective body clothing such as, but not limited to, gowns, aprons, lab coats, clinic jackets, or similar outer garments, shall be worn in occupational exposure situations. The type and characteristics will depend on the task and degree of exposure anticipated. Surgical caps or hoods or shoe covers must be worn in situations in which "gross contamination" can reasonably be anticipated (eg, autopsies, orthopedic surgery).

HOUSEKEEPING

Employers must ensure that the worksite is maintained in a clean and sanitary condition and shall develop and implement a written schedule for cleaning and method of decontamination based on the location within the facility, type of surface to be cleaned, type of soil present, and tasks or procedures being performed in the area. All equipment and working surfaces shall be cleaned and decontaminated after contact with blood or other potentially infectious materials.

Contaminated work surfaces shall be decontaminated with an appropriate disinfectant after tasks and procedures are completed; immediately or as soon as feasible when surfaces are contaminated or after any spill of blood or other potentially infectious materials; and at the end of the work shift if the surface may have become contaminated since the last cleaning. Protective covering (eg, plastic wrap, aluminum foil, or imperviously backed absorbent paper used to cover equipment and environmental surfaces) must be removed and replaced as soon as feasible upon contamination or at the end of the work shift if they may have become contaminated during the shift. All bins, pails, cans, and similar containers intended for reuse shall be inspected and decontaminated on a regularly scheduled basis and cleaned immediately or as soon as feasible on visible contamination.

Broken glassware that may be contaminated must not be picked up directly with the hands; it must be cleaned up using a brush and dustpan, tongs, or forceps. Contaminated reusable sharp objects must not be stored or processed in a manner that requires employees to reach by hand into the containers in which these sharp objects have been placed. Containers for contaminated sharp objects must be closable, puncture resistant, leakproof on the sides and bottom, and labeled or color coded in accordance with the regulations. During use, containers for contaminated sharp objects shall be easily accessible to personnel and located as close as possible to the immediate area where sharp objects are used. Additionally, these containers must be maintained upright throughout use, replaced routinely, and not be allowed to be overfilled. Reusable containers shall not be opened, emptied, or cleaned manually or in any other manner that would expose employees to the risk of percutaneous injury. Containers of contaminated disposable sharp objects and personal protective equipment are defined as regulated waste; such containers must prevent the spillage or protrusion of contents during handling, storage, transport, or shipping.

Contaminated laundry shall be handled as little as possible and must be placed in bags or containers at the location where it was used; it must not be sorted or rinsed in the location of use. Contaminated laundry shall be transported in clearly labeled or color-coded bags or containers in accordance with the regulations. Employers shall ensure that employees who have contact with contaminated laundry wear protective gloves and other appropriate personal protective equipment. When a facility ships contaminated laundry offsite to a second facility that does not use universal precautions in handling all laundry, the facility generating the contaminated laundry must clearly mark or color code the bags or containers with appropriate biohazard labels.

HEPATITIS B VACCINATION

Employers are required to provide the vaccination for HBV free of charge to all employees who are at risk for occupational exposure. The vaccine must be provided within 10 days of an employee's initial assignment, except in the following cases:

- The employee has previously received the complete HBV vaccination series.
- Antibody testing has revealed that the employee is immune.
- The vaccine is contraindicated for medical reasons.

The regulations prohibit employers from making employees participate in a prescreening program as a prerequisite for receiving the vaccination. Employees who refuse the vaccination must sign a "Hepatitis B Vaccine Declination" form stating that they have declined the vaccine. If the U.S. Public Health Service ever recommends booster doses of HBV vaccine, they also must be provided to employees free of charge. The employee, however, is allowed to change his or her mind and elect to receive the vaccine at any time at the employer's expense.

POSTEXPOSURE EVALUATION AND FOLLOW-UP

Following a report of an employee exposure incident, the employer must make immediately available to the exposed employee a confidential medical evaluation and follow-up, including at least the following information:

1. Documentation of the route(s) of exposure and the circumstances under which the exposure occurred

2. Identification and documentation of the individual who is the source of the blood or potentially infectious material, unless the employer can establish that such identification is not feasible or is prohibited by state or local law. The source individual's blood shall be tested as soon as possible and after consent is obtained, to determine HBV or HIV infectivity. If consent is not obtained, the employer must document that legally required consent cannot be obtained. If the source individual's consent is not required by law, the source individual's blood if available shall be tested and the results documented. However, when the source individual is already known to be infected with HBV or HIV, blood testing for HBV or HIV is not required. Results of the source individual's blood test shall be made available to the exposed employee, and the employee shall be informed of all applicable laws concerning the disclosure of the source individual's identity and infectious status.

3. Collection and testing of the exposed employee's blood for HBV and HIV serologic status as soon as feasible after the employee gives consent. If the employee consents to baseline blood collection but does not give consent at that time for HIV serologic testing, the sample shall be preserved for 90 days. Testing of the blood shall take place within the 90 days if the employee decides to do so.

4. Postexposure prophylaxis when medically indicated, as recommended by the U.S. Public Health Service

5. Counseling

6. Evaluation of reported illnesses

The employer must ensure that the health professional responsible for the employee's HBV vaccination is provided a copy of the OSHA regulation on bloodborne pathogens. In the case of a health professional evaluating an exposed employee, the employer shall ensure that the health professional is provided the following information:

- A copy of the OSHA bloodborne pathogens regulations
- A description of the exposed employee's duties as they relate to the exposure incident
- Documentation of the routes of exposure and circumstances under which exposure occurred
- Results of the source individual's blood testing, if available
- All medical records relevant to the appropriate treatment of the exposed employee, including vaccination status, which is the employer's responsibility to maintain

The employer must obtain and provide the employee with a copy of the evaluating health professional's written opinion within 15 days of completion. The health professional's written opinion for HBV vaccination shall be limited to whether HBV vaccination is indicated for the employee and if the employee has received such vaccination. The health professional's written opinion for postexposure evaluation and follow-up shall be limited to the following information:

- The employee has been informed of the results of the evaluation.
- The employee has been told about any medical conditions resulting from exposure to blood or other potentially infectious materials that require further evaluation or treatment.

All other findings or diagnoses must remain confidential and shall not be included in the written report.

COMMUNICATIONS OF HAZARDS TO EMPLOYEES

Warning Labels and Signs

The regulations require warning labels on containers of regulated waste and refrigerators and freezers containing blood or other potentially infectious materials. Warning labels also must be affixed to containers used to store, transport, or ship blood or other potentially infectious materials. The warnings must be fluorescent orange or orange-red; however, red bags or red containers may be substituted for labels.

Employee Training

Employers must ensure that all employees at risk for occupational exposure participate in a training program at no cost to employees and during working hours. Training shall take place at the time of an employee's initial assignment to tasks that risk exposure and at least annually thereafter. Annual training for employees shall be provided within 1 year of their previous training. Additional training must be provided when changes such as modifications of tasks or procedures or introduction of new tasks and procedures affect the worker's exposure risk. The training must be conducted by a person knowledgeable about the subject matter, and the material shall be presented at an educational level appropriate to the employees. The training program at a minimum must include:

1. A copy of the bloodborne pathogens regulations and an explanation of their contents

2. A general explanation of the epidemiology and symptoms of bloodborne diseases

3. An explanation of the modes of transmission of bloodborne diseases

4. An explanation of the employer's Exposure Control Plan and information on how the employee can obtain a copy of the plan

5. An explanation of the appropriate methods for identifying tasks and other activities that may involve exposure

6. An explanation of the methods that will prevent or reduce exposure (including appropriate engineering controls, work practices, and personal protective equipment)

7. Information on the types, proper use, location, removal, handling, decontamination, and disposal of personal protective equipment

8. An explanation of the basis for selection of personal protective equipment

9. Information on the HBV vaccine (efficacy, safety, method of administration, benefits of being vaccinated, and that the vaccine will be offered free of charge)

10. Information on the appropriate actions to take and persons to contact in an emergency involving blood or other infectious materials

11. An explanation of the procedure for follow-up if an exposure incident occurs (including the method for reporting incident and the medical follow-up that may be available)

12. Information on the postexposure evaluation and follow-up that the employer is required to provide for the employee

13. An explanation of the signs and labels and/or color-coding requirements

14. An opportunity for interactive questions and answers with the person conducting the training session

Record-Keeping Requirements

The employer shall maintain an accurate record for each employee at risk for occupational exposure that includes the following information:

- The name and social security number of employee
- The employee's HBV vaccination status (dates and any medical information relative to the employee's ability to receive the vaccination)
- The results of examinations, medical testing, and follow-up procedures
- The employer's copy of the health professional's written evaluation as required following an exposure incident
- A copy of the information provided to the health professional as required following an exposure incident

The employer shall ensure the confidentiality of employee records; information shall not be disclosed without the employee's written consent. The employer is required to maintain records for the duration of employment plus 30 years. The employer also must maintain records of the training sessions that include the dates, the names and qualifications of persons who conducted training sessions, and the names and job titles of employees who attended sessions. These records shall be maintained for 3 years from the date the training session occurred.

All records shall be made available to the assistant secretary of OSHA for examination and copying, including employee medical records, for which the employee's consent is not needed. In the event of an employer going out of business, these records must be transferred to the new owner or must be offered to the National Institute for Occupational Safety and Health.

Sharps Injury Log

An employer with more than 10 employees shall maintain a "sharps injury log" to record percutaneous injuries from contaminated sharps. The information in the log shall be kept in a way to protect the confidentiality of the injured employee. The log must contain:

- The type and brand of device involved in the incident
- The department or work area where the exposure incident occurred
- An explanation of how the incident occurred

The bloodborne pathogens regulations are just one of the OSHA standards that physician offices must follow to be in compliance. Other OSHA regulations include standards on the hazards of chemicals in the workplace, compressed gases, office equipment, and an action plan in case of fire. An emergency hotline number has been established by OSHA to report emergencies: 800-321-OSHA.

AAP Policy Statements and ACOG Committee Opinions, Educational Bulletins, and Practice Bulletins

American Academy of Pediatrics Policy Statements

AD HOC TASK FORCE ON DEFINITION OF THE MEDICAL HOME

American Academy of Pediatrics. Ad Hoc Task Force on Definition of the Medical Home. The medical home. Pediatrics 1992;90:774. Current w addendum 11-93 AAP News RE9262 (revised July 2002)

COMMITTEE ON ADOLESCENCE

American Academy of Pediatrics, Committee on Adolescence. Adolescent pregnancy. Pediatrics 1999;103:516–20.

American Academy of Pediatrics, Committee on Adolescence. Counseling the adolescent about pregnancy options. Pediatrics 1998;101:938–40. (reaffirmed January 2001)

COMMITTEE ON BIOETHICS

American Academy of Pediatrics, Committee on Bioethics. Ethics and the care of critically ill infants and children. Pediatrics 1996;98:149–52. (reaffirmed October 1999)

American Academy of Pediatrics, Committee on Bioethics. Fetal therapy—ethical considerations. Pediatrics 1999;103:1061–3. (reaffirmed May 1999)

American Academy of Pediatrics, Committee on Bioethics. Guidelines on foregoing life-sustaining medical treatment. Pediatrics 1994;93:532-6. (reaffirmed October 2000)

COMMITTEE ON CHILDREN WITH DISABILITIES

American Academy of Pediatrics, Committee on Children with Disabilities. Guidelines for home care of infants, children, and adolescents with chronic disease. Pediatrics 1995;96:161-4. (reaffirmed April 2000)

COMMITTEE ON DRUGS

American Academy of Pediatrics, Committee on Drugs. Guidelines for monitoring and management of pediatric patients during and after sedation for diagnostic and therapeutic procedures. Pediatrics 1992;89:1110-5. (reaffirmed June 1998)

American Academy of Pediatrics, Committee on Drugs. Neonatal drug withdrawal. Pediatrics 1998;101:1079-88. (reaffirmed May 2001)

American Academy of Pediatrics, Committee on Drugs. Transfer of drugs and other chemicals into human milk. Pediatrics 2001;108:776-89.

COMMITTEE ON FETUS AND NEWBORN

American Academy of Pediatrics, Committee on Fetus and Newborn. Advanced practice in neonatal nursing (RE9257). AAP News 1992;8:17. (reaffirmed 1995; reaffirmed October 1998)

American Academy of Pediatrics, Committee on Fetus and Newborn. Hospital stay for healthy term newborns. Pediatrics 1995;96:788-90. (reaffirmed October 1999)

American Academy of Pediatrics, Committee on Fetus and Newborn. The initiation or withdrawal of treatment for high-risk newborns. Pediatrics 1995;96:362-3. (reaffirmed June 2001)

American Academy of Pediatrics, Committee on Fetus and Newborn and American College of Obstetricians and Gynecologits. Perinatal care at the threshold of viability. Pediatrics 1995;96:974-6. (reaffirmed October 1998)

American Academy of Pediatrics, Committee on Fetus and Newborn. Surfactant replacement therapy for respiratory distress syndrome. Pediatrics 1999;103:684-5.

American Academy of Pediatrics, Committee on Fetus and Newborn, and American College of Obstetricians and Gynecologists. Use and abuse of the Apgar score. Pediatrics 1996;98:141–2. (reaffirmed October 2000)

COMMITTEE ON GENETICS

American Academy of Pediatrics, Committee on Genetics. Folic acid for the prevention of neural tube defects. Pediatrics 1999;104:325–7.

American Academy of Pediatrics, Committee on Genetics. Maternal phenylketonuria. Pediatrics 2001;107:427–8.

American Academy of Pediatrics, Committee on Genetics. Newborn screening fact sheets. Pediatrics 1996;98:473–501.

American Academy of Pediatrics, Committee on Genetics. Prenatal genetic diagnosis for pediatricians. Pediatrics 1994;93:1010–5.

COMMITTEE ON INFECTIOUS DISEASES

American Academy of Pediatrics. Pickering LK, editor. 2000 Red book: report of the Committee on Infectious Diseases. 25th ed. Elk Grove Village (IL): AAP, 2000.

American Academy of Pediatrics, Committee on Infectious Diseases. Reassessment of the indications for ribavirin therapy in respiratory syncytial virus infections. Pediatrics 1996;97:137–40. (reaffirmed February 1999)

American Academy of Pediatrics, Committee on Infectious Diseases and Committee on Fetus and Newborn. Respiratory syncytial virus immune globulin intravenous: indications for use. Pediatrics 1997;99:645–50. (reaffirmed February 2000)

American Academy of Pediatrics, Committee on Infectious Diseases and Committee on Fetus and Newborn. Revised guidelines for prevention of early-onset group B streptococcal (GBS) infection. Pediatrics 1997;99: 489–96. (reaffirmed February 2000)

COMMITTEE ON INJURY AND POISON PREVENTION

American Academy of Pediatrics, Committee on Injury and Poison Prevention. Safe transportation of newborns at hospital discharge. Pediatrics 1999; 104:986–7.

American Academy of Pediatrics, Committee on Injury and Poison Prevention and Committee on Fetus and Newborn. Safe transportation of premature and low birth weight infants. Pediatrics 1996;97:758–60. (reaffirmed September 1999)

COMMITTEE ON NUTRITION

American Academy of Pediatrics, Committee on Nutrition. Aluminum toxicity in infants and children. Pediatrics 1996;97:413–6. (reaffirmed April 2000)

American Academy of Pediatrics, Committee on Nutrition. Hypoallergenic infant formulas. Pediatrics 2000;106:346–9.

American Academy of Pediatrics, Committee on Nutrition. Iron fortification of infant formulas. Pediatrics 1999;104:119–23.

American Academy of Pediatrics, Committee on Nutrition. Pediatric nutrition handbook. 4th ed. Elk Grove Village (IL): AAP; 1998.

American Academy of Pediatrics, Committee on Nutrition. Soy protein-based formulas: recommendations for use in infant feeding. Pediatrics 1998;101: 148–53. (reaffirmed April 2001)

COMMITTEE ON PEDIATRIC AIDS

American Academy of Pediatrics, Committee on Pediatric AIDS. Human milk, breastfeeding, and transmission of human immunodeficiency virus in the United States. Pediatrics 1995;96:977–9. (reaffirmed 2000)

COMMITTEE ON PRACTICE AND AMBULATORY MEDICINE

American Academy of Pediatrics, Committee on Practice and Ambulatory Medicine and Section on Ophthalmology. Eye examination and vision screening in infants, children, and young adults. Pediatrics 1996;98:153–7.

American Academy of Pediatrics, Committee on Practice and Ambulatory Medicine. Recommendations for preventive pediatric health care. Pediatrics 1995;96:373–4. (revised March 2000)

American Academy of Pediatrics, Committee on Practice and Ambulatory Medicine and Committee on Fetus and Newborn. The role of the primary care pediatrician in the management of high-risk newborn infants. Pediatrics 1996;98:786–8.

COMMITTEE ON PSYCHOSOCIAL ASPECTS OF CHILD AND FAMILY HEALTH

American Academy of Pediatrics, Committee on Psychosocial Aspects of Child and Family Health. Guidelines for health supervision III. Elk Grove Village (IL): AAP; 2002.

American Academy of Pediatrics, Committee on Psychosocial Aspects of Child and Family Health. The prenatal visit. Pediatrics 2001;107:1456–8.

COMMITTEE ON STATE GOVERNMENT AFFAIRS

American Academy of Pediatrics. Post-delivery care for mothers and newborns act. Available at http://www.aap/org/policy/968.html. Retrieved July 1, 2002. (reaffirmed January 2000)

COMMITTEE ON SUBSTANCE ABUSE

American Academy of Pediatrics, Committee on Substance Abuse. Alcohol use and abuse: a pediatric concern. Pediatrics 2001;108:185–9.

American Academy of Pediatrics, Committee on Substance Abuse and Committee on Children with Disabilities. Fetal alcohol syndrome and alcohol-related neurodevelopmental disorders. Pediatrics 2000;106:358–61.

JOINT COMMITTEE ON INFANT HEARING

American Academy of Pediatrics, Joint Committee on Infant Hearing. Year 2000 position statement: principles and guidelines for early hearing detection and intervention programs. Pediatrics 2000;106:798–817.

NEONATAL RESUSCITATION STEERING COMMITTEE

American Academy of Pediatrics, American Heart Association. Neonatal resuscitation textbook. 4th ed. Elk Grove Village (IL): AAP; Dallas (TX): AHA; 2000.

PROVISIONAL COMMITTEE ON PEDIATRIC AIDS

American Academy of Pediatrics, Provisional Committee on Pediatric AIDS. Technical report: perinatal human immunodeficiency virus testing and prevention of transmission. Pediatrics 2000;106:e88.

Provisional Committee on Quality Improvement

American Academy of Pediatrics, Provisional Committee on Quality Improvement and Subcommittee on Hyperbilirubinemia. Practice Parameter: management of hyperbilirubinemia in the healthy term newborn. Pediatrics 1994;94:558–65.

Section on Endocrinology

American Academy of Pediatrics, AAP Section on Endocrinology and Committee on Genetics, and American Thyroid Association Committee on Public Health. Newborn screening for congenital hypothyroidism: recommended guidelines. Pediatrics 1993;91:1203–9. (reaffirmed 1996)

Section on Ophthalmology

American Academy of Pediatrics, Section on Ophthalmology, American Association for Pediatric Ophthalmology and Strabismus, and American Academy of Ophthalmology. Screening examination of premature infants for retinopathy of prematurity. Pediatrics 2001;108:809–11.

Task Force on Circumcision

American Academy of Pediatrics, Task Force on Circumcision. Circumcision policy statement. Pediatrics 1999;103:686–93.

Task Force on Infant Positioning and SIDS

American Academy of Pediatrics, Task Force on Infant Sleep Positioning and Sudden Infant Death Syndrome. Changing concepts of sudden infant death syndrome: implications for infant sleeping environment and sleep position. Pediatrics 2000;105:650–96.

Task Force on Interhospital Transport

American Academy of Pediatrics, Task Force on Interhospital Transport. Guidelines for air and ground transport of neonatal and pediatric patients. 2nd ed. Elk Grove Village (IL): AAP; 1999.

TASK FORCE ON PROLONGED INFANTILE APNEA

American Academy of Pediatrics, Task Force on Prolonged Infantile Apnea. Prolonged infantile apnea: 1985. Pediatrics 1985;76:129–31. (reaffirmed 1995)

VITAMIN K AD HOC TASK FORCE

American Academy of Pediatrics, Vitamin K Ad Hoc Task Force. Controversies concerning vitamin K and the newborn. Pediatrics 1993;91:1001–3.

ACOG Committee Opinions

COMMITTEE ON GENETICS

161   Fragile X Syndrome (October 1995; reaffirmed 2000)

162   Screening for Tay–Sachs Disease (November 1995; reaffirmed 2000)

183   Routine Storage of Umbilical Cord Blood for Potential Future Transplantation (joint with Committee on Obstetric Practice) (April 1997; reaffirmed 2000)

189   Advanced Paternal Age: Risks to the Fetus (October 1997; reaffirmed 2000)

192   Genetic Screening of Gamete Donors (October 1997; reaffirmed 2001)

212   Screening for Canavan Disease (November 1998; reaffirmed 2002)

223   First-Trimester Screening for Fetal Anomalies with Nuchal Translucency (October 1999; reaffirmed 2001)

230   Maternal Phenylketonuria (January 2000)

238   Genetic Screening for Hemoglobinopathies (July 2000; reaffirmed 2002)

239   Breast–Ovarian Cancer Screening (August 2000)

257   Genetic Evaluation of Stillbirths and Neonatal Deaths (May 2001)

COMMITTEE ON OBSTETRIC PRACTICE

125   Placental Pathology (July 1993; reaffirmed 2000)

138   Utility of Umbilical Cord Blood Acid–Base Assessment (April 1994; reaffirmed 2000)

PRACTICE BULLETINS

Obstetrics

ACOG EDUCATIONAL BULLETINS

General

255 Psychosocial Risk Factors: Perinatal Screening and Intervention (November 1999)

258 Breastfeeding: Maternal and Infant Aspects (July 2000)

Obstetrics

207 Fetal Heart Rate Patterns: Monitoring, Interpretation, and Management (July 1995)

218 Dystocia and the Augmentation of labor (December 1995)

227 Management of Isoimmunization in Pregnancy (August 1996)

230 Assessment of Fetal Lung Maturity (November 1996)

244 Antiphospholipid Syndrome (February 1998)

248 Viral Hepatitis in Pregnancy (July 1998)

251 Obstetric Aspects of Trauma Management (September 1998)

253 Special Problems of Multiple Gestation (November 1998)

260 Smoking Cessation During Pregnancy (September 2000)

ACOG TECHNOLOGY ASSESSMENTS

Genetics

1 Genetics and Molecular Diagnostic Testing (July 2002)

Scope of Services for Uncomplicated Obstetric Care

Global obstetric care comprises services normally provided in uncomplicated obstetric care. These include antepartum care, intrapartum care, and postpartum care.

- Antepartum Care
  - The first prenatal visit with initial history and physical examination
  - Generally, a woman with an uncomplicated pregnancy is examined every 4 weeks for the first 28 weeks of gestation, every 2 weeks until 36 weeks of gestation, and weekly thereafter. The frequency of follow-up visits is determined by the individual needs of the woman and the assessment of her risks.

- Intrapartum Care
  - Supervision of uncomplicated labor
  - Uncomplicated vaginal delivery (with or without episiotomy, and/or forceps/vacuum delivery)

- Postpartum Care
  - Hospital visits
  - Outpatient (office, routine, uncomplicated visits)

Web Site Resources

Agency for Healthcare Research and Quality	www.ahcpr.gov
AIDS Clinical Trials Information Service	www.actis.org
AIDS/HIV Treatment Information Service	www.hivatis.org
American Academy of Pediatrics	www.aap.org
The American College of Obstetricians and Gynecologists	www.acog.org
American Medical Association (Practice Guidelines Partnership)	www.ama-assn.org
Association of Women's Health, Obstetric and Neonatal Nurses	www.awhonn.org
The Centers for Disease Control and Prevention	www.cdc.gov
Cochrane Collaboration	hiru.mcmaster.ca/cochrane/default.htm
Joint Commission on Accreditation of Healthcare Organizations	www.jcaho.org
March of Dimes	www.modimes.com/
Medem	medem.com
The National Academies	www.nas.edu

National Center for Health Statistics	www.cdc.gov/nchswww/index.htm
National Institutes of Health	www.nih.gov
Occupational Safety and Health Administration	www.osha.gov/oshstats
Pediatric Infectious Diseases Society	www.pids.org
U.S. Food and Drug Administration	www.hivatis.org
U.S. Public Health Service	phs.os.dhhs.gov/phs/phs.html